AF615853

Therapeutic Strategies

METABOLIC SYNDROME

Therapeutic Strategies

METABOLIC SYNDROME

Edited by

Vivian Fonseca

CLINICAL PUBLISHING

OXFORD

Clinical Publishing
an imprint of Atlas Medical Publishing Ltd

Oxford Centre for Innovation
Mill Street, Oxford OX2 0JX, UK
Tel: +44 1865 811116
Fax: +44 1865 251550
Email: info@clinicalpublishing.co.uk
Web: www.clinicalpublishing.co.uk

Distributed in USA and Canada by:

Clinical Publishing
30 Amberwood Parkway
Ashland OH 44805 USA
Tel: 800-247-6553 (toll free within USA and Canada)
Fax: 419-281-6883
Email: order@bookmasters.com

Distributed in UK and Rest of World by:

Marston Book Services Ltd
PO Box 269
Abingdon
Oxon OX14 4YN, UK
Tel: +44 1235 465500
Fax: +44 1235 465555
Email: trade.orders@marston.co.uk

First published 2008

A catalogue record for this book is available from the British Library.

ISBN–13 978 1 904392 99 6
ISBN e-book 978 1 846952 592 4

Project manager: Gavin Smith, GPS Publishing Solutions, Hertfordshire, UK
Typeset by Mizpah Publishing Services Private Limited, Chennai, India
Printed by Biddles Ltd, King's Lynn, Norfolk

Cover image kindly donated by Tayeba Khan, Albert Einstein College of Medicine, Department of Cell Biology, Bronx, NY, USA

Contents

Editor and Contributors vii

Preface ix

1 Lifestyle intervention to reduce metabolic and cardiovascular risks 1
S. Dagogo-Jack

2 Dietary controversies in treatment of the metabolic syndrome 13
N. Davis, N. Tomuta, J. Wylie-Rosett

3 An exercise prescription for the metabolic syndrome 29
R. Bentley-Lewis, M. Pendergrass

4 Impact of hypoglycemic agents on the metabolic syndrome 43
T. K. Thethi, S. Singh, V. Fonseca

5 Weight loss agents and the metabolic syndrome 55
W. T. Cefalu, C. Champagne, F. Greenway

6 Blockage of the renin–angiotensin system in metabolic syndrome: implications for the prevention of diabetes 69
K. Vijayaraghavan, P. C. Deedwania

7 Lipid management in the metabolic syndrome 93
O. P. Ganda

8 A potential role for insulin in management of the metabolic syndrome 111
P. Dandona, A. Chaudhuri, P. Mohanty, H. Ghanim

9 Suppressing inflammation: a novel approach to treating the metabolic syndrome 125
A. D. Rao, V. Fonseca

10 GLP-1 analogues, DPP-IV inhibitors and the metabolic syndrome 137
A. H. Stonehouse, J. H. Holcombe, D. M. Kendall

List of Abbreviations 159

Index 165

Editor

VIVIAN FONSECA, MD, FRCP, Professor of Medicine and Pharmacology, Tullis Tulane Alumni Chair in Diabetes; Chief, Section of Endocrinology, Department of Medicine, Tulane University Health Sciences Center, New Orleans, Louisiana, USA

Contributors

RHONDA BENTLEY-LEWIS, MD, MBA, MMSc, Instructor in Medicine, Harvard Medical School; Associate Physician, Division of Endocrinology, Diabetes and Hypertension, Brigham and Women's Hospital, Boston, Massachusetts, USA

WILLIAM T. CEFALU, MD, Douglas L. Manship Senior Professor of Diabetes; Chief, Division of Nutrition and Chronic Diseases, Pennington Biomedical Research Center, Louisiana State University System, Baton Rouge, Louisiana, USA

CATHERINE M. CHAMPAGNE, PhD, RD, Professor and Chief, Nutritional Epidemiology, Pennington Biomedical Research Center, Louisiana State University System, Baton Rouge, Louisiana, USA

AJAY CHAUDHURI, MD, Division of Endocrinology, State University of New York at Buffalo, Millard Fillmore Hospital, Buffalo, New York, USA

SAMUEL DAGOGO-JACK, MD, FACC, FACP, FAHA, Professor of Medicine, Department of Medicine and General Clinical Research Center, University of Tennessee Health Science Center, Memphis, Tennessee, USA

PARESH DANDONA, MD, PhD, FRCP, FACP, FACC, FACE, Director, Diabetes-Endocrinology Center of WNY; Chief, Division of Endocrinology SUNY at Buffalo; Distinguished Professor of Medicine, Division of Endocrinology, State University of New York at Buffalo, Millard Fillmore Hospital, Buffalo, New York, USA

NICHOLA J. DAVIS, MD, MS, Assistant Professor, Department of Medicine, Albert Einstein College of Medicine/Montefiore Medical Center, Department of Epidemiology, Bronx, New York, USA

PRAKASH C. DEEDWANIA, MD, FACC, FAHA, Chief, Cardiology Division, Veterans Administration Central California Health Care System, Fresno; Professor of Medicine, UCSF School of Medicine, San Francisco, California, USA

VIVIAN FONSECA, MD, FRCP, Professor of Medicine and Pharmacology, Tullis Tulane Alumni Chair in Diabetes; Chief, Section of Endocrinology, Department of Medicine, Tulane University Health Sciences Center, New Orleans, Louisiana, USA

OM P. GANDA, MD, Director, Lipid Clinic, Joslin Diabetes Center; Associate Clinical Professor of Medicine, Harvard Medical School, Boston, Massachusetts, USA

HUSAM GHANIM, PhD, Division of Endocrinology, State University of New York at Buffalo, Millard Fillmore Hospital, Buffalo, New York, USA

FRANK L. GREENWAY, MD, Professor and Director of Outpatient Clinical Research, Pennington Biomedical Research Center, Louisiana State University System, Baton Rouge, Louisiana, USA

JOHN H. HOLCOMBE, MD, Medical Fellow, Lilly Research Laboratories, Eli Lilly and Company, Indianapolis, Indiana, USA

DAVID M. KENDALL, MD, Executive Director, Medical Affairs, Amylin Pharmaceuticals, Inc., San Diego, California, USA

PRIYA MOHANTY, MD, Division of Endocrinology, State University of New York at Buffalo, Millard Fillmore Hospital, Buffalo, New York, USA

MERRI PENDERGRASS, MD, PhD, Associate Professor of Medicine, Harvard Medical School; Director of Clinical Diabetes, Brigham and Women's Hospital, Boston, Massachusetts, USA

AJAY D. RAO, MD, Fellow, Endocrinology, Section of Endocrinology, Tulane University Health Sciences Center, New Orleans, Louisiana, USA

SHIPRA SINGH, MBBS, MPH, Section of Endocrinology, Department of Medicine, Tulane University, New Orleans, Louisiana, USA

ANTHONY H. STONEHOUSE, PhD, Medical Affairs Scientist, Amylin Pharmaceuticals, Inc., San Diego, California, USA

TINA K. THETHI, MD, MPH, Assistant Professor of Medicine, Section of Endocrinology, Department of Internal Medicine, Tulane University Health Sciences Center, New Orleans, Louisiana, USA

NORICA TOMUTA, MD, Research Associate, Department of Epidemiology and Population Health, Division of Behavioral and Nutrition Research, General Clinic Research Center, Albert Einstein College of Medicine, Bronx, New York, USA

KRISHNASWAMI VIJAYARAGHAVAN, MD, FACP, FACC, Director of Cardiovascular Research, Scottsdale Healthcare, Scottsdale, Arizona; Consultant Cardiologist, Scottsdale Cardiovascular Center; Clinical Professor of Medicine, Midwestern University School of Medicine, Glendale, Arizona, USA

JUDITH WYLIE-ROSETT, EdD, RD, Professor, Department of Epidemiology and Population Health, Albert Einstein College of Medicine, Bronx, New York, USA

Preface

We are in the midst of a worldwide epidemic of obesity and its consequences, in particular type 2 diabetes and cardiovascular disease. Clinical studies have recognized that risk factors for these conditions frequently cluster in individuals, leading to the development of the concept of the metabolic syndrome. This was soon followed by considerable controversy as to whether the syndrome is a distinct entity or not. In addition, multiple definitions and diagnostic criteria have made interpretation of data occasionally problematic. I expect that this controversy will continue, though all parties on both sides of the argument are clearly in agreement on one thing – we need action to halt the progression from risk factor development to clinical events and death. Despite the controversies on terminology, therefore, it is important to focus on the goal of effective treatment, hence the development of this book.

Although our goal is to have an in-depth analysis of treatment strategies, we felt it important to first review the epidemiology and pathophysiology of the syndrome, in order to lay the groundwork for developing treatment concepts. We have also strongly emphasized the importance of lifestyle (and perhaps societal) change that is needed to halt this epidemic. Clearly, preventing and treating obesity effectively should liberate us from the syndrome. However, whether we use population strategies or individualized pharmacotherapy for obesity, the greatest impact is likely to be seen in treatments that alleviate risk factors involved in the pathogenesis of cardiovascular events such as blood pressure, lipids, inflammation and thrombogenesis. To that end, we have focused on the impact of treatment on these factors.

It is also important to recognize the impact of current treatments for individual risk factors on other components of the syndrome. This is most clearly recognizable in the effect of glucose-lowering drugs, particularly insulin sensitizers if insulin resistance is an important underlying feature of the syndrome. Some of these drugs, as well as insulin itself, paradoxically cause weight gain, yet favorably impact other features of the syndrome. Is that good or bad? The answers are currently surrounded by controversy, the essence of which we hope we have captured adequately in the text. We look forward to further clarification from ongoing clinical trials.

I am most grateful to the outstanding group of authors who have contributed scholarly and up-to-date reviews in a timely fashion.

Finally, I would like to dedicate this book to the city of New Orleans and to its fragile recovery from disaster.

Vivian Fonseca
June 2008

1

Lifestyle intervention to reduce metabolic and cardiovascular risks

S. Dagogo-Jack

INTRODUCTION

More than 75% of deaths in people with diabetes are attributable to cardiovascular disease (CVD). Compared with non-diabetic persons, the CVD risk rises exponentially among patients with type 1 and type 2 diabetes [1–3]. Cardiometabolic risk factors, including insulin resistance and its associated manifestations, predispose to the 2–4-fold increased risk for CVD in type 2 diabetes. Strikingly, coronary artery disease (CAD) is ten times more prevalent among patients with type 1 diabetes than age- and gender-matched persons without diabetes [2, 3]. Clearly, insulin resistance is not a characteristic feature of type 1 diabetes, at least not during the initial years. Therefore, the mechanisms underlying the 10-fold increased risk of CAD in type 1 diabetes must involve factors beyond insulin resistance, and hyperglycemia appears to be a mediator. The role of hyperglycemia as a major CVD risk mediator in type 1 diabetes has been strengthened by new data [4] from the Diabetes Control and Complications Trial/Epidemiology of Diabetes Interventions and Complications (DCCT/EDIC). The strategy for reduction of CVD risk in patients with type 1 or type 2 diabetes must necessarily be comprehensive and multifaceted. At the least, such strategy should include bio-behavioral interventions (smoking cessation, weight reduction, dietary modification, increased physical activity) and pharmacological therapies to control hyperglycemia, hypertension, dyslipidemia, dysfibrinolysis, and other comorbid conditions. This review focuses on the role of lifestyle modification as a primary or adjunctive intervention to prevent or decrease CVD and cardiometabolic risks in persons with diabetes and prediabetes.

CHRONIC COMPLICATIONS OF DIABETES

The prevalence and incidence rates for both type 1 and type 2 diabetes are increasing worldwide, although the rates for type 2 diabetes are disproportionately greater. Diabetes is a major public health problem, largely because of its long-term complications. These complications include microvascular (retinopathy, nephropathy and neuropathy) and macrovascular (CAD, cerebrovascular disease and peripheral vascular disease) categories. Hyperglycemia is the driving force for the development of microvascular complications in patients with type 1 or type 2 diabetes, as has been confirmed in landmark studies [5, 6]. Hyperglycemia is also one of several major etiological factors for macrovascular disease in

---

Samuel Dagogo-Jack, MD, FACC, FACP, FAHA, Professor of Medicine, Department of Medicine and General Clinical Research Center, University of Tennessee Health Science Center, Memphis, Tennessee, USA

type 2 diabetes. Diabetes leads to accelerated atherosclerosis through a variety of mutually reinforcing mechanisms [7]. For patients with type 2 diabetes, the risk of first myocardial infarction (MI) is similar to that of recurrent MI in non-diabetic persons who have had a previous heart attack [8]. Although no exactly similar data have been reported for type 1 diabetes, the pattern is likely identical or worse, given the known 10-fold increased prevalence of CVD in patients with type 1 diabetes [2, 3].

MECHANISMS OF THE CVD RISK IN DIABETES

Cardiometabolic risk factors, including insulin resistance, dysmetabolic syndrome and associated manifestations, predispose to the increased CVD in type 2 diabetes [9]. Features of the dysmetabolic syndrome include visceral obesity, insulin resistance, hypertension, hypertriglyceridemia, decreased high-density lipoprotein (HDL)-cholesterol levels, small dense low-density lipoprotein (LDL)-cholesterol levels, pro-inflammatory state, endothelial dysfunction and a pro-coagulant state, among others [1, 10]. In contrast, insulin resistance is not the dominant feature of type 1 diabetes, at least not during the initial years. It must be noted, though, that a phenotype of insulin resistance can be superimposed upon pre-existing type 1 diabetes, particularly in persons with a family history of type 2 diabetes and those who develop abdominal obesity [11, 12]. Conceptually, the mechanisms underlying the 10-fold increased CVD risk in type 1 diabetes must involve at least two sets of factors: those expressed during the initial years that may be independent of insulin resistance, and factors arising from the insulin resistance that is superimposed in later years. Of course, there is also a multiplicative effect from non-glycemic risk factors (e.g., hypertension, dyslipidemia, smoking etc.).

The pathogenesis of diabetes-specific long-term complications is not fully understood. Some suggested mechanisms include genetic predisposition; hyperglycemia-induced abnormalities in the polyol pathway; toxic effects of advanced glycated end-products; glomerular hyperfiltration; aberrant growth factor expression, inflammation, altered redox state, and abnormal endothelial function [13–18]. Thus, the mechanisms responsible for the initiation of macrovascular complications in type 1 diabetes could well involve hyperglycemia as a direct mediator or trigger. Despite the existing gaps in our knowledge, one can argue that lifestyle measures that decrease CVD risk in type 2 diabetes should prove beneficial in type 1 diabetes also, despite mechanistic differences in the pathophysiology of CVD in the two forms of diabetes. Therefore, the specific lifestyle interventions to be discussed later in this review (consisting of smoking cessation, weight optimization, dietary modification and increased physical activity) constitute a generic strategy for cardiometabolic risk reduction.

PREDIABETES AND THE CONTINUUM OF CARDIOMETABOLIC RISK

The term 'prediabetes' refers to impaired glucose tolerance (IGT) and impaired fasting glucose (IFG), two intermediate metabolic states between normal glucose tolerance and diabetes. IGT is defined by a plasma glucose level of 140 mg/dl to 199 mg/dl, 2 h following ingestion of a 75 g oral solution. IFG is defined by a fasting plasma glucose of 100 mg/dl to 125 mg/dl [19]. IFG and IGT are risk factors for type 2 diabetes, and persons with these conditions progress to type 2 diabetes at variable rates. The prediabetic state is associated with numerous CVD risk markers that overlap considerably with components of the metabolic syndrome. Among several definitions of the metabolic syndrome, the one proposed by the National Cholesterol Education Program, Adult Treatment Panel III (NCEP, ATP III) [20] that focuses on abdominal obesity, low HDL-cholesterol (<40 mg/dl in men and <50 mg/dl in women), triglycerides (>150 mg/dl), blood pressure (>130/80 mmHg) and fasting plasma glucose (>100 mg/dl) has the merits of simplicity and specific numerical cut-off points. Estimates using the NCEP criteria for the metabolic syndrome have indicated an alarming prevalence of the syndrome [21]. Components of the metabolic syndrome can

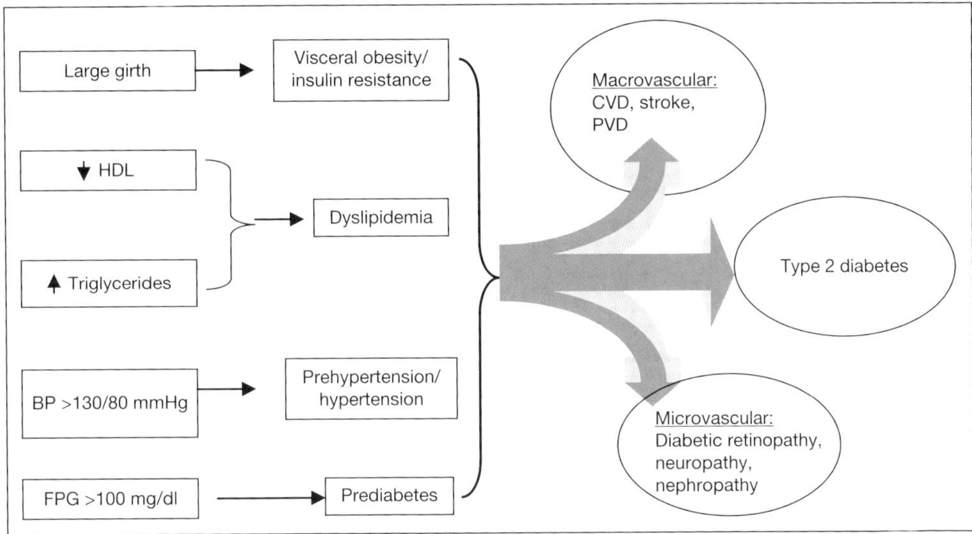

Figure 1.1 Sequelae of the metabolic syndrome. Individual components of the syndrome are risk factors for type 2 diabetes and CVD. Progression to diabetes initiates susceptibility to microvascular complications and further exacerbates the risk for CVD. Lifestyle prevents or delays progression to type 2 diabetes and ameliorates each of the cardiometabolic risk factors. BP = blood pressure; CVD = cardiovascular disease; FPG = Fasting plasma glucose; PVD = Peripheral vascular disease.

be identified in prediabetic subjects several years before the diagnosis of type 2 diabetes, are significantly associated with expression of pro-inflammatory cytokines, and are predictive of future risk of incident diabetes and CVD [22].

Furthermore, the individual components of the metabolic syndrome represent pre-nosologic or prodromal states for subsequent disease states (Figure 1.1). Thus, dyslipidemia and hypertension lead to CVD; obesity and IGT/IFG lead to type 2 diabetes, and also predict increased CVD risk. In the Paris Prospective Study [23], a prediabetes status at baseline conferred a doubling of the 10-year risk for CVD mortality. In the EPIC-Norfolk study [24], the degree of glycemia (as assessed by glycosylated hemoglobin [HbA1c]) emerged as an independent predictor of CVD mortality. The relationship between HbA1c and CVD mortality was evident as a continuum of risk, beginning well before the glycemic threshold for the diagnosis of diabetes is reached (Figure 1.2). These data indicate that macrovascular disease manifests during the prediabetic stage, thus arguing for early intervention. The insulin resistance (metabolic) syndrome appears to be the link between prediabetes and macrovascular disease. Therefore, interventions that reduce insulin resistance and attenuate expression of the metabolic syndrome can be expected to reduce the metabolic and cardiovascular consequences of the syndrome. The stark reality from long-term follow-up of prediabetic subjects assigned to a placebo arm is that spontaneous recovery from prediabetes rarely occurs [25]. This realization makes early lifestyle intervention a clinical imperative and a compelling public health priority.

LIFESTYLE INTERVENTION FOR PREVENTION OF CVD IN DIABETES

The multifactorial origin of CVD in diabetes compels a comprehensive approach that incorporates lifestyle modification with an appropriate selection of medications for glucoregulation, control of hypertension, dyslipidemia, antiplatelet therapy and other comorbid conditions [26] (Table 1.1).

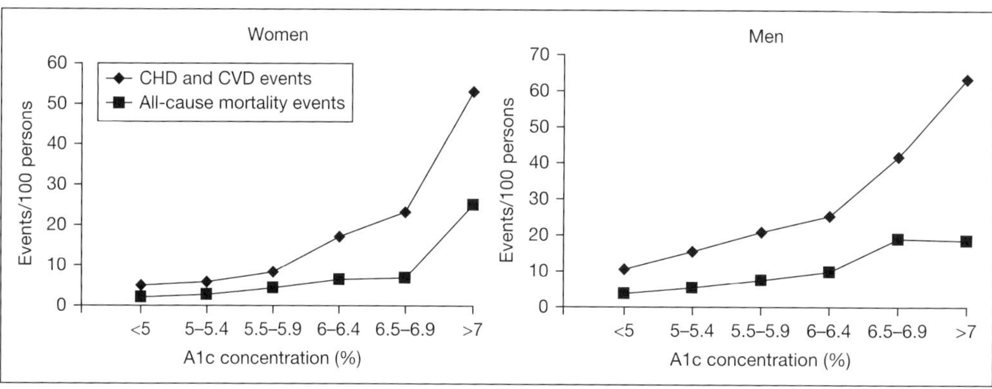

Figure 1.2 Hemoglobin A1c and CVD events and mortality in the EPIC-Norfolk study. An increase in A1c of 1% was associated with a 20% to 30% increase in cardiovascular events or mortality. CHD = coronary heart disease; CVD = cardiovascular disease. Reproduced with permission from [7].

Table 1.1 Targets of intervention for CVD risk reduction

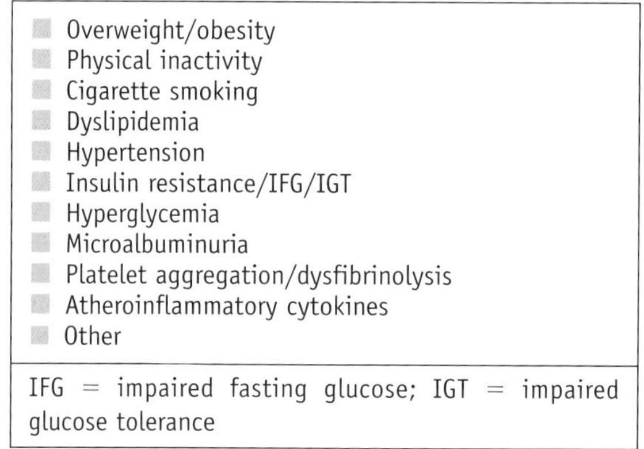

- Overweight/obesity
- Physical inactivity
- Cigarette smoking
- Dyslipidemia
- Hypertension
- Insulin resistance/IFG/IGT
- Hyperglycemia
- Microalbuminuria
- Platelet aggregation/dysfibrinolysis
- Atheroinflammatory cytokines
- Other

IFG = impaired fasting glucose; IGT = impaired glucose tolerance

Smoking cessation

The use of tobacco products exacerbates adverse metabolic and cardiovascular outcomes among diabetic patients [7, 9, 27]. Studies have found that cigarette smoking is associated with up to four-fold additional increase in the risk of cardiovascular death among people with diabetes, depending on the amount smoked [7]. Diabetic patients with a current history of cigarette smoking have been reported to have higher HbA1c and lipoprotein levels compared with non-smokers [9, 27]. Cigarette smoking is also a risk factor for the metabolic syndrome [28]. The mechanisms for the association between smoking and increased metabolic and CVD risks include induction of insulin resistance, increased hepatic lipase activity and dyslipidemia [29–31]. Other contributory factors include the chronic elevation of stress hormones, endothelial dysfunction and the vasoconstrictive effect of nicotine [30]. It is reasonable to expect that smoking cessation would improve cardiometabolic risk through the amelioration of these noxious effects of nicotine.

Despite evidence supporting their efficacy, smoking cessation counseling and interventions are offered to only about 50% of diabetic smokers [32]. Clearly, smoking cessation counseling must become standard practice in the management and prevention of CVD and diabetes complications. As already discussed, there are several putative mechanisms whereby smoking cessation could improve cardiometabolic risk. The observation that blood pressure, heart rate, blood flow and skin temperature of hands and feet return to normal within 20 min after smoking cessation suggests rapid reversal of the acute vasoconstrictive effects of nicotine. However, rigorous intervention studies testing the effect of smoking cessation on progression of prediabetes and metabolic endpoints are yet to be reported. Nonetheless, there are compelling reasons for promoting smoking cessation counseling in clinical practice. These include the expected reduction in the risks for emphysema, lung cancer, CAD and stroke following smoking cessation; cleaner air and improved blood oxygenation; and overall improvement in quality of life [33]. Furthermore, exercise tolerance is expected to improve in ex-smokers, which should improve fitness and potentiate adherence to the exercise habit.

Interestingly, the standard lifestyle interventions (increased physical activity and caloric restriction) have been shown to enhance successful abstinence from smoking. In one randomized controlled trial, a regimen of three exercise sessions per week for 12 weeks plus a cognitive behavioral program improved continuous abstinence from smoking at 12 months compared with behavioral program alone [34]. The actual approach to smoking cessation in a given patient should be individualized. However, common elements of any specific approach include application of the transtheoretical model of readiness for change [35], periodic reinforcement of key messages, cognitive behavioral therapy, use of tapered transdermal or buccal nicotine, and prescription medications (bupropion, varenicline) to decrease craving during the transitional period. Referral to a specialized smoking cessation center, where available, is an efficient way of accomplishing the desired goal.

Physical activity and dietary modification

Increased physical activity and dietary modification are the cornerstones of non-pharmacological intervention for glycemic control. These lifestyle measures also provide broad benefits toward reducing cardiometabolic risk. Regular physical activity improves insulin action, blood pressure and lipid levels, and decreases obesity, among other benefits. Notably, the pro-atherogenic visceral fat compartment has been reported to be quite sensitive to physical activity [36], and decreases in waist circumference often occur early during lifestyle change. Moreover, exercise conditioning that improves cardiorespiratory fitness significantly predicts longevity [37]. The recommended goal for most people is 30–60 min of moderate-intensity aerobic exercise, repeated three or more times per week. Programs should be tailored to individual patients' physical condition, and should always include warm-up and cool-down periods. Cardiac screening is advisable for patients aged 35 years or older, especially if they have been sedentary.

Dietary practices that restrict saturated fat intake, with augmentation of dietary fiber, fruits and vegetables, offer distinct metabolic and cardiovascular benefits [38]. Fat intake should be limited to ~30% of total calories (saturated fat should be <7%). The intake of trans fatty acids should be reduced drastically to <1% of energy consumption [26]. The so-called Mediterranean diet, based on generous servings of fruits, vegetables and nuts, has been shown to reduce CVD risk factors, reverse components of the metabolic syndrome, and improve morbidity and mortality [39–41]. Although lifestyle interventions that target the metabolic syndrome are most germane to type 2 diabetes, the cardioprotective benefits of exercise and dietary modification should extend to patients with type 1 diabetes and even persons without diabetes. Despite the intuitive appeal of the lifestyle approach, it must be acknowledged that randomized controlled trials are needed to demonstrate unique, independent benefits on CVD. One such study is the ongoing LOOK-Ahead project, funded by

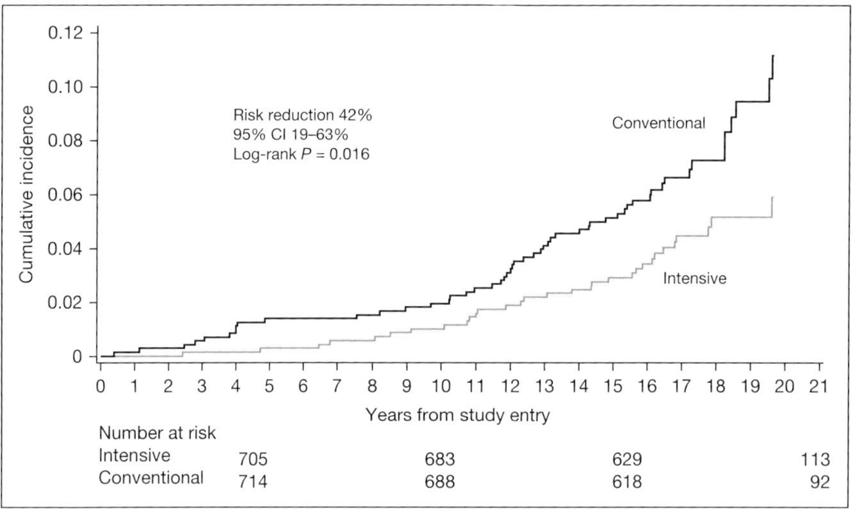

Figure 1.3 Cumulative incidence of the first of any cardiovascular disease event in the DCCT/EDIC cohort. CI = confidence interval. Reproduced with permission from [4].

the National Institutes of Health. LOOK-Ahead is a multicenter longitudinal study that has enrolled persons with type 2 diabetes with two or more additional CVD risk factors. The study subjects are randomized to a lifestyle intervention to induce ~10% weight loss vs no weight loss intervention, on a background of optimized pharmacotherapy for diabetes and comorbid conditions. The primary goal of the study is to determine whether weight loss *per se* results in CVD risk reduction in persons with diabetes.

REDUCTION OF CVD RISK THROUGH CONTROL OF HYPERGLYCEMIA IN DIABETES

The DCCT [4] showed that achievement of near-normoglycemia using insulin therapy prevented long-term microvascular complications in patients with type I diabetes. The United Kingdom Prospective Diabetes Study (UKPDS) [6] demonstrated similar benefits of intensive glycemic control on microvascular endpoints in type 2 diabetes. However, the effect of glycemic control on the occurrence of CVD in type 1 or type 2 diabetes has been an unsettled question. *Post hoc* analysis of the UKPDS data demonstrated a linear relationship between glycemic control and the rate of MI [42]. In the DCCT/EDIC study, intensive glycemic control significantly reduced the risk of any CVD event by 42% (Figure 1.3) and the risk of non-fatal MI, stroke, or death from CVD by 57% [4]. In a multivariate analysis, the decrease in HbA1c values significantly predicted the cardioprotective effect of intensive treatment, and the cardiovascular benefits persisted after adjusting for blood pressure, proteinuria, use of angiotensin inhibitors or lipid-lowering medication [4].

The patients assigned to intensive therapy in the DCCT used a regimen of multiple (four or more) daily insulin injections or continuous subcutaneous insulin infusion, whereas the control group used a conventional insulin regimen comprising two daily injections of a mixture of regular insulin and intermediate-acting insulin. Thus, improved control of post-prandial glucose among patients in the intensive therapy arm possibly contributed to the cardiovascular benefits. In the STOP-NIDDM trial, reduction of post-prandial glycemia with acarbose treatment in subjects with IGT was associated with a reduction in CVD risk

[43]. Although long-term maintenance of glycemic control is not feasible using lifestyle measures alone, the adjunctive role of dietary modification and physical activity in optimizing glycemic control cannot be overstated. At every stage of the disease, institution of the dietary principles discussed earlier leads to improvement in glycemic control, whereas *ad libitum* feeding escalates hyperglycemia. Similarly, exercise improves glycemic control in patients with type 1 or type 2 diabetes, in addition to the other well-known metabolic and cardiovascular benefits.

LIFESTYLE INTERVENTION FOR PRIMARY PREVENTION OF DIABETES

Three landmark studies have demonstrated the efficacy of lifestyle intervention in preventing the development of type 2 diabetes in high-risk individuals [44–46]. All studies targeted persons with prediabetes (IGT). The lifestyle interventions applied in these studies generally involved a modest weight loss (~5% to <10%) through dietary modification and increased physical activity. The dietary modification involved reduction in caloric consumption, selective reduction in saturated fat calories, and increased intake of complex carbohydrates. The physical activity component involved accrual of additional 150–240 min per week of voluntary, moderate-intensity (~55% VO_2 max) physical activity above routine levels [44–46]. The primary outcome measure was the rate of progression from IGT to type 2 diabetes over a defined period (~3–6 years) of observation in the intervention arm versus a comparison group.

Investigators in the Da Qing study [44] enrolled 577 Chinese adults (mean age 45 years; mean body mass index [BMI] 26 kg/m^2) who had IGT at baseline. The subjects were randomized by clinic to a control group or to one of three active treatment groups: diet only, exercise only, or diet plus exercise. The dietary policy had a target BMI of <23 kg/m^2; the exercise goal was an increase in physical activity of 210 min per week (30 min daily). The follow-up schedule was approximately every 2 weeks during the initial 3 months and quarterly thereafter. The cumulative incidence of diabetes at 6 years was 67.7% in the control group compared with 43.8% in the diet group, 41.1% in the exercise group and 46.0% in the diet-plus-exercise group. Cox's proportional hazards analysis, adjusted for differences in baseline BMI and fasting glucose, showed that the diet, exercise, and diet-plus-exercise interventions resulted in 31%, 46% and 42% reductions in risk of developing diabetes, respectively, compared with the control group. Surprisingly, the Da Qing study failed to show an additive effect of diet plus exercise on the primary endpoint.

In the Finnish Diabetes Prevention Study [45], 522 middle-aged IGT subjects (172 men and 350 women; mean age 55 years; mean BMI 31 kg/m^2) were randomly assigned to either an intervention or control group. Each subject in the intervention group received individualized lifestyle counseling aimed at inducing ~5% weight loss and increasing physical activity by ~210 min per week. The mean weight loss by the end of the second year was ~3.5 kg in the intervention group and ~0.8 kg in the control group. The cumulative incidence of diabetes after 4 years was 11% in the intervention group and 23% in the control group, a significant 58% reduction in diabetes incidence.

THE DIABETES PREVENTION PROGRAM

The lifestyle intervention arm of the Diabetes Prevention Program (DPP) enrolled 1079 subjects with IGT (out of the 3234 participants enrolled in the study) drawn from all ethnic and racial groups in the US population [46]. The goals for the participants assigned to the intensive lifestyle intervention were to achieve and maintain a weight reduction of at least 7% of initial body weight through modest caloric restriction (500–700 fewer calories per day) and to engage in physical activity of moderate intensity, such as brisk walking, for at least 150 min per week. After an average follow-up period of 2.8 years, the participants randomized to lifestyle intervention showed a 58% reduction in the incidence of diabetes, as compared with placebo [46]. This beneficial effect of lifestyle intervention was seen in all age, gender, racial and ethnic subgroups of the DPP participants. Furthermore, reversion to normal glucose tolerance (NGT) occurred in ~30% of subjects in the lifestyle intervention arm, as compared with ~18% in the control arm. Thus, caloric restriction and increased physical activity not only prevented progression from IGT to diabetes but were also effective in restoring NGT in a substantial proportion of subjects with initial IGT [46].

PRIMARY PREVENTION OF CVD IN PREDIABETES

The DPP investigators [47] assessed the effects of lifestyle intervention, metformin and placebo on CVD risk factors and markers of the metabolic syndrome among subjects with IGT. Compared with the placebo and metformin arms, subjects assigned to lifestyle intervention showed decreased blood pressure, increased HDL-cholesterol levels, and lower triglyceride levels during approximately 3 years of follow-up. Moreover, there was a reduced need for antihypertensive and lipid-lowering medications among subjects assigned to the intensive lifestyle arm. Besides reducing the need for antihypertensive medications, lifestyle intervention reduced the crude incidence of hypertension by 33% in the DPP lifestyle group [47, 48]. The level of LDL-cholesterol was not significantly altered by lifestyle intervention, although a reduction in the more atherogenic small, dense LDL particles was observed [47]. Because total LDL particles, rather than subclasses, have been the standard measurement for landmark outcome trials, early initiation of therapy with an HMG-CoA reductase inhibitor (statin) may be indicated, to reach protective levels of LDL in high-risk subjects. The favorable effects of lifestyle intervention on blood pressure and the levels of HDL-cholesterol, triglycerides, and small dense LDL particles suggest that the overall risk for CVD ought to be decreased. The DPP Outcomes Study is tracking the original cohort for another decade, to determine whether the aforementioned improvements in risk factors would translate to reduction in clinical events.

EMERGING MOLECULAR MECHANISMS

The emerging data on the interactions between lifestyle intervention and incident diabetes suggest possible epigenetic effects at the molecular level that translate to prevention of diabetes [49, 50]. In the Finnish Diabetes Prevention Study, a significant interaction was reported among weight change, progression from IGT to type diabetes, and the G308A polymorphism of the tumor necrosis factor alpha (TNF-α) gene among subjects randomized to the intensive lifestyle intervention arm [49]. Also, the DPP investigators have reported intriguing data that suggest possible epigenetic interactions between lifestyle modification on the transcription factor 7-like 2 gene (*TCF7L2*) [50]. Previously, genotyping of microsatellite markers throughout a 10.5-Mb interval on chromosome 10q in an Icelandic cohort with type 2 diabetes had revealed a microsatellite within intron 3 of *TCF7L2* (formerly known as *TCF4*) that was associated with diabetes [51]. Compared with non-carriers, heterozygous and homozygous carriers of the at-risk alleles (38% and 7% of the Icelandic population, respectively) have relative risks of 1.45 and 2.41 (population attributable risk of 21%) [52]. The TCF7L2 gene product has been implicated in blood glucose homeostasis, probably through the regulation of proglucagon gene expression in enteroendocrine cells [51].

Two of the most strongly associated *TCF7L2* variants (rs12255372 and rs7903146) have been examined in the DPP, to determine whether they predict progression from IGT to type 2 diabetes [50]. Both variants were genotyped in 3548 DPP participants, and Cox regression analysis was performed using genotype, intervention, and their interactions as predictors. During ~3 years of follow-up, subjects harbouring the rs7903146 risk-conferring TT genotype were more likely to have progressed from IGT to type 2 diabetes than were CC homozygotes (hazard ratio [HR] 1.55; confidence interval [CI] 1.20–2.01; $P < 0.001$). Interestingly, the predictive effect of the TT genotype was strongest in the placebo group (HR 1.81) and weakest among subjects randomized to intensive lifestyle modification (HR 1.15). Further analysis revealed that the TT genotype was associated with decreased insulin secretion but not increased insulin resistance at baseline [50]. The data obtained from analysis of the rs12255372 variant were concordant with the findings from analysis of the rs7903146 variant.

SUMMARY

Dietary modification, regular physical activity, smoking cessation and other lifestyle changes have been shown to exert favorable effects on glycemia, blood pressure, body weight, fat distribution, lipid and lipoprotein profiles, among other metabolic and psychological benefits. Lifestyle interventions have also been demonstrated to be effective in primary prevention of type 2 diabetes. These consistent metabolic and cardiovascular benefits make the implementation of lifestyle intervention a public health imperative. In the DPP, the benefits of lifestyle change were observed universally across all age and BMI groups, whereas the effect of metformin was restricted to young obese persons [46, 52]. The fascinating observations that suggest possible modulation of pro-inflammatory and glucoregulatory genes by lifestyle intervention [49, 50] provide a novel insight into how behavioral interventions can alter the expression of genetic diseases. This area of study into epigenetic influences in behavioral metabolism is still in its infancy, and can be expected to advance rapidly in coming years. Among patients with isolated diabetes, hypertension, dyslipidemia, or the metabolic syndrome, lifestyle change is an important adjunct to medications. For the millions of people who have prediabetes, lifestyle modification is especially compelling because of its non-toxicity and superb efficacy, compared with medications.

REFERENCES

1. Beckman JA, Creager MA, Libby P. Diabetes and atherosclerosis: epidemiology, pathophysiology, and management. *JAMA* 2002; 287:2570–2581.
2. Dorman JS, LaPorte RE, Kuller LH *et al.* The Pittsburgh insulin-dependent diabetes mellitus (IDDM) morbidity and mortality study: mortality results. *Diabetes* 1984; 33:271–276.
3. Laing SP, Swerdlow AJ, Slater SD *et al.* Mortality from heart disease in a cohort of 23,000 patients with insulin-treated diabetes. *Diabetologia* 2003; 46:760–765.
4. DCCT/EDIC Research Group. Intensive diabetes treatment and cardiovascular disease in type 1 diabetes in the DCCT/EDIC. *N Eng J Med* 2005; 353:2643–2653.
5. The Diabetes Control and Complications Trial Research Group. The effect of intensive treatment of diabetes on the development and progression of long-term complications in insulin-dependent diabetes mellitus. *N Engl J Med* 1993; 329:978–986.
6. United Kingdom Prospective Diabetes Study Group. Intensive blood-glucose control with sulfophonylurea or insulin compared with conventional treatment and risk of complications in patients with type 2 diabetes (UKPDS 33). *Lancet* 1998; 352:837–853.
7. Khaw KT, Wareham N, Bingham S, Luben R, Welch A, Day N. Association of hemoglobin A1c with cardiovascular disease and mortality in adults: the European prospective investigation into cancer in Norfolk. *Ann Intern Med* 2004; 141:413–420.
8. Haffner SM, Lehto S, Ronnemaa T *et al.* Mortality from coronary heart disease in subjects with type 2 diabetes and in nondiabetic subjects with and without prior myocardial infarction. *N Engl J Med* 1998; 339:229–234.
9. Stamler J, Vaccaro O, Neaton JD *et al.* Diabetes, other risk factors, and 12-year mortality for men screened in the Multiple Risk Factor Intervention Trial. *Diabetes Care* 1993; 16:434–444.
10. Zimmet P, Shaw J, Alberti KGMM. Preventing type 2 diabetes and the dysmetabolic syndrome in the real world: a realistic view. *Diabet Med* 2003; 20:693–702.
11. Sibley SD, Palmer JP, Hirsch IB, Brunzell JD.Visceral obesity, hepatic lipase activity, and dyslipidemia in type 1 diabetes. *J Clin Endocrinol Metab* 2003; 88:3379–3384.

12. Sibley SD, Hokanson JE, Steffes MW *et al*. Increased small dense LDL and intermediate-density lipoprotein with albuminuria in type 1 diabetes. *Diabetes Care* 1999; 22:1165–1170.
13. Pettitt DJ, Saad MF, Bennett PM, Nelson RG, Knowler WC. Familial predisposition to renal disease in two generations of Pima Indians with type II (non-insulin dependent) diabetes mellitus. *Diabetologia* 1990; 33:438–443.
14. Greene DA, Lattimer SA, Sima AAF. Sorbitol, phosphoinosotides, and sodium-potassium-ATPase in the pathogenesis of diabetic complications. *N Engl J Med* 1987; 316:599–606.
15. Vlassara H. Receptor-mediated interaction of advanced glycosylation end products with cellular components within diabetic tissues. *Diabetes* 1992; 41(suppl 2):52–56.
16. Hostetter TH. Diabetic nephropathy, metabolic versus hemodynamic considerations. *Diabetes Care* 1992; 15:1205–1215.
17. Sharp PS. Growth factors in the pathogenesis of diabetic retinopathy. *Diabetes Rev* 1995; 3:164–176.
18. Pacher P, Szabo C. Role of poly(ADP-ribose) polymerase-1 activation in the pathogenesis of diabetic complications: endothelial dysfunction, as a common underlying theme. *Antioxid Redox Signal* 2005; 7:1568–1580.
19. American Diabetes Association. Standards of medical care in diabetes – 2007. *Diabetes Care* 2007; 30(suppl 1):S4–S41.
20. Expert Panel on Detection, Evaluation, and Treatment of High Blood Cholesterol in Adults: Executive summary of the Third Report of the National Cholesterol Education Program (NCEP) Expert Panel on Detection, Evaluation, and Treatment of High Blood Cholesterol in Adults (Adult Treatment Panel III). *JAMA* 2001; 285:2486–2497.
21. Ford ES, Giles WH, Dietz WH. Prevalence of the metabolic syndrome among US adults: findings from the Third National Health and Nutrition Examination Survey. *JAMA* 2002; 287:356–359.
22. Ridker PM, Buring JE, Cook NR, Rifai N. C-reactive protein, the metabolic syndrome, and risk of incident cardiovascular events: an 8-year follow-up of 14 719 initially healthy American women. *Circulation* 2003; 107:391–397.
23. Eschwege E, Richard JL, Thibult N *et al*. Coronary heart disease mortality in relation with diabetes, blood glucose and plasma insulin levels. The Paris Prospective Study, ten years later. *Horm Metab Res* 1985; 15(suppl):41–46.
24. Khaw K-T, Wareham N, Luben R *et al*. Glycated haemoglobin, diabetes, and mortality in men in Norfolk cohort of European Prospective Investigation of Cancer and Nutrition (EPIC-Norfolk). *Br Med J* 2001; 322:15–28.
25. DREAM (Diabetes REduction Assessment with ramipril and rosiglitazone Medication) Trial Investigators. Effect of rosiglitazone on the frequency of diabetes in patients with impaired glucose tolerance or impaired fasting glucose: a randomised controlled trial. *Lancet* 2006; 368:1096–1105.
26. Buse JB, Ginsgerg HN, Bakris GL *et al*. Primary prevention of cardiovascular diseases in people with type 2 diabetes mellitus. A scientific statement from the American Heart Association and the American Diabetes Association. *Circulation* 2007; 115:114–126.
27. Sharrett AR, Heiss G, Chambless LE *et al*. Metabolic and lifestyle determinants of postprandial lipemia differ from those of fasting triglycerides: The Atherosclerosis Risk in Communities (ARIC) Study. *Arterioscler Thromb Vasc Biol* 2001; 21:275–281.
28. Miyatake N, Wada J, Kawasaki Y, Nishii K, Makino H, Numata T. Relationship between metabolic syndrome and cigarette smoking in the Japanese population. *Intern Med* 2006; 45:1039–1043.
29. Facchini FS, Hollenbeck CB, Jeppesen J, Chen YD, Reaven GM. Insulin resistance and cigarette smoking. *Lancet* 1992; 339:1128–1130.
30. Heitzer T, Yla-Herttuala S, Luoma J *et al*. Cigarette smoking potentiates endothelial dysfunction of forearm resistance vessels in patients with hypercholesterolemia: role of oxidized LDL. *Circulation* 1996; 9:1346–1353.
31. Kong C, Nimmo L, Elatrozy T *et al*. Smoking is associated with increased hepatic lipase activity, insulin resistance, dyslipidaemia and early atherosclerosis in type 2 diabetes. *Atherosclerosis* 2001; 156:373–378.
32. Law M, Tang JL. An analysis of the effectiveness of interventions intended to help people stop smoking. *Arch Intern Med* 1995; 155:1933–1941.
33. Solberg LI, Boyle RG, Davidson G *et al*. Patient satisfaction and discussion of smoking cessation during clinical visits. *Mayo Clin Proc* 2001; 76:138–143.
34. Marcus BH, Albrecht AE, King TK *et al*. The efficacy of exercise as an aid for smoking cessation in women. *Arch Intern Med* 1999; 159:1229–1234.

35. Prochaska JO, Velicer WF, Prochaska JM, Johnson JL. Size, consistency, and stability of stage effects for smoking cessation. *Addict Behav* 2004; 29:207–213.
36. Despres J-P, Pouliot M-C, Moorjani S *et al.* Loss of abdominal fat and metabolic response to exercise training in obese women. *Am J Physiol* 1991; 261:E159–E167.
37. Katzmarzyk PT, Church TS, Blair SN. Cardiorespiratory fitness attenuates the effects of the metabolic syndrome on all-cause and cardiovascular disease mortality in men. *Arch Intern Med* 2004; 164:1092–1097.
38. Hu FB, Willett WC. Optimal diets for prevention of coronary heart disease. *JAMA* 2002; 288:2569–2578.
39. Esposito K, Marfella R, Ciotola M *et al.* Effect of a Mediterranean-style diet on endothelial dysfunction and markers of vascular inflammation in the metabolic syndrome: a randomized trial. *JAMA* 2004; 292:1440–1446.
40. Estruch R, Martinez-Gonzalez MA, Corella D *et al.* Effects of a Mediterranean-style diet on cardiovascular risk factors. A randomized trial. *Ann Intern Med* 2006; 145:1–11.
41. Knoops KT, de Groot LC, Kromhout D *et al.* Mediterranean diet, lifestyle factors, and 10-year mortality in elderly European men and women: the HALE project. *JAMA* 2004; 292:1433–1439.
42. Stratton IM, Adler AI, Neil HA *et al.* Association of glycaemia with macrovascular and microvascular complications of type 2 diabetes (UKPDS 35): prospective observational study. *Br Med J* 2000; 321:405–412.
43. Chiasson JL, Josse RG, Gomis R, Hanefeld M, Karasik A, Laakso M, STOP-NIDDM Trial Research Group: Acarbose treatment and the risk of cardiovascular disease and hypertension in patients with impaired glucose tolerance: the STOP-NIDDM trial. *JAMA* 2003; 290:486–494.
44. Pan XR, Li GW, Hu YH *et al.* Effects of diet and exercise in preventing NIDDM in people with impaired glucose tolerance. The Da Qing IGT and Diabetes Study. *Diabetes Care* 1997; 20:537–544.
45. Tuomilehto J, Lindstrom J, Eriksson JG *et al.* Finnish Diabetes Prevention Study Group. Prevention of type 2 diabetes mellitus by changes in lifestyle among subjects with impaired glucose tolerance. *N Engl J Med* 2001; 344:1343–1350.
46. The Diabetes Prevention Program Research Group. Reduction in the incidence of type 2 diabetes with lifestyle intervention or metformin. *N Engl J Med* 2002; 346:393–403.
47. The Diabetes Prevention Program Research Group: Impact of intensive lifestyle and metformin therapy on cardiovascular disease risk factors in the Diabetes Prevention Program. *Diabetes Care* 2005; 28:888–894.
48. Dagogo-Jack S. Primary prevention of cardiovascular disease in pre-diabetes: The glass is half-full and half-empty (editorial). *Diabetes Care* 2005; 28:971–972.
49. Kubaszek A, Pihlajamaki J, Komarovski V *et al.* Finnish Diabetes Prevention Study. Promoter polymorphisms of the TNF-alpha (G-308A) and IL-6 (C-174G) genes predict the conversion from impaired glucose tolerance to type 2 diabetes: the Finnish Diabetes Prevention Study. *Diabetes* 2003; 52:1872–1876.
50. Diabetes Prevention Program Research Group; Crandall J, Schade D, Ma Y *et al.* The influence of age on the effects of lifestyle modification and metformin in prevention of diabetes. *J Gerontol A Biol Sci Med Sci* 2006; 61:1075–1081.
51. Florez JC, Jablonski KA, Bayley N *et al.* Diabetes Prevention Program Research Group. TCF7L2 polymorphisms and progression to diabetes in the Diabetes Prevention Program. *N Engl J Med* 2006; 355:241–250.
52. Grant SF, Thorleifsson G, Reynisdottir I *et al.* Variant of transcription factor 7-like 2 (TCF7L2) gene confers risk of type 2 diabetes. *Nat Genet* 2006; 38:320–323.

2

Dietary controversies in treatment of the metabolic syndrome

N. Davis, N. Tomuta, J. Wylie-Rosett

INTRODUCTION

Weight loss plays an integral role in the treatment of metabolic syndrome. Modest weight loss defined as 5–10% reduction in body weight has many beneficial effects including reduction of the metabolic syndrome, risk of type 2 diabetes and blood pressure. Hallmark features of the metabolic syndrome including obesity, insulin resistance and a pro-inflammatory state are all modifiable through lifestyle intervention [1–3]. Pharmacotherapy can successfully treat each of the individual risk factors of the metabolic syndrome, but lifestyle intervention through diet and exercise can provide an integrated strategy to improve all aspects of the metabolic syndrome [4, 5]. There is, however, significant debate both about the role of dietary intake in contributing to the prevalence of metabolic syndrome, and about the optimal dietary composition for weight loss and treatment of the metabolic syndrome.

The role of macronutrient composition in the development and treatment of metabolic syndrome is uncertain, and the role of dietary fat and dietary carbohydrate is frequently debated. Dietary fat has been hypothesized to contribute to the increasing rates of obesity and diabetes [6, 7]. High-fat diets are associated with increased caloric consumption, and long-term reduction of total dietary fat has been shown to result in weight loss [8–10]. Dietary carbohydrate has similarly been hypothesized to contribute to increasing rates of obesity and diabetes, and reduction in carbohydrates can stimulate weight loss and reduce insulin resistance [11, 12]. Additionally, the role of low glycemic index foods in achieving weight loss and reducing metabolic risk is unclear.

This chapter will review the current evidence exploring dietary factors in the development and the treatment of the metabolic syndrome (Figure 2.1). We will specifically review epidemiologic and clinical trial evidence of the roles of dietary fat, dietary carbohydrate, fructose and high glycemic index foods in the development of the metabolic syndrome. Finally, we will explore the roles of low-fat, low-carbohydrate, low-calorie, diets with low glycemic index, and diets that emphasize dietary patterns as strategies for weight reduction and treatment of the metabolic syndrome.

Nichola J. Davis, MD, MS, Assistant Professor, Department of Medicine, Albert Einstein College of Medicine/Montefiore Medical Center, Department of Epidemiology, Bronx, New York, USA

Norica Tomuta, MD, Research Associate, Department of Epidemiology and Population Health, Division of Behavioral and Nutrition Research, General Clinic Research Center, Albert Einstein College of Medicine, Bronx, New York, USA

Judith Wylie-Rosett, EdD, RD, Professor, Department of Epidemiology and Population Health, Albert Einstein College of Medicine, Bronx, New York, USA

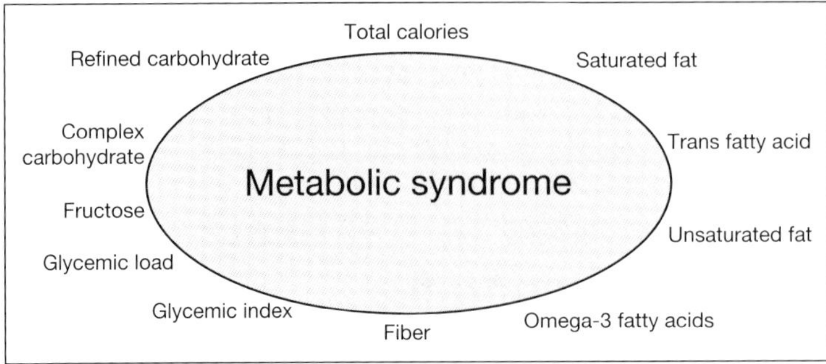

Figure 2.1 Dietary factors that may impact the metabolic syndrome.

THE CONTROVERSY OF DIETARY FAT

OVERVIEW

Obesity is a primary risk in development of the metabolic syndrome and is usually accompanied by increased body fat and visceral fat accumulation. Increased visceral fat can contribute to the development of insulin resistance and inflammation, which are hallmark features of the metabolic syndrome. Although the mechanisms of developing insulin resistance and inflammation are not clearly elucidated, there are several key hypotheses. One such hypothesis is that as a consequence of increasing body fat, there is increasing overload of lipid-filled tissue which primarily deposits in the liver and skeletal muscle [13]. This increased visceral fat reduces the ability of peripheral tissues to utilize insulin effectively resulting in insulin resistance. Adipocytes, which were previously believed to be inactive storage depots for fat cells, appear to play a key role in the development of insulin resistance through the release of adipokines such as adiponectin [14, 15]. Additionally, adipocytes may play key roles in the underlying state of chronic inflammation through their release of inflammatory cytokines such as tumor necrosis factor alpha (TNF-α) and interleukin-6 (IL-6) [16, 17]. What role then does dietary fat play in this cycle? Does dietary fat contribute to increased body weight and visceral fat? Does dietary fat contribute to inflammation and development of insulin resistance? Are there differential effects on inflammation and insulin resistance depending on the type of dietary fat, i.e. saturated fat, unsaturated fat, and trans fatty acids? And importantly, is there evidence to support modulating dietary fat in the treatment of the metabolic syndrome?

ROLE OF DIETARY FAT IN THE DEVELOPMENT OF METABOLIC SYNDROME

Although the percentage of calories from dietary fat has declined since the 1950s, unprecedented rates of obesity have occurred since then [18]. Between the 1970s and 1980s dietary fat intake decreased by 11% with a concomitant decrease of caloric intake by 4%. Despite this, however, the prevalence of overweight increased by 31% [19]. These changes in dietary trends and increases in overweight prevalence have stimulated questions about whether dietary fat contributes to obesity. High-fat diets are thought to be associated with overconsumption of energy and weight gain, however dietary strategies such as low-carbohydrate diets, which are high in fat, can result in weight loss. Conflicting evidence also exists as to the role of dietary fat in inducing insulin resistance and inflammation. Animal feeding studies have demonstrated an increase in visceral fat and insulin resistance with high-fat diets [20], however this is not as conclusive in human studies. Higher intake of dietary fat predicts type 2 diabetes incidence, and is associated with increased fasting hyperinsulinemia in some human studies [21, 22]. Analysis of over 80 000 women enrolled in the Nurse's Health Study, however, found no association between type of dietary fat and body mass index (BMI) [23], and after controlling for known risk factors of type 2 diabetes, total dietary fat was not found to be related to an increased risk of type 2 diabetes.

While there are debates about the effects of total dietary fat intake, there is substantial evidence regarding the effects of specific dietary fatty acids. Saturated fatty acids and trans fatty acids can increase low-density lipoprotein (LDL)-cholesterol, which is recognized as an important predictor of cardiovascular disease in patients with type 2 diabetes [13, 24]. Conversely, diets rich in unsaturated fats and omega-3 fatty acids are associated with lower rates of cardiovascular disease in both observation and randomized clinical trials [25].

Serum level of fatty acids may additionally be an important predictor in the development of the metabolic syndrome. Warensjo *et al.* [26] examined fatty acid composition in 1558 men enrolled in the Uppsala Longitudinal Study of Adult Men, a population cohort study in Uppsala, Sweden. The men were enrolled at age 50, and without a diagnosis of hypertension, diabetes, or hyperlipidemia at the time of enrollment. Serum fatty acid composition was measured at baseline and at follow-up 20 years later. Levels of saturated fatty acids including myristic acid (14:0), and palmitic acid (16:0) were significantly higher at baseline in men who later developed the metabolic syndrome [26]. Levels of omega-3 fatty acids did not differ between men who developed the metabolic syndrome, compared to those who did not.

Interestingly, this study further highlighted differences among types of saturated fatty acids, which may reflect the effects that specific saturated fatty acids may have on LDL concentration. Unlike myristic and palmitic acid, levels of the saturated fatty acid, stearic acid (18:0), did not predict development of metabolic syndrome [26]. This may be related to differences in absorption of saturated fatty acids, as well as their effects on LDL concentration. Diets high in myristic and palmitic acid have been demonstrated to increase serum LDL more significantly than diets high in stearic acid, which may be partially due to conversion of stearic acid (18:0) to oleic acid (18:1), which has hypocholesterolemic effects [27].

Feeding studies have demonstrated that saturated fat and trans fatty acids may induce inflammation and insulin resistance in the post-prandial state. In a randomized study, Esposito *et al.* [28] compared healthy subjects to obese patients with type 2 diabetes and meals with varied fat, carbohydrate and fiber content were given to all subjects. Consumption of a high-fat meal resulted in increases in interleukin-18 levels (a marker of inflammation) and decreased adiponectin, suggesting post-prandial increases in inflammation and reduced insulin sensitivity following high-fat meals. In contrast, a low-fat/high-carbohydrate meal resulted in decreases of IL-18 levels in both patients with and without type 2 diabetes [28]. In healthy patients given a high-fat meal, increases in TNF-α and IL-6 were observed 2–4 h after ingestion and these increases were greater in patients with diabetes [29] also suggesting that high-fat meals induce inflammation.

ROLE OF REDUCING DIETARY FAT IN THE TREATMENT OF METABOLIC SYNDROME

Statements by the American Heart Association, the American Diabetes Association and the National Cholesterol Education Adult Treatment Panel III (ATP III) recommend reducing saturated fat intake to 7% of calories of fat to control cardiovascular risk factors [24, 30, 31]. Reducing dietary fat can play an important role in controlling body weight and reducing the risk of developing diabetes [32] (Table 2.1). Results of meta-analyses indicate that *ad libitum* diets which reduce energy intake from dietary fat by 10% can result in a weight loss of 4–5 kg in obese patients [33].

The Diabetes Prevention Program (DPP) and the Finnish Diabetes Prevention Study (FDPS) investigated the efficacy of a low-fat diet as part of a lifestyle intervention in reducing

Table 2.1 Intervention studies: low-fat diets in treatment of metabolic syndrome

Authors	*Intervention*	*n*	*Length of intervention*	*Effect on metabolic syndrome*
Diabetes Prevention Program [3]	Low-fat diet; <25% energy from fat, physical activity 180 min/week compared to metformin or control	Total $n = 3234$, $n = 1711$ with metabolic syndrome at baseline	3.5 years	Weight reduction by 7%; reduction in waist circumference, triglycerides, fasting glucose, blood pressure and inflammation. Increase in HDL. Resolution of metabolic syndrome in 38% of participants in lifestyle intervention
Finnish Diabetes Prevention Study [34]	Low-fat diet; <30% of energy from fat, increased fiber, whole grains	522 adults with impaired fasting glucose	4 years	Weight reduction; reduction in waist circumference, triglycerides, fasting glucose, blood pressure. Increase in HDL
Muzio *et al.* [39]	ATP III low-fat diet; 30% energy from fat, <7% from saturated fat, 55% energy from carbohydrate	41 patients with metabolic syndrome	2 years	Weight reduction by 9.9%. Resolution of metabolic syndrome in 37% of participants

the incidence of diabetes [3, 34]. While both studies focused on diabetes prevention in patients at risk for diabetes, a significant percentage of participants at baseline met criteria for the metabolic syndrome.

The DPP was a multicentered US study that evaluated the effects of a lifestyle intervention compared with placebo or treatment with metformin in reducing diabetes in adults at risk for developing type 2 diabetes [9]. This study randomized 3234 adults with impaired glucose tolerance to receive an intensive lifestyle intervention, metformin, or placebo. Fifty-three percent ($n = 1711$) of participants in DPP at baseline met criteria for the metabolic syndrome as defined by ATP III criteria [3]. The intensive lifestyle intervention included a low-fat (<25% of energy) reduced calorie diet and physical activity of 150 min per week and was designed to achieve and maintain a 7% reduction of body weight. The lifestyle intervention was found to improve all components of the metabolic syndrome (reduce prevalence of low HDL, reduce waist circumference, fasting glucose, blood pressure, and triglycerides.) In contrast, treatment with metformin reduced the prevalence of low HDL, waist circumference and fasting glucose only [3]. Following 3.2 years of the intervention, 38% of participants in the lifestyle intervention, compared with 23% in metformin and 18% in the placebo group no longer met criteria for the metabolic syndrome. Among participants without the metabolic syndrome at baseline, incidence of developing metabolic syndrome over three years was lowest in the lifestyle intervention (38%) compared to the metformin (47%) and placebo (53%) groups [3]. Among all participants, the lifestyle intervention reduced the risk of type 2 diabetes by 58% [9]. Further analysis of the DPP data examined the effect of each intervention on inflammation as measured by C-reactive protein (CRP). Results indicated approximately a 30% reduction in CRP levels following the lifestyle intervention [35]. Interestingly, following the initial 6 months of the intervention, CRP levels continued to decline independent of weight changes, suggesting that the reduction in inflammation may have been secondary to other aspects of the intervention [35].

The FDPS also evaluated the effects of a weight loss lifestyle intervention on the incidence of diabetes as well as the metabolic syndrome [34]. This study randomized 522 overweight adults with impaired fasting glucose to a lifestyle intervention or placebo [34, 36]. Seventy-eight percent of this population met criteria for metabolic syndrome at baseline [37]. The lifestyle intervention in this study similarly included a low-fat diet with <30% of calories from fat and <10% from saturated fat [36]. Additional features of the lifestyle intervention included increased fiber intake, increased intake of whole grains, fruits and vegetables, and use of oils with monounsaturated fats. Following one year of the intervention, a mean reduction in weight of 4.2 kg was achieved and a 58% reduction in incidence of diabetes was observed in participants following the lifestyle intervention. When individual components of the metabolic syndrome are examined in this population, significant reductions in waist circumference, plasma glucose, blood pressure and triglycerides, and significant elevations in HDL were observed [36]. After controlling for other risk factors for developing diabetes, reduced dietary fat and fiber intake were found to be significant predictors of both sustained weight loss and development of type 2 diabetes [10].

The low-fat diet in DPP restricted fat to <25% of energy, to correspond to a calorie reduction to achieve a one pound weight loss per week [38]. The FDPS restricted total fat to <30% and saturated fat to <10%. The ATP III diet recommends a restriction of total fat to 25–35% with <7% saturated fat. In a smaller study, 41 patients with metabolic syndrome were treated with the ATP III diet for two years [39]. This diet consisted of 30% of energy from fat, with less than 7% from saturated fat and 55% of energy from carbohydrates. Following 2 years of this intervention, there was a mean reduction of body weight of 9.9%, and 37% of participants no longer fulfilled the criteria for metabolic syndrome. Two-thirds of participants who lost more than 10% of their body weight had resolution of the metabolic syndrome. In comparison, 19% of participants who lost less than 10% of their body weight had resolution of the metabolic syndrome [39]. In all patients with resolution of the metabolic syndrome, the BMI remained in the obese range, emphasizing the importance of achieving modest weight loss.

Although the contribution of dietary fat to the development of obesity and metabolic syndrome remains debatable, it is evident that reducing dietary fat in the setting of a weight loss lifestyle intervention is effective in reducing weight and treating the metabolic syndrome. One consequence of reducing total dietary fat intake, however, is the reduction in polyunsaturated and monounsaturated fats, which may have beneficial effects on insulin resistance and inflammation, as well as beneficial effects on levels of high-density lipoprotein (HDL). Increasing polyunsaturated and monounsaturated fats as part of a weight loss strategy usually accompanies reduction in carbohydrates, and these diets will be discussed in greater detail in the sections on carbohydrate restriction. Beyond the concern of reducing polyunsaturated and unsaturated fats, there are no studies to our knowledge that have demonstrated adverse outcomes when following a low-fat diet. Therefore, we can conclude from the current evidence that reduction in dietary fat as part of a weight loss strategy is an important strategy in the treatment of metabolic syndrome.

THE CONTROVERSY OF DIETARY CARBOHYDRATE

The optimal level and type of carbohydrate intake for patients with the metabolic syndrome is unknown and continues to be a source of controversy. The reduction in dietary fat that has occurred in the US has been replaced by increased carbohydrate intake and has paralleled the rise in obesity rates and the metabolic syndrome. Between the years of 1980 and 1997, there was a general increase in dietary carbohydrate consumption from 48% to 54% of total energy, an increase in total energy of >500 kcal/day, an 80% increase in obesity and a 47% increase in type 2 diabetes [12]. Eighty percent of the increase in total energy during this time period was from dietary carbohydrate. As a result of this trend, many questions concerning the role of carbohydrates in both the development and the treatment of metabolic syndrome have developed. How do carbohydrates differ in their effect on metabolic syndrome? Does the type of carbohydrate matter, i.e. simple vs complex carbohydrates, low vs high glycemic index carbohydrates, glucose vs fructose? Finally, does reducing dietary carbohydrate improve the metabolic syndrome? To better understand this debate, we will first examine the role that carbohydrates may play in the development of metabolic syndrome, and then examine their potential role in treatment.

THE ROLE OF CARBOHYDRATES IN THE DEVELOPMENT OF METABOLIC SYNDROME

Longitudinal data suggest that a high-carbohydrate diet, particularly of refined carbohydrates, is associated with the development of obesity and metabolic syndrome [12]. Gross *et al.* performed an ecologic analysis of the use of refined carbohydrates and the prevalence of obesity and type 2 diabetes. In this analysis, intake of refined carbohydrates (corn syrup), protein, fat, and total energy were correlated with the prevalence of type 2 diabetes from 1909 to 1997 in the US population. While higher intake of each of these variables was significantly correlated with the prevalence of type 2 diabetes in univariate analyses, multivariate modeling resulted in positive associations between corn syrup and type 2 diabetes, while high fiber intake was negatively associated [12].

Fructose and the metabolic syndrome

Dietary carbohydrate provides an essential source of fuel for normal body function including normal brain and muscle function. However, the increased intake of carbohydrates in combination with dramatic changes in carbohydrate sources from whole grains in 1909 to refined carbohydrates and fructose may have metabolic consequences [12, 40]. Since the mid-1960s, corn has been refined to produce corn-based syrups which are now among the leading sweeteners used in the US. High fructose corn syrup, a refined carbohydrate, is consumed in high quantities through soft drinks, baked goods, and canned goods [11, 41].

It is hypothesized that the metabolism of fructose may contribute to the development of metabolic syndrome. The metabolism of fructose, which is a monosaccharide, differs from that of sucrose, which is a disaccharide of glucose plus fructose. Fructose, unlike glucose, does not depend on insulin for uptake into cells, does not stimulate insulin secretion, and was therefore believed to be an alternative to glucose and an advantage for patients with diabetes [41]. However the association between fructose and weight gain, and its worsening effects on insulin resistance has changed this theory.

Fructose does not directly stimulate insulin or increase insulin levels. However, it has been hypothesized that high intake of fructose may contribute to obesity with concomitant insulin resistance and hyperinsulinemia through various proposed mechanisms. Fructose is metabolized by the liver and consumption in large quantities (e.g. 85–100 g daily) may increase lipogenesis and triglyceride accumulation which in turn reduces insulin sensitivity, contibuting to glucose intolerance [40, 41]. Fructose additionally does not appear to turn on satiety signals in the brain [41], potentially resulting in increased consumption and weight gain, obesity and metabolic syndrome.

Epidemiologic and ecologic studies support the link between fructose, refined carbohydrates, obesity and type 2 diabetes [12, 40, 41]. Animal models as well as human studies demonstrate that increased consumption of fructose results in increased weight gain [41]. Schulze *et al.* [42] examined women prospectively in the Nurse's Health Study and demonstrated that over four years, weight gain was highest among women who increased their consumption from one or fewer sweetened soft drinks per week to more than one per day. Whether specifically reducing dietary fructose improves metabolic syndrome is not well studied, and is an area for future research. Based on the physiologic effects of fructose, however, it is plausible that dietary reductions

Table 2.2 Low-carbohydrate diets and treatment of metabolic syndrome

Authors	*Intervention*	*n*	*Length of intervention*	*Effect on metabolic syndrome*
Foster *et al.* [44]	Low-carbohydrate compared to low-fat diet	63 obese adults	1 year	Weight reduction in both groups, without significant differences between dietary groups. Significant increases in insulin sensitivity at 6 months, but no significant improvement in insulin sensitivity at one year
Samaha *et al.* [48]	Low-carbohydrate compared to low-fat diet	132 adults; 43% with metabolic syndrome	6 months	Significant weight loss and significant improvements in insulin sensitivity in participants following low-carbohydrate diet
Stern *et al.* [45]	Low-carbohydrate compared to low-fat diet	132 adults; 43% with metabolic syndrome	1 year	Significant weight reduction in each dietary group, with similar weight loss between dietary groups. Significant reduction in triglycerides and increase in HDL in low-carbohydrate arm only
Poppit *et al.* [53]	Low-fat diet with high simple carbohydrates, compared to low-fat diet with high complex carbohydrates, compared to control	46 adults with metabolic syndrome	6 months	Significant weight reduction only in low-fat, high complex carbohydrates. Higher triglycerides in the low-fat, high simple carbohydrate group
Muzio *et al.* [50]	High-carbohydrate diet (65% of calories), compared to low-carbohydrate (48% of calories)	100 patients with metabolic syndrome	5 months	Significant weight reduction in both groups and improved metabolic syndrome in both groups. Greater reductions in LDL in the high-carbohydrate group. Greater reductions in blood pressure and triglycerides in the low-carbohydrate diet

in fructose may have favorable effects on weight and insulin resistance, and may be a potential dietary target in the treatment of the metabolic syndrome.

Carbohydrate restriction and the metabolic syndrome

A daily intake of 130 g of carbohydrate is recommended by the Institute of Medicine to address overall health needs [43]. The increased popularity of low-carbohydrate diets has prompted research to study the metabolic effects of such diets. Recently, this weight loss strategy has been compared to more traditional dietary approaches. In addition, several studies have specifically examined low-carbohydrate diets in patients with the metabolic syndrome (Table 2.2). Randomized clinical trials of low-carbohydrate diets (defined as carbohydrate restriction of <20 g carbohydrate daily) compared to low-fat diets have demonstrated more rapid weight loss within the first 6 months of a low-carbohydrate diet, and equivalent weight loss after one year of each intervention [44, 45].

Stern *et al.* [45] evaluated the one-year effects of a low-carbohydrate diet compared to a low-fat diet in 132 obese subjects. In this population, 44% of subjects in the low-carbohydrate arm and 40% in the low-fat arm had the metabolic syndrome. There were no significant differences in weight loss between the two groups after one year, however the low-carbohydrate arm did result in significant decreases in triglycerides and increases in HDL [45]. These favorable changes in triglycerides and HDL, however, may be accompanied by a modest unfavorable increase in LDL-cholesterol [46]. Independent of weight loss, the role of carbohydrate restriction is very provocative because of its potential effect on insulin sensitivity, a hallmark feature of the metabolic syndrome. In obese patients with type 2 diabetes ($n = 10$), Boden *et al.* [47] found improvements in insulin sensitivity secondary to increased peripheral glucose uptake following 2 weeks of a low-carbohydrate (<20 g carbohydrate daily) diet, but this study did not have a dietary comparison group. Samaha *et al.* [48] reported greater insulin sensitivity in non-diabetic participants following a low-carbohydrate diet when compared to a low-fat diet, but after controlling for weight loss the difference was not statistically significant.

Low-carbohydrate diets are often criticized because of the potential metabolic effects of unlimited fat intake, particularly saturated fat intake, and the difficulty with long-term adherence. Aude *et al.* [49] studied the effects of a modified low-carbohydrate diet, which was low in carbohydrates (ranges of 10–33% of total calories, high in protein (ranges of 28–33% of total calories), and high in fat (ranges from 39–62% of total fat). Unique features of this study included the high percentage of monounsaturated and polyunsaturated fats, and the use of complex carbohydrates. The effect of weight loss following the modified low-carbohydrate diet was compared to a control isocaloric ATP III diet. Following 12 weeks of dietary intervention, greater weight loss was observed in the modified low-carbohydrate arm (13.6 lbs), compared to the NCEP group (7.5 lbs) [49]. This study did not specifically examine the metabolic syndrome, but there was a significant reduction in triglycerides in both treatment groups.

Specifically studying the metabolic syndrome, Muzio *et al.* [50] randomized 100 patients with the metabolic syndrome to two reduced-calorie diets with varying carbohydrate and fat composition. The 'high-carbohydrate' diet had 65% of calories from carbohydrate and 22% of calories from fat. The 'low-carbohydrate' diet reduced carbohydrates to 48% of calories and had 33% of calories from fat. Following 5 months of each diet, participants in both groups had similar weight reduction (approximately 10%) and significant improvements in all components of the metabolic syndrome. However, the groups differed slightly in the magnitude of improvement in individual components of the metabolic syndrome. The 'high-carbohydrate' dietary group had more significant reductions in LDL-cholesterol, while the 'low-carbohydrate' group had more significant reductions in systolic blood pressure and triglycerides. These findings suggest that it may be important to consider the individual components of the metabolic syndrome when thinking about the optimal dietary strategy.

Simple versus complex carbohydrates

Carbohydrates have been classified according to the complexity of their biochemical structure. Sugars (simple carbohydrates) refer to monosaccharides such as glucose and fructose and disaccharides such as sucrose and lactose. Refined carbohydrates may be used to describe the sugars, or processes, polysaccharides such as starches, or in some cases highly processed flours [51]. The term complex carbohydrate is used to refer to the longer chain carbohydrates, but is sometimes used to refer to unrefined whole grains and legumes. Several studies have investigated the role of different simple compared to complex carbohydrates in the treatment of obesity and the metabolic syndrome. The CARMEN Study was a controlled multicenter study, which randomized 398 overweight and obese adults

(BMI 26–35 mg/m^2) to one of two experimental diets or a control group. Each experimental diet reduced fat intake by 10% of energy. The experimental diets however differed in the type of carbohydrates. One experimental group had a higher intake of simple carbohydrates, while the comparison diet had a higher intake of complex carbohydrates [52]. Following 6 months of the intervention, both dietary groups lost significantly more weight than the control arm, which received no dietary intervention. The low-fat complex carbohydrate diet had a significantly greater decrease in energy intake than the low-fat simple carbohydrate diet. However, when weight loss was compared, the differences between the two diet treatment arms were similar, with a 2.6 kg reduction in the low-fat complex carbohydrate group, and a 1.7 kg reduction in the low-fat simple carbohydrate [52]. Poppitt *et al.* [53] evaluated 46 subjects with the metabolic syndrome and randomized them to the dietary interventions outlined in the CARMEN Study. Following 6 months of the intervention, only participants in the low-fat with complex carbohydrates had significant weight loss of 4.3 kg. The low-fat simple carbohydrate group did not have any change in weight, and were noted to have significantly higher triglyceride concentration [53], leading to the conclusion that complex carbohydrates may be more beneficial than simple carbohydrates in weight loss and management of metabolic risk factors.

Glycemic index and glycemic load

Carbohydrates are additionally classified according to their glycemic index or glycemic load, which are both ways of explaining the post-prandial glycemic excursion [11]. Glycemic index was initially proposed in 1981 by Jenkins *et al.* [54] and compares foods to a reference standard of glucose or white bread. Over a 2-h period, the area under the glucose response curve after consuming a 50 g load of a particular food is compared to the area under the glucose response curve after consuming 50 g of the reference standard [11, 54]. Based on comparisons in the glucose response from the test food to the reference standard, an index is developed. Noted concerns about the glycemic index include the wide glycemic index range given to many foods and difficulty translating its use into clinical practice [11, 54]. Despite this limitation, several studies have emerged utilizing the glycemic index that offer some insights to its potential role in the metabolic syndrome.

Glycemic load is calculated from the glycemic index and can be determined by multiplying the glycemic index of a food by the carbohydrate content of the food [54]. Foods that have a high glycemic index, however, may not necessarily have a high glycemic load. For example, carrots have a high glycemic index, but because they contain relatively little carbohydrates, the glycemic load is modest [11].

Theoretically, consuming diets with lower glycemic index and lower glycemic load should reduce post-prandial hyperglycemia and reduce insulin levels. This may in turn result in reduced insulin resistance and may improve elements of the metabolic syndrome. Epidemiologic studies have supported the association between dietary glycemic index, glycemic load and metabolic syndrome, however interventional studies have contradictory results. Several prospective cohort studies in patients without metabolic syndrome have further demonstrated an association between the dietary glycemic index and incidence of type 2 diabetes [54, 55].

Specifically, studying the metabolic syndrome, McKeown *et al.* [56] examined the associations between dietary glycemic index and the prevalence of metabolic syndrome among 2834 participants in the Framingham Offspring Study. Results from this analysis demonstrated a significant positive association between high dietary glycemic index and metabolic syndrome. When quintiles of dietary glycemic index were compared, participants with the highest dietary glycemic index were 40% more likely to have the metabolic syndrome when compared to participants with the lowest dietary glycemic index [56]. Higher whole grain and cereal fiber intake was also associated with lower prevalence of metabolic syndrome.

To examine the effects of glycemic index on weight, several studies have compared isocaloric high vs low glycemic index diets. [54, 57]. Millan-Price *et al.* [58] randomized 129 overweight and obese young adults (age range 18–40 years) to one of four different diets for 12 weeks. Each diet contained 30% of energy from fat, and differed according to the quantity and glycemic index of carbohydrates. The first two diets contained 55% carbohydrates and 15% protein, and differed according to the glycemic index of the source of carbohydrates, high vs low glycemic index foods. The third and fourth diets had a macronutrient composition of 45% carbohydrates with 25% protein and differed according to the glycemic index of each diet [58]. Following 12 weeks of each diet, weight reduction, improvement in insulin sensitivity, and reduced levels of CRP were observed in each group, without significant differences between groups.

Low-calorie diets

Regardless of macronutrient composition, calorie reduction is an important goal in weight loss. Although *ad libitum* low-fat and low-carbohydrate diets do not primarily restrict the calories, the reduction in fat or carbohydrates usually results in decreased caloric intake. Because of independent metabolic effects of nutrients, it is not certain if weight loss with caloric restriction alone without any emphasis on macronutrient composition is as effective as diets which focus on macronutrient composition.

Dietary strategies that incorporate liquid meal replacements may reduce calories without emphasis on macronutrient composition. Hong *et al.* [59] examined the metabolic syndrome in patients enrolled in a self-paid weight management program. In this retrospective chart review of 304 enrolled patients, 40% were found to meet criteria for the metabolic syndrome. The weight management program utilized meal replacements as components of very low-calorie diets, which provided 500–800 kcal daily. Following 12 weeks of this very low-calorie diet, mean weight loss among participants was approximately 9% of body weight. This was accompanied by significant improvements in systolic and diastolic blood pressure, total cholesterol and triglycerides. The metabolic syndrome resolved in 39% of patients, and developed in 8% of patients who did not initially meet criteria for the metabolic syndrome [59]. Similarly, Xydakis *et al.* [60] examined the use of protein-sparing very low-calorie diets in 40 patients with the metabolic syndrome enrolled in a medically supervised weight loss program. The meal replacement comprised 600–800 kcal daily. Following 4–6 weeks of this diet, the average weight loss was a 7% reduction from initial body weight. There was resolution in all components of the metabolic syndrome except HDL, which was significantly decreased. Insulin sensitivity and inflammation were both demonstrated to improve over 4–6 weeks.

Few studies have compared the effects of reduced calorie diets to diets with specific dietary compositions in treating the metabolic syndrome (Table 2.3). Azabdakht *et al.* [61] randomized 116 patients to a control diet, a reduced calorie diet, and a reduced calorie DASH (Dietary Approaches to Stop Hypertension) diet. The reduced calorie diet did not emphasize any specific nutrient composition or food groups. The reduced calorie DASH diet, however, emphasized low-fat dairy products, vegetables, fruits, whole grains and legumes. Caloric reduction in both intervention groups was a 500 kcal deficit. Following 6 months of each diet, the control diet did not have any changes in weight, waist circumference, blood pressure or lipids. The reduced calorie group and the reduced calorie DASH group had similar weight reductions over 6 months, (12 kg in the reduced calorie and 14 kg in the reduced calorie DASH group). Both intervention groups also had similar reductions in waist circumference, and in serum triglycerides [61]. The reduced calorie DASH group also had significant increases in HDL, significant reductions in systolic and diastolic blood pressure and reductions in fasting blood sugar. These findings suggest that although weight loss improves many elements of the metabolic syndrome, obtaining a similar weight loss through emphasis of dietary components such as fruits, vegetables and fiber may be more

Table 2.3 Low-calorie dietary interventions and treatment of the metabolic syndrome

Authors	*Intervention*	*n*	*Length of intervention*	*Effect on metabolic syndrome*
Hong *et al.* [59]	Meal replacement of 500–800 kcal daily	304 adults, 40% with metabolic syndrome	12 weeks	9% reduction in weight; significant improvement in triglycerides and blood pressure. Resolution of metabolic syndrome in 39% of patients; 8% developed metabolic syndrome. Significant reductions in HDL
Xydakis *et al.* [60]	Meal replacement 600–800 kcal daily	40 patients with metabolic syndrome	4–6 weeks	Resolution in all components of metabolic syndrome, except HDL which was also reduced. Reduction in inflammation; improved insulin sensitivity
Azadbakht *et al.* [61]	Reduced-calorie Dietary Approaches to Stop Hypertension (DASH) diet compared to reduced-calorie diet, and control diet	116 patients	6 months	Reduction in weight, waist circumference and triglycerides in reduced calorie DASH diet and reduced-calorie diet. Reduced-calorie DASH group had significant reductions in systolic and diastolic BP, increases in HDL, and reductions in fasting glucose

beneficial. Increased fiber and vitamin intake in patients following the DASH diet may explain this finding [62].

ADDITIONAL DIETARY CONSIDERATIONS

Dietary patterns and the metabolic syndrome

Several epidemiologic studies have examined the effects of dietary patterns on the metabolic syndrome. Millen *et al.* [63] prospectively studied 300 healthy women without metabolic syndrome or risks for metabolic syndrome enrolled in the Framingham Offspring Study. Participants were followed for a mean of 12 years, during which data on nutrient intake were taken every 4 years. Results of this study demonstrated that participants with lower intake of total carbohydrates, fiber, micronutrients, and higher intake of dietary lipids (including total, saturated and monounsaturated fats) had an increased (2–3-fold) risk of developing abdominal obesity and metabolic syndrome [64]. These findings were independent of smoking, age and physical activity. Additional data from the Framingham Offspring Study evaluated the dietary patterns of women ($n = 1615$) and classified their nutrient intake into one of five distinct patterns: heart healthier, lighter eating, wine and moderate eating, higher fat, and empty calories. Participants with the empty calorie-eating pattern were found to have the highest intake of dietary fat, calories and sweetened beverages, and the lowest intake of fiber and vegetables. Both obese and non-obese participants with the empty calorie pattern had the greatest risk of developing metabolic syndrome [64].

Intervention studies have further emphasized the importance of considering whole dietary patterns in the treatment of metabolic syndrome. Esposito *et al.* [65] randomized 180 patients with metabolic syndrome to receive a Mediterranean-style diet consisting of increased whole grains, fruits, vegetables, nuts, and olive oil, or to a prudent diet, which consisted of total fat intake of <30%. Following two years of the intervention, participants receiving the Mediterranean-style diet had a higher intake of polyunsaturated and monounsaturated fat, increased intake of complex carbohydrates, higher intake of fiber, lower intake of saturated fat and lower energy intake than controls. Significant reductions in components of the metabolic syndrome including decreased body weight, decreased waist circumference, improved insulin sensitivity, reduced blood pressure and reduced triglycerides were observed in the intervention group [65]. At the end of two years, only 40 participants in the intervention, compared to 78 in the control group met criteria for the metabolic syndrome.

Fiber

Dietary fiber consists of the edible components of plant foods and is found in abundance in cereals, fruits, vegetables and nuts. Dietary fiber has been demonstrated to promote satiety, potentially through its effects on appetite-regulating hormones such as ghrelin and glucagon-like peptide-1 [66]. Additionally, it slows the absorption of food resulting in reduced post-prandial hyperglycemia [66]. Several epidemiologic studies have demonstrated an inverse relationship between high fiber intake and type 2 diabetes [67]. Analysis of over 2000 participants in the Framingham Offspring Study revealed inverse relationships between high whole grain intake and cereal fiber intake with lower prevalence of the metabolic syndrome [56]. Similarly, Sahyoun *et al.* [68] demonstrated an inverse relationship between whole grain intake and metabolic syndrome, among 535 elderly adults, after controlling for other dietary factors.

Many foods rich in dietary fiber may also have a low glycemic index. This has resulted in further debate regarding which factor may be more important in the treatment and prevention of the metabolic syndrome. Laaksonen *et al.* [69] examined this question in a prospective study comparing different carbohydrate sources of dietary fiber on metabolic parameters. In this study, 72 overweight or obese adults with the metabolic syndrome were randomized to a diet high in rye bread and pasta, compared to a diet high in oat or wheat bread and potatoes. The diets were similar in fiber intake, but the glycemic index of the pasta/rye diet was lower than that of the oat/wheat/potato diet. Following 12 weeks of each diet, there were no significant changes in weight, fasting glucose or insulin concentrations between groups. However, early insulin secretion was found to be higher in the rye bread and pasta group when compared to the oat, wheat and potato group, inferring a lower risk of developing type 2 diabetes in this group. This suggests that both fiber content and the glycemic index of foods from which the fiber is obtained may have independent effects on insulin resistance.

There is clearly substantial epidemiologic evidence to support the relationship between high intake of dietary fiber and reduced weight and metabolic syndrome. Several of these studies further point to the effects of different sources of fiber, i.e. cereal fiber such as oat or barley compared to other sources of fiber such as fruit. Associations between high intake of cereal fiber and insulin resistance and type 2 diabetes appear stronger than the associations between other sources of fiber [55, 67]. Few intervention studies exist, however, that test the effects of different sources of fiber on development or treatment of the metabolic syndrome, and this may be a focus for future research.

SUMMARY

Much work has been accomplished in understanding the integral relationship between diet, obesity and the metabolic syndrome. It is clear that dietary fat and carbohydrates play key

Table 2.4 Dietary treatment of the metabolic syndrome

- Weight reduction of 5-10% of body weight.
- Reduction in saturated fat intake to <7%. Potential benefit in increasing monounsaturated fat intake.
- Reduction in refined carbohydrates.
- Increased fiber intake.
- Adoption of dietary patterns rich in fruits, vegetables, fiber and monounsaturated fats, while low in saturated fats and refined carbohydrates.

roles in the development as well as in the treatment of the metabolic syndrome. While more research will be needed to define the optimal diet, several conclusions can be made based on research to date (Table 2.4). It is evident that lifestyle interventions, which include a low-fat (<30% of total energy) diet are successful in reducing weight and features of the metabolic syndrome. There is overall cardiovascular benefit in reducing saturated fat intake and there is potential benefit in substituting saturated fat with polyunsaturated or monounsaturated fats.

Low-carbohydrate diets achieve weight reduction that is comparable to traditional low-fat diets. Low-carbohydrate diets may have an advantage in improving insulin sensitivity, but there is limited long-term (greater than one year) data in patients with metabolic syndrome. Because of their varying effects on blood glucose, intake of carbohydrates that are higher in fiber and may also have a lower glycemic index and load appears to be more beneficial in reducing type 2 diabetes risk, and may be effective as part of a weight loss strategy. There is a lack of clinical trial evidence addressing specific carbohydrates, such as fructose, and future research will need to be conducted in this area.

Low-calorie diets are successful in achieving weight loss, however the rapid weight loss observed in studies utilizing very low-calorie diets may result in decreased HDL, and further study will be needed to determine the long-term efficacy of such interventions in the treatment of the metabolic syndrome.

Diets that emphasize healthy dietary patterns such as the DASH and Mediterranean diets show great promise in the treatment of the metabolic syndrome. These dietary patterns are high in fruits, vegetables and fiber, low in saturated fat, and may be high in monounsaturated fats. When used as part of a weight loss diet, these patterns appear to reduce many risk factors of the metabolic syndrome, including features of insulin resistance and inflammation. Future studies should focus on adaptation of such dietary patterns on a population level for reduction of obesity and the metabolic syndrome.

REFERENCES

1. Grundy SM, Hansen B, Smith SC, Jr, Cleeman JI, Kahn RA. Clinical management of metabolic syndrome: report of the American Heart Association/National Heart, Lung, and Blood Institute/American Diabetes Association conference on scientific issues related to management. *Circulation* 2004; 109:551–556.
2. Grundy SM, Cleeman JI, Daniels SR *et al.* Diagnosis and management of the metabolic syndrome: an American Heart Association/National Heart, Lung, and Blood Institute Scientific Statement. *Circulation* 2005; 112:2735–2752.
3. Orchard TJ, Temprosa M, Goldberg R *et al.* The effect of metformin and intensive lifestyle intervention on the metabolic syndrome: the Diabetes Prevention Program randomized trial. *Ann Intern Med* 2005; 142:611–619.
4. Grundy SM. Metabolic syndrome: therapeutic considerations. *Handb Exp Pharmacol* 2005; 170: 107–133.
5. Ford ES, Giles WH, Dietz WH. Prevalence of the metabolic syndrome among US adults: findings from the third National Health and Nutrition Examination Survey. *JAMA* 2002; 287:356–359.

6. Howard BV. Dietary fat as a risk factor for type 2 diabetes. *Ann N Y Acad Sci* 2002; 967:324–328.
7. Ludwig DS. Dietary glycemic index and obesity. *J Nutr* 2000; 130(suppl):280S–283S.
8. Giugliano D, Ceriello A, Esposito K. The effects of diet on inflammation: emphasis on the metabolic syndrome. *J Am Coll Cardiol* 2006; 48:677–685.
9. Knowler WC, Barrett-Connor E, Fowler SE *et al.* Reduction in the incidence of type 2 diabetes with lifestyle intervention or metformin. *N Engl J Med* 2002; 346:393–403.
10. Lindstrom J, Peltonen M, Eriksson JG *et al.* High-fibre, low-fat diet predicts long-term weight loss and decreased type 2 diabetes risk: the Finnish Diabetes Prevention Study. *Diabetologia* 2006; 49:912–920.
11. Wylie-Rosett J, Segal-Isaacson CJ, Segal-Isaacson A. Carbohydrates and increases in obesity: does the type of carbohydrate make a difference? *Obes Res* 2004; 12(suppl 2):124S–129S.
12. Gross LS, Li L, Ford ES, Liu S. Increased consumption of refined carbohydrates and the epidemic of type 2 diabetes in the United States: an ecologic assessment. *Am J Clin Nutr* 2004; 79:774–779.
13. Grundy SM, Abate N, Chandalia M. Diet composition and the metabolic syndrome: what is the optimal fat intake? *Am J Med* 2002; 113(suppl 9B):25S–29S.
14. Sowers JR. Obesity as a cardiovascular risk factor. *Am J Med* 2003; 115(suppl 8A):37S–41S.
15. Fantuzzi G. Adipose tissue, adipokines, and inflammation. *J Allergy Clin Immunol* 2005; 115:911–919.
16. Caballero AE. Endothelial dysfunction in obesity and insulin resistance: a road to diabetes and heart disease. *Obes Res* 2003; 11:1278–1289.
17. Kahn BB, Flier JS. Obesity and insulin resistance. *J Clin Invest* 2000; 106:473–481.
18. Stephen AM, Wald NJ. Trends in individual consumption of dietary fat in the United States, 1920–1984. *Am J Clin Nutr* 1990; 52:457–469.
19. Heini AF, Weinsier RL. Divergent trends in obesity and fat intake patterns: the American paradox. *Am J Med* 1997; 102:259–264.
20. Howard BV. Dietary fat as a risk factor for type 2 diabetes. *Ann N Y Acad Sci* 2002; 967:324–328.
21. Mayer-Davis EJ, Monaco JH, Hoen HM *et al.* Dietary fat and insulin sensitivity in a triethnic population: the role of obesity. The Insulin Resistance Atherosclerosis Study (IRAS). *Am J Clin Nutr* 1997; 65:79–87.
22. Marshall JA, Bessesen DH, Hamman RF. High saturated fat and low starch and fibre are associated with hyperinsulinaemia in a non-diabetic population: the San Luis Valley Diabetes Study. *Diabetologia* 1997; 40:430–438.
23. Salmeron J, Hu FB, Manson JE *et al.* Dietary fat intake and risk of type 2 diabetes in women. *Am J Clin Nutr* 2001; 73:1019–1026.
24. Lichtenstein AH, Appel LJ, Brands M *et al.* Diet and lifestyle recommendations revision 2006: a scientific statement from the American Heart Association Nutrition Committee. *Circulation* 2006; 114:82–96.
25. Kris-Etherton PM, Harris WS, Appel LJ. Fish consumption, fish oil, omega-3 fatty acids, and cardiovascular disease. *Arterioscler Thromb Vasc Biol* 2003; 23:e20–e30.
26. Warensjo E, Riserus U, Vessby B. Fatty acid composition of serum lipids predicts the development of the metabolic syndrome in men. *Diabetologia* 2005; 48:1999–2005.
27. Emken EA. What is the metabolic fate of dietary long-chain fatty acids (especially stearic acid) in normal physiological states, and how might this relate to thrombosis? *Am J Clin Nutr* 1992; 56 (4 suppl):798S.
28. Esposito K, Nappo F, Giugliano F *et al.* Meal modulation of circulating interleukin 18 and adiponectin concentrations in healthy subjects and in patients with type 2 diabetes mellitus. *Am J Clin Nutr* 2003; 78:1135–1140.
29. Nappo F, Esposito K, Cioffi M *et al.* Postprandial endothelial activation in healthy subjects and in type 2 diabetic patients: role of fat and carbohydrate meals. *J Am Coll Cardiol* 2002; 39:1145–1150.
30. Expert Panel on Detection, Evaluation, and Treatment of High Blood Cholesterol in Adults: Executive summary of the Third Report of the National Cholesterol Education Program (NCEP) Expert Panel on Detection, Evaluation, and Treatment of High Blood Cholesterol in Adults (Adult Treatment Panel III). *JAMA* 2001; 285:2486–2497.
31. Buse JB, Ginsberg HN, Bakris GL *et al.* Primary prevention of cardiovascular diseases in people with diabetes mellitus: a scientific statement from the American Heart Association and the American Diabetes Association. *Circulation* 2007; 115:114–126.
32. Bantle JP, Wylie-Rosett J, Albright AL *et al.* Nutrition recommendations and interventions for diabetes – 2006: a position statement of the American Diabetes Association. *Diabetes Care* 2006; 29:2140–2157.

33. Astrup A, Astrup A, Buemann B, Flint A, Raben A. Low-fat diets and energy balance: how does the evidence stand in 2002? *Proc Nutr Soc* 2002; 61:299–309.
34. Lindstrom J, Louheranta A, Mannelin M *et al.* The Finnish Diabetes Prevention Study (DPS): Lifestyle intervention and 3-year results on diet and physical activity. *Diabetes Care* 2003; 26:3230–3236.
35. Haffner S, Temprosa M, Crandall J *et al.* Intensive lifestyle intervention or metformin on inflammation and coagulation in participants with impaired glucose tolerance. *Diabetes* 2005; 54:1566–1572.
36. Tuomilehto J, Lindstrom J, Eriksson JG *et al.* Prevention of type 2 diabetes mellitus by changes in lifestyle among subjects with impaired glucose tolerance. *N Engl J Med* 2001; 344:1343–1350.
37. Ilanne-Parikka P, Eriksson JG, Lindstrom J *et al.* Prevalence of the metabolic syndrome and its components: findings from a Finnish general population sample and the Diabetes Prevention Study cohort. *Diabetes Care* 2004; 27:2135–2140.
38. The Diabetes Prevention Program (DPP): description of lifestyle intervention. *Diabetes Care* 2002; 25:2165–2171.
39. Muzio F, Mondazzi L, Sommariva D, Branchi A. Long-term effects of low-calorie diet on the metabolic syndrome in obese nondiabetic patients. *Diabetes Care* 2005; 28:1485–1486.
40. Bray GA, Nielsen SJ, Popkin BM. Consumption of high-fructose corn syrup in beverages may play a role in the epidemic of obesity. *Am J Clin Nutr* 2004; 79:537–543.
41. Basciano H, Federico L, Adeli K. Fructose, insulin resistance, and metabolic dyslipidemia. *Nutr Metab (Lond)* 2005; 2:5.
42. Schulze MB, Manson JE, Ludwig DS *et al.* Sugar-sweetened beverages, weight gain, and incidence of type 2 diabetes in young and middle-aged women. *JAMA* 2004; 292:927–934.
43. Dietary Reference Intakes for Energy, Carbohydrate, Fiber, Fat, Fatty Acids, Cholesterol, Protein, and Amino Acids. 2002.
44. Foster GD, Wyatt HR, Hill JO *et al.* A randomized trial of a low-carbohydrate diet for obesity. *N Engl J Med* 2003; 348:2082–2090.
45. Stern L, Iqbal N, Seshadri P *et al.* The effects of low-carbohydrate versus conventional weight loss diets in severely obese adults: one-year follow-up of a randomized trial. *Ann Intern Med* 2004; 140:778–785.
46. Nordmann AJ, Nordmann A, Briel M *et al.* Effects of low-carbohydrate vs low-fat diets on weight loss and cardiovascular risk factors: a meta-analysis of randomized controlled trials. *Arch Intern Med* 2006; 166:285–293.
47. Boden G, Sargrad K, Homko C, Mozzoli M, Stein TP. Effect of a low-carbohydrate diet on appetite, blood glucose levels, and insulin resistance in obese patients with type 2 diabetes. *Ann Intern Med* 2005; 142:403–411.
48. Samaha FF, Iqbal N, Seshadri P *et al.* A low-carbohydrate as compared with a low-fat diet in severe obesity. *N Engl J Med* 2003; 348:2074–2081.
49. Aude YW, Agatston AS, Lopez-Jimenez F *et al.* The national cholesterol education program diet vs a diet lower in carbohydrates and higher in protein and monounsaturated fat: a randomized trial. *Arch Intern Med* 2004; 164:2141–2146.
50. Muzio F, Mondazzi L, Harris WS, Sommariva D, Branchi A. Effects of moderate variations in the macronutrient content of the diet on cardiovascular disease risk factors in obese patients with the metabolic syndrome. *Am J Clin Nutr* 2007; 86:946–951.
51. Howard BV, Wylie-Rosett J. Sugar and cardiovascular disease: A statement for healthcare professionals from the Committee on Nutrition of the Council on Nutrition, Physical Activity, and Metabolism of the American Heart Association. *Circulation* 2002; 106:523–527.
52. Saris WH, Astrup A, Prentice AM *et al.* Randomized controlled trial of changes in dietary carbohydrate/fat ratio and simple vs. complex carbohydrates on body weight and blood lipids: the CARMEN study. The Carbohydrate Ratio Management in European National diets. *Int J Obes Relat Metab Disord* 2000; 24:1310–1318.
53. Poppitt SD, Keogh GF, Prentice AM *et al.* Long-term effects of ad libitum low-fat, high-carbohydrate diets on body weight and serum lipids in overweight subjects with metabolic syndrome. *Am J Clin Nutr* 2002; 75:11–20.
54. Livesey G. Low-glycaemic diets and health: implications for obesity. *Proc Nutr Soc* 2005; 64:105–113.
55. Schulze MB, Liu S, Rimm EB, Manson JE, Willett WC, Hu FB. Glycemic index, glycemic load, and dietary fiber intake and incidence of type 2 diabetes in younger and middle-aged women. *Am J Clin Nutr* 2004; 80:348–356.

56. McKeown NM, Meigs JB, Liu S, Saltzman E, Wilson PW, Jacques PF. Carbohydrate nutrition, insulin resistance, and the prevalence of the metabolic syndrome in the Framingham Offspring Cohort. *Diabetes Care* 2004; 27:538–546.
57. Ebbeling CB, Leidig MM, Sinclair KB, Seger-Shippee LG, Feldman HA, Ludwig DS. Effects of an ad libitum low-glycemic load diet on cardiovascular disease risk factors in obese young adults. *Am J Clin Nutr* 2005; 81:976–982.
58. Millan-Price J, Petocz P, Atkinson F *et al.* Comparison of 4 diets of varying glycemic load on weight loss and cardiovascular risk reduction in overweight and obese young adults: a randomized controlled trial. *Arch Intern Med* 2006; 166:1466–1475.
59. Hong K, Li Z, Wang HJ, Elashoff R, Heber D. Analysis of weight loss outcomes using VLCD in black and white overweight and obese women with and without metabolic syndrome. *Int J Obes (Lond)* 2005; 29:436–442.
60. Xydakis AM, Case CC, Jones PH *et al.* Adiponectin, inflammation, and the expression of the metabolic syndrome in obese individuals: the impact of rapid weight loss through caloric restriction. *J Clin Endocrinol Metab* 2004; 89:2697–2703.
61. Azadbakht L, Mirmiran P, Esmaillzadeh A, Azizi T, Azizi F. Beneficial effects of a Dietary Approaches to Stop Hypertension eating plan on features of the metabolic syndrome. *Diabetes Care* 2005; 28:2823–2831.
62. Ard JD, Grambow SC, Liu D, Slentz CA, Kraus WE, Svetkey LP. The effect of the PREMIER interventions on insulin sensitivity. *Diabetes Care* 2004; 27:340–347.
63. Millen BE, Pencina MJ, Kimokoti RW *et al.* Nutritional risk and the metabolic syndrome in women: opportunities for preventive intervention from the Framingham Nutrition Study. *Am J Clin Nutr* 2006; 84:434–441.
64. Sonnenberg L, Pencina M, Kimokoti R *et al.* Dietary patterns and the metabolic syndrome in obese and non-obese Framingham women. *Obes Res* 2005; 13:153–162.
65. Esposito K, Marfella R, Ciotola M *et al.* Effect of a Mediterranean-style diet on endothelial dysfunction and markers of vascular inflammation in the metabolic syndrome: a randomized trial. *JAMA* 2004; 292:1440–1446.
66. Delzenne NM, Cani PD. A place for dietary fibre in the management of the metabolic syndrome. *Curr Opin Clin Nutr Metab Care* 2005; 8:636–640.
67. Meyer KA, Kushi LH, Jacobs DR, Jr, Slavin J, Sellers TA, Folsom AR. Carbohydrates, dietary fiber, and incident type 2 diabetes in older women. *Am J Clin Nutr* 2000; 71:921–930.
68. Sahyoun NR, Jacques PF, Zhang XL, Juan W, McKeown NM. Whole-grain intake is inversely associated with the metabolic syndrome and mortality in older adults. *Am J Clin Nutr* 2006; 83:124–131.
69. Laaksonen DE, Toppinen LK, Juntunen KS *et al.* Dietary carbohydrate modification enhances insulin secretion in persons with the metabolic syndrome. *Am J Clin Nutr* 2005; 82:1218–1227.

3

An exercise prescription for the metabolic syndrome

R. Bentley-Lewis, M. Pendergrass

INTRODUCTION

Exercise, especially when associated with weight loss, improves all of the components of the metabolic syndrome [1]. Exercise may also decrease the risk of developing type 2 diabetes mellitus (T2DM) [2] and cardiovascular disease (CVD) [3], the two major sequelae of metabolic syndrome [4]. Disappointingly, in the US, only about 27% of women and 34% of men exercise for at least 30 min each day [5]. Furthermore, according to national survey data from 2004, 26% of women and 21% of men do not engage in any leisure-time physical activity at all [6].

There may be several reasons why people are not more active. Some may not realize the many benefits of exercise. Others may feel they do not have the time or the expertise to begin an exercise program. Ultimately, significant societal change will be required in order to increase the average levels of physical activity in the US. Until this change takes place, there is general agreement that physicians should counsel patients to begin and maintain exercise programs.

The idea of counseling patients to exercise may be a daunting task for many physicians. Unfortunately, availability of an exercise specialist to whom they can refer patients for counseling tends to be the exception, rather than the rule. Personal trainers may be expensive and may not have sufficient training to tailor an exercise program to an individual patient's medical needs. Certain healthcare providers, such as exercise physiologists and physical therapists, may be well qualified to provide instruction about exercise. However, their services frequently are not available or not reimbursed by insurance plans.

Fortunately, a well-informed physician should be able to prescribe and monitor exercise regimens for most patients. In this chapter we have outlined issues a physician should consider when counseling patients to increase their level of physical activity. We begin with a brief review of the literature supporting the use of exercise in the treatment of the metabolic syndrome. Next, we discuss the pre-exercise evaluation and outline a strategy for initiating a simple walking program during a brief patient encounter. We conclude with a discussion of the components of a more comprehensive exercise prescription. The terms 'exercise' and 'physical activity' are used interchangeably throughout the chapter.

Rhonda Bentley-Lewis, MD, MBA, MMSc, Instructor in Medicine, Harvard Medical School; Associate Physician, Division of Endocrinology, Diabetes and Hypertension, Brigham and Women's Hospital, Boston, Massachusetts, USA

Merri Pendergrass, MD, PhD, Associate Professor of Medicine, Harvard Medical School; Director of Clinical Diabetes, Brigham and Women's Hospital, Boston, Massachusetts, USA

Table 3.1 Potential benefits of exercise

- Reduces risk of developing diabetes
- Reduces risk of cardiovascular disease and stroke
- Lowers blood glucose
- Lowers blood pressure
- Improves lipid profile
- Promotes weight loss/maintenance
- Helps build and maintain healthy bones, muscles and joints
- Increases strength and flexibility
- Reduces risk of falls in older persons
- Reduces risk of breast and colon cancer
- Improves psychological well-being

BENEFITS OF EXERCISE

Potential benefits of exercise are outlined in Table 3.1. A review of prospective studies published between 1990 and 2000 concluded that T2DM and CVD could potentially be reduced 30–50% through a physically active, compared with a sedentary, lifestyle [7].

There are several potential mechanisms by which increased physical activity may promote positive heath effects. These include favorable effects on body weight, insulin sensitivity, blood glucose, endothelial function, fibrinolysis, the inflammatory response, blood pressure and lipids [3, 8]. For example, an investigation of non-dieting, overweight men and women revealed that activity produced weight and fat loss in a dose-dependent manner, with greater amounts of exercise associated with greater losses [9]. Similarly, in a study of obese and overweight exercising subjects, exercise improved insulin sensitivity in a dose-dependent manner [10]. Physical activity, even in the absence of changes in body weight, has also been shown to reduce both visceral and total abdominal fat, key components of the metabolic syndrome [11]. Improvements in endothelial function have been demonstrated with physical activity [8], which may, in part, be attributed to benefits in fibrinolytic and inflammatory factors. Blood pressure benefits have been observed in both normotensive and hypertensive patients [12]. Reductions are most significant in hypertensive patients, with blood pressure-lowering of approximately 5–7 mmHg after an isolated endurance exercise session. These reductions can endure up to 22 h [13]. Finally, lipid benefits of exercise have also been observed. In the Health, Risk Factors, Exercise Training, and Genetics (HERITAGE) study of normolipidemic participants, 5 months of exercise training in men resulted in reductions in triglycerides of 2.7% and in low-density lipoprotein (LDL) of 0.8%; women demonstrated reductions in triglycerides of 0.6% and in LDL of 4.4%. High-density lipoprotein (HDL) increased after the exercise intervention by 3% in both men and women [14]. Benefits in hyperlipidemic patients may be even greater.

WEIGHT LOSS

The effect of exercise on weight loss deserves special mention. Many physicians and patients mistakenly believe that if they eat the same amount, but exercise more, they will lose weight. If the patient's primary goal is to lose weight, they must be counseled to reduce caloric intake in addition to becoming more active. This is illustrated in the following discussion. It requires a deficit of approximately 3500 calories in order for a patient to lose a single pound of fat. Therefore, a deficit of 500 calories per day, attained through exercise, dietary restriction or a combination of the two, would be expected to lead to a weight loss of about one

Table 3.2 Physical activities with approximately 150 calories of energy expenditure

Common Activities	*Sports*
Walking for 30 min	Running for 15 min
Climbing stairs for 15 min	Bicycling for 15 min
Pushing a stroller for 30 min	Jumping rope for 15 min
Washing windows for 45–60 min	Swimming laps for 20 min
Gardening for 30–45 min	Playing volleyball for 45–60 min
Raking leaves for 30 min	Playing basketball for 15–20 min
Shoveling snow for 15 min	Dancing fast for 30 min

pound per week. This means, as illustrated in Table 3.2, a patient would have to participate in unrealistic amounts of exercise in order to expend sufficient calories to lose substantial weight through exercise alone [15]. For example, in order for an average person to lose a single pound, they would need to jog for nearly 6 hours! It is important that patients understand this so they will not have unrealistic goals related to exercise.

It is, however, important to note that metabolic benefits of lifestyle modification may occur with even modest amounts of exercise and weight loss. Furthermore, benefits may be achieved despite relatively small effects on a patient's perception of their physical appearance. For example, in the Diabetes Prevention Program (DPP), patients in the lifestyle intervention group had an average baseline weight of about 94 kg and a body mass index (BMI) of 34 kg/m^2. Following an intervention designed to achieve a 7% reduction in body weight (diet and approximately 150 min per week of exercise), patients lost an average of about 5.6 kg. Even though most patients would still be considered obese following this small amount of weight loss, they experienced a dramatic 58% reduction in the onset of type 2 diabetes [16].

In summary, exercise has multiple metabolic benefits, as shown in Table 3.1. Metabolic benefits may occur with exercise, even in the absence of significant weight loss. Although exercise alone is unlikely to result in significant weight loss, when combined with caloric restriction it will assist patients in achieving and maintaining weight loss.

OPTIMAL EXERCISE TYPE/VOLUME

The American College of Sports Medicine (ACSM), in conjunction with the American Heart Association (AHA), recently updated physical activity guidelines for healthy adults [17]. Summarized in Table 3.3 are recommendations for the type as well as the volume of exercise. In terms of exercise type, the guidelines recommend that both cardiorespiratory (aerobic) and strength-developing (resistance) exercises be included in the exercise regimen. Two options are offered for aerobic exercise volume, which is a function of exercise intensity, duration, and frequency. It is recommended that *either* vigorous exercise be performed at least 20 min on 3 days a week *or* moderate exercise be performed at least 30 min on 5 days per week. While the optimal volume of exercise continues to be debated, it appears likely that 'some' exercise is better than 'no' exercise, and the more exercise the better [18]. This is illustrated by the results of the Studies of a Targeted Risk Reduction Intervention through Defined Exercise (STRRIDE) trial.

In the STRRIDE trial [19], sedentary patients were randomized to one of four levels of physical activity: no exercise; low-dose/moderate-intensity exercise equivalent to walking 12 miles per week; low-dose/vigorous-intensity exercise equivalent to jogging 12 miles per week; or high-dose/vigorous-intensity exercise equivalent to jogging 20 miles per week. Weight change was 3.5% loss in the high-dose/vigorous-intensity group and approximately

Table 3.3 Summary of exercise recommendations by American College of Sports Medicine/American Heart Association

Intensity	*Level description*	*Example*	*Frequency/duration*
Aerobic training			
Light	No major increase in pulse or breathing rate	Walking slowly around home; sitting or standing in normal daily activities	Normal daily routine
AND			
Moderate	Increase in pulse/heart rate and breathing but can comfortably engage in conversation	Walking at very brisk pace; bicycling (flat surface); swimming (leisurely); shooting baskets	5 days/week, 30 min/day,
OR			
Vigorous	Rapid pulse and breathing	Walking at very fast pace; jogging; running	3 days/week, 20 min/day,
AND			
Srength and endurance training			
	Substantial fatigue after 8–12 repetitions	Exercise with weights, crunches	8–12 repetitions of 8–10 exercises using major muscle groups, 2 non-consecutive days/weeks

1% loss in the two low-dose exercise groups, compared to 1.1% weight gain in the control group. The two low-exercise groups lost both weight and fat, while those in the more intensive exercise group lost more of each in a dose–response manner. The equivalent of 11 miles of exercise per week at low or high intensity prevented significant accumulation of visceral fat, a key component of metabolic syndrome. The highest volume of exercise resulted in decreases in both visceral and subcutaneous abdominal fat.

It is important to note that different doses of exercise may be required to achieve different benefits. It has been estimated that approximately 150 min per week of exercise are required to facilitate weight loss and to improve glucose control; 300 min per week are required to improve blood pressure and lipid parameters; and 450 min per week may be required for long-term maintenance of major weight loss [20]. Moreover, mean aerobic fitness, defined as peak absolute oxygen consumption, improves in a dose-dependent fashion [21]. In a recent study, mean aerobic fitness was increased compared to a non-exercise control group by 4.2%, 6.0% and 8.2% as the mean minutes of exercise per week increased from 72.2, 135.8 and 191.7 min, respectively.

PRE-EXERCISE EVALUATION

Low- to moderate-intensity exercise, such as walking, has been shown to have significant benefits and minimal associated risks. Before recommending that patients begin an exercise program more vigorous than a brisk walk, they should be evaluated for potential conditions that may predispose them to injury or which require treatment.

Table 3.4 Pre-exercise evaluation

A complete medical history, physical examination, and laboratory evaluation should be performed with special attention to the following:

1. Exercise history including information on readiness for change and baseline activity
2. Presence of one of the following conditions that may require special consideration:
   - Cardiovascular disease
   - Hypertension
   - Diabetes with or without complications (e.g. retinopathy, neuropathy, nephropathy)
   - Osteoporosis
3. Medications, e.g. insulin or anti-hypertensives, that may require adjustment in relation to the exercise program

Components of a pre-exercise evaluation are outlined in Table 3.4. The evaluation should address medical and psychosocial issues that may pose barriers to successful execution of the program. A complete medical history, physical examination, and laboratory evaluation should be obtained to determine whether the patient has any medical condition that may constitute a contraindication for certain exercises. An exercise history that includes information on readiness for exercise and habitual level of activity should be included in this evaluation. Attention also should be given to any medications, such as anti-hyperglycemic agents, that may need to be adjusted or timed in relation to the exercise regimen.

Special considerations will be required if the patient has a diagnosed chronic medical condition such as diabetes, hypertension, CVD or osteoporosis. These have been the subject of prior reviews and will not be discussed in detail here. A summary of these considerations is provided in Table 3.5 [13, 20, 22–24].

Since patients with metabolic syndrome have increased risk for CVD, screening for asymptomatic CVD should always be considered. However, despite the increased risk, not all patients with metabolic syndrome will require formal cardiac testing. The US Preventive Services Task Force advises that stress tests *not* be recommended for asymptomatic individuals with low coronary artery disease risk, defined as men <50 years of age, women <60 years of age, and <10% risk of a cardiac event over 10 years. The rationale is that the risk of invasive follow-up testing outweighs the anticipated benefit from detecting undiagnosed disease [25]. The estimation of a person's risk for a CVD event in the subsequent 10 years is based on risk factors for heart disease, such as age, gender, cholesterol level and smoking. A risk calculator can be accessed at http://hin.nhlbi.nih.gov/atpiii/calculator.asp?usertype=prof [20]. Those at increased risk, including older adults or young adults with 15–20% 10-year risk for CVD, may be considered for screening evaluation in the context of other risk factors.

THE EXERCISE PRESCRIPTION

Table 3.6 summarizes an approach to formulating an exercise prescription. An ideal exercise prescription should specifically address questions of what type (mode), how much (intensity and duration), and how often (frequency) exercise should be performed. The rate of progression, as well as strategies to promote safety, should also be addressed in the exercise prescription. These topics will be discussed in the section below titled *Beyond Walking*.

For many clinicians, it may be unrealistic to provide detailed recommendations regarding mode, intensity, duration and frequency. Fortunately, significant benefits have been demonstrated when patients are counseled simply to increase their walking. A 2007 systematic review of randomized and non-randomized studies found that counseling targeted at motivated sedentary patients could significantly increase walking (6 weeks to 12 months) follow-up [26].

Table 3.5 Special considerations with common chronic medical problems

Chronic Condition	*Considerations*
Cardiovascular disease	■ May need to limit exercise intensity ■ Before initiating an exercise program, perform graded exercise testing to assess risk, prognosis, and functional capacity
Hypertension	■ Increased risk for CVD ■ Intense exercise or exercise using valsalva maneuvers (e.g. lifting heavy weights) may significantly increase the blood pressure ■ Certain blood pressure-lowering drugs, such as β-blockers and diuretics may impair the ability to regulate body temperature or can cause dehydration ■ Certain blood pressure-lowering drugs, such as α-blockers calcium, channel blockers and vasodilators may cause blood pressure levels to drop after abruptly ending exercise
Diabetes	■ Increased risk for CVD ■ Need to coordinate timing of exercise, meals, medications, glucose testing
Diabetes complications	
Retinopathy	■ Caution with exercises that involve valsalva (e.g. lifting heavy weights), pounding (e.g. tennis), or contact sports
Peripheral neuropathy	■ Caution with repetitive stepping exercise (e.g. jogging, step classes)
Autonomic neuropathy	■ Very high risk for CVD ■ Caution with activities requiring temperature regulation (e.g. running in hot weather), changes in posture (e.g. certain yoga poses), or night vision
Osteoporosis	■ Caution with exercises that may increase risk for falls ■ High-impact exercises (e.g. jogging) may increase compression in the spine and lower extremities and can lead to fractures in weakened bones ■ Exercises which involve bending forward and twisting the waist (e.g. touching toes, doing sit-ups, using a rowing machine, or some yoga poses) may compress the bones in the spine and be harmful

Table 3.6 Approach to formulating the exercise prescription

- Discuss the patient's expectations
- Establish realistic goals
- Review safety considerations
  - Specific types of exercises that may be contraindicated
  - When to take medications in relation to exercise
  - When to eat or check the blood glucose in relation to exercise (diabetes only)
  - Plan to have water and snacks available during activity
  - Plan for appropriate footwear
  - Plan to wear a medical identification bracelet or necklace
- Discuss mode, frequency, duration, intensity, and rate of progression of activity to be performed
- Develop a plan to monitor progress

INITIATING A WALKING PROGRAM DURING A ROUTINE OFFICE VISIT

The most important step for sedentary patients initiating an exercise regimen is the first step. Even if they do nothing more than take a walk around the block or do a single set on the bench press, it is all progress! There are an increasing number of community and internet resources available for assisting healthcare providers in advising patients on how to initiate simple programs. Patients can be referred to fitness programs at a local recreation center, health club, workplace or place of worship for help initiating and maintaining a comprehensive exercise program. However, since most patients may not follow up those referrals, physicians can help their patients take that first step by providing instruction on how to get started.

Even very busy physicians with only rudimentary knowledge about an exercise prescription should be able to prescribe a simple walking program. Walking is easy to do and is effective at reducing metabolic syndrome [27]. As long as there are no contraindications, such as severe peripheral neuropathy, the potential benefits of walking outweigh potential risks in the vast majority of patients. Common popular programs are based on either: (1) the number of steps walked in a day or (2) the number of minutes of exercise in a day.

Step (pedometer)-based exercise program

Pedometers have become popular as a tool for motivating physical activity. Numerous studies have demonstrated that physical activity is increased by pedometer use. In order for this strategy to be effective, (1) patients must be provided with a step goal, (2) patients must be asked to keep a record of their daily steps, and (3) the record of steps must be regularly reviewed during physician visits.

A recent review examined studies that investigated the efficacy of a pedometer-based program in motivating physical activity [28]. Pedometer users increased their physical activity 27% above baseline, a magnitude equal to about 2000 steps or about 1 mile of walking per day. Moreover, the use of pedometers was associated with clinically relevant reductions in weight and blood pressure. Pedometer users decreased their BMI by 0.38 kg/m^2 (95% CI 0.05–0.72) and decreased their systolic blood pressure by 3.8 mmHg (95% CI 1.7–5.9 mmHg). An important predictor of increased physical activity was having a step goal. Those pedometer users who were given a goal, whether it was the commonly used 10 000 step goal or an individualized step goal, significantly increased their physical activity, whereas those users who weren't given a goal did not.

An outline of a pedometer-based program is shown in Table 3.7. The objective of a pedometer-based strategy is to increase the total number of steps a patient takes each day. The number of steps is quantified by having the patient wear a pedometer during their waking hours and keeping a daily record of the results (Table 3.8). After a baseline number of steps is established, the patient should gradually increase the number of daily steps. For instance, if they take an average of 3000 steps per day during the first three days of wearing the pedometer, during the next week they should increase by 500 steps (equivalent to approximately 5 min of walking) to achieve 3500 steps per day. The interim goal for the number of daily steps should be increased on a regular (e.g. weekly) basis until the final goal is reached. A goal of 10 000 steps per day has been commonly recommended [29] because this quantity approximated the Surgeon General's recommendation to accumulate at least 30 min of activity beyond normal daily life most days of the week [30].

Time-based exercise program

Another strategy for initiating an exercise program is to ask the patient to engage in some form of physical activity for a certain number of minutes each day. Typically, 30 to 60 min per day of activity is recommended. The minutes can be consecutive, or they can be the sum of multiple shorter 'bouts' of activity. The minimum duration of each 'bout' of exercise should be 10 min. The exercise can be of any type, including walking. If patients choose walking as an exercise, it is helpful to state recommendations in a way that provides the patient with a concrete and attainable goal. For example, rather than advise a sedentary patient to walk 30 min a day, it may be preferable to advise them to walk for 15 min 'out' from their starting

Table 3.7 Initiating a pedometer-based walking program

1. Determine the baseline number of daily steps
   - Have the patient wear the pedometer on most days of the week and record the number of steps/day in a pedometer diary
   - Determine the average number of steps/day during the first week. This should be considered the baseline
2. Provide patient with a daily step goal
   - The initial step goal should be about 500 steps/day (approximately 5 min) more than the baseline
   - At regular (e.g. weekly) intervals, increase the goal number of steps/day by about 500 until the final goal is reached. A final goal of 10 000 steps/day is commonly recommended
3. Review pedometer diary and daily step goals at each patient visit

Table 3.8 Examples of physical activity logs

A: Time-based activity log
Goal = *150 mins per week*

Date	*Activity*	*Monday*	*Tuesday*	*Wednesday*	*Thursday*	*Friday*	*Saturday*	*Sunday*	*Total*
	Type	Walking	Walking	Swimming	Walking		Tennis		
	Number of minutes	10+ 10+ 10	20+ 10	30	30	–	30	–	150 mins/week

B: Pedometer-based activity log
Goal = *10 000 steps per day*

Date	*Activity*	*Monday*	*Tuesday*	*Wednesday*	*Thursday*	*Friday*	*Saturday*	*Sunday*	*Average*
	Number of steps	6487	12 364	8978	8692	–	14 302	9177	10 000 steps/day

point and then turn around and walk back to that starting point. An alternative would be to ask them to walk for 10 min, three times per day.

BEYOND WALKING

A more detailed approach to developing an exercise prescription is described in this section. The ideal prescription should specify what type, intensity, duration, and frequency of exercise should be performed. These components are interrelated and will vary depending on each patient's interests, needs, exercise experience, health status, and goals for physical activity. The rate of progression, as well as strategies to promote safety, should also be addressed in the exercise prescription.

TYPE OF EXERCISE

For most patients, the exercise program should include both aerobic and resistance exercises as recommended (Table 3.3).

Aerobic exercises include activities that use rhythmic repeated and continuous movements of the same large muscle groups over at least 10 min at a time. Typical examples include walking, jogging, swimming, bicycling, and stair climbing. For a given level of energy expenditure, the health benefits are independent of the mode of aerobic activity. Unless there are precautions against engaging in specific exercises, such as in the setting of chronic diseases (Table 3.5), the type of exercise an individual performs is a matter of personal preference.

Resistance exercise refers to forms of exercise that use muscular strength to move a weight or work against a resistive load. Examples include abdominal crunches and exercises using free weights, weight machines, and various types of springs, rubber bands or elastic tubing. Exercises should be selected for each of the muscle groups, i.e. hips and legs, chest, shoulders, back, arms and abdomen. Resistance exercise training, by increasing muscle mass and endurance may cause changes in functional status and body composition more rapidly than aerobic training alone. Contrary to common belief, resistance exercise improves insulin sensitivity to approximately the same extent as aerobic exercise [31].

AEROBIC EXERCISE

Intensity

Aerobic exercise intensity is the most difficult part of the exercise prescription to determine. Various techniques can be used to prescribe and monitor exercise intensity [32]. The most commonly used technique is the heart rate method, which is based on the linear relationship that exists between heart rate and exercise intensity. Exercise intensity typically is prescribed as a percentage of a patient's maximal heart rate (HR_{max}). Ideally, the HR_{max} should be determined during graded exercise testing. From a practical standpoint, since the true HR_{max} is usually unknown, it can be estimated by the equation $HR_{max} = 220 -$ (the patient's age in years). While this estimate may be reasonably accurate in sedentary people, it may not be as accurate in individuals who exercise regularly and/or intensely; have autonomic neuropathy; or who are taking medications known to alter HR_{max} such as β-blockers.

The American College of Sports Medicine recommends an intensity of exercise for healthy adults corresponding to 55–90% of the HR_{max} [32]. Since higher-intensity exercise is associated with a greater risk of cardiovascular or musculoskeletal injury than exercise programs emphasizing low- to moderate-intensity (55–70% of the HR_{max}), low- to moderate-intensity exercise may be preferable for most people with metabolic syndrome. On the other hand, progression of exercise to a vigorous intensity (>70% of HR_{max}) may be acceptable for patients with a low risk for cardiovascular complications.

Regardless of the intensity of exercise prescribed, patients should be advised to include adequate warm-up and cool-down periods. These periods can be accomplished by performing the prescribed aerobic activity at a lower intensity for the initial and final 5 min of each exercise period. For example, this lower intensity can be defined as the target heart rate −20 beats/min.

Volume

The concepts of *frequency, duration,* and/or *intensity* of exercise are commonly combined to describe a recommended *volume* of exercise. The appropriate frequency and duration of each exercise session is inversely related to the intensity at which the exercise is performed. Thus, low-intensity exercises should generally be conducted more frequently and for a longer duration than high-intensity exercises. The current recommendations from the ACSM/AHA [17] are summarized in Table 3.3. Moderate-intensity aerobic exercise is advised on 5 days per week for at least 30 min each day. Alternatively, vigorous activity can be performed for 20 min on three days each week. Bouts of exercise, with a minimum of 10 min/bout, can be accumulated toward the recommended minimum weekly amount of

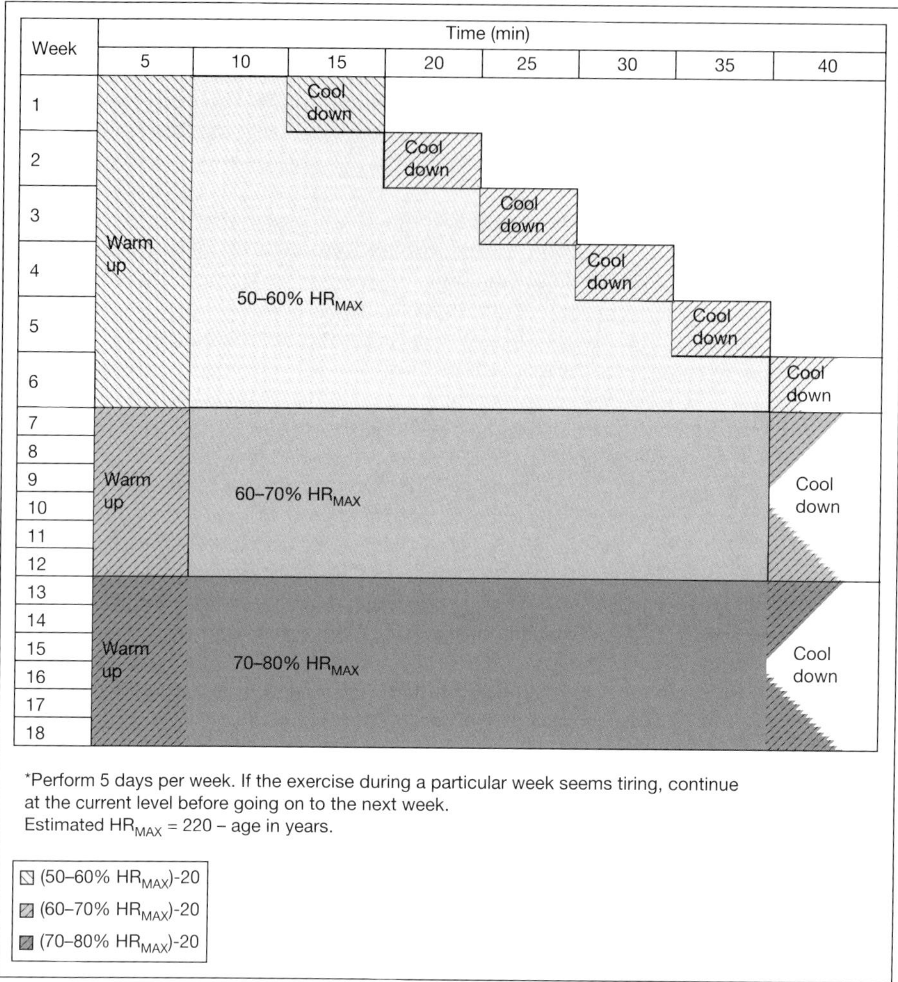

Figure 3.1 Sample advancement of an aerobic exercise program.* HR$_{max}$ = maximal heart rate.

physical activity. Since the duration of improvement in insulin sensitivity after the last bout of aerobic exercise is generally between 24 and 72 h [28], it seems reasonable to recommend aerobic exercise on at least three non-consecutive days each week, and ideally, on at least 5 days per week.

Rate of progression

Exercise should be initiated at a comfortable intensity that is well within the individual's current capacity. In general, sessions initially should last no more than 10–15 min. If the patient tolerates the activity, the duration of exercise should gradually be increased at a rate that is comfortable for the patient. Once a desired duration is achieved, exercise intensity may then be gradually increased. A sample aerobic exercise progression strategy is shown in Figure 3.1.

RESISTANCE EXERCISE

Resistance training should be performed at regular intervals in order to improve cardiovascular and musculoskeletal health, to maintain independence in performing the activities of daily life, and to reduce the risk of falling in older patients. In order to ensure resistance exercises are performed in a fashion that maximizes benefits and minimizes the risk for injury, resistance exercises initially should be performed under the supervision of a qualified exercise specialist. Although exercise specialists are often not available through healthcare system referrals, they usually can be located through gyms or community programs. The National Strength and Conditioning Association (www.nsca-lift.org), which certifies exercise professionals competent in planning and supervising resistance training programs, may be helpful in providing a list of certified trainers.

The current ACSM/AHA guidelines recommend that resistance exercise should be performed on a minimum of 2 non-consecutive days per week [17]. Resistance exercise is typically quantified in terms of the number of repetitions that are performed. Repetitions are performed in groups or 'sets', which typically consist of 8–12 repetitions of 8–10 exercises. A conservative approach is to begin with the lightest possible weight for each exercise and to monitor the patient's response for one set. If the patient tolerates this well, they can gradually progress to three sets of 8–12 repetitions at a weight that cannot be lifted more than 8–12 times. Although one set of each exercise may be sufficient to increase muscle strength, data suggest that performing three sets of each exercise produces greater metabolic benefit [33].

Each resistance-training workout should be preceded by approximately 5 min of warm-up and followed by approximately 5 min of cool-down. These periods should consist of light aerobic activity with or without flexibility (stretching) exercises. Rest periods between sets should be adequate to allow successful completion of the next set. Periods typically range between 15 s for moderate-intensity exercise and 5 min for high-intensity exercise.

ADHERENCE TO EXERCISE REGIMEN

Specific steps should be taken to maximise adherence to the exercise regimen [34]. Factors that may help individuals maintain an exercise program include setting realistic expectations and goals, encouraging self-rewards, identifying alternative exercises to reduce boredom, using appropriate training and equipment, progressing slowly in exercise intensity and duration, reviewing the person's performance on a regular basis, and providing feedback on the patient's progress. Appropriately timing the exercise routine may also facilitate adherence to the program. Ideally, physical activity should be performed at the time of day that is most convenient for the participant. In special circumstances, such as in patients with diabetes, exercise may need to be timed in relation to meals, medications, and glucose monitoring [22].

MONITORING PROGRESS

Regardless of the strategy used, patients should always be advised to record their daily activity and bring this documentation with them to their physician visits. A weekly log (Table 3.8) should be provided to patients for this purpose. The physician should review the records, provide feedback at regular intervals, and modify the exercise prescription as necessary.

SUMMARY

Physical activity is an essential part of a healthy lifestyle. Exercise has multiple potential benefits, including improving the metabolic syndrome. Since many patients depend on their physicians to counsel them about ways to improve their health, physicians have both the opportunity and the responsibility to help their patients initiate and maintain a more physically active lifestyle. With minimal time, an informed physician can provide appropriate recommendations for most sedentary patients to begin a safe and effective exercise program, such as walking. After patients become more active, they may become motivated to seek more extensive instruction from other sources, such as gym personnel or a personal trainer. It is imperative that primary care physicians begin the dialogue regarding exercise because they are often the only physicians many patients with metabolic syndrome will encounter. Carpe diem!

REFERENCES

1. Orchard T *et al.* Diabetes Prevention Program Research Group. The effect of metformin and intensive lifestyle intervention on the metabolic syndrome: the Diabetes Prevention Program randomized trial. *Ann Intern Med* 2005; 142:611–619.
2. Diabetes Prevention Program Research Group. Reduction in the incidence of type 2 diabetes with lifestyle intervention or metformin. *N Engl J Med* 2002; 346:393–403.
3. Thompson PD, Buchner D, Pina IL *et al.*; American Heart Association Council on Clinical Cardiology Subcommittee on Exercise, Rehabilitation, and Prevention; American Heart Association Council on Nutrition, Physical Activity, and Metabolism Subcommittee on Physical Activity. Exercise and physical activity in the prevention and treatment of atherosclerotic cardiovascular disease: a statement from the Council on Clinical Cardiology (Subcommittee on Exercise, Rehabilitation, and Prevention) and the Council on Nutrition, Physical Activity, and Metabolism (Subcommittee on Physical Activity). *Circulation* 2003; 107: 3109–3116.
4. Sattar N, Gaw A, Scherbakova O *et al.* Metabolic syndrome with and without C-reactive protein as a predictor of coronary heart disease and diabetes in the West of Scotland Coronary Prevention Study. *Circulation* 2003; 108:414–419.
5. Bassuk S, Manson J. Physical activity and cardiovascular disease prevention in women: how much is good enough? *Exercise & Sport Sciences Reviews* 2003; 31:176–181.
6. Centers for Disease Control and Prevention (CDC). Trends in leisure-time physical inactivity by age, sex, and race/ethnicity – United States, 1994–2004. *MMWR Morb Mortal Wkly Rep* 2005; 54:991–994.
7. Bassuk S, Manson J. Epidemiological evidence for the role of physical activity in reducing risk of type 2 diabetes and cardiovascular disease. *J Appl Physiol* 2005; 99:1193–1204.
8. Paterick TE, Fletcher GF. Endothelial function and cardiovascular prevention: role of blood lipids, exercise, and other risk factors. *Cardiol Rev* 2001; 9:282–286.
9. Slentz CA, Duscha BD, Johnson JL *et al.* Effects of the amount of exercise on body weight, body composition, and measures of central obesity: STRRIDE – a randomized controlled study. *Arch Intern Med* 2004; 164:31–39.
10. Houmard JA, Tanner CJ, Slentz CA, Duscha BD, McCartney JS, Kraus WE. Effect of the volume and intensity of exercise training on insulin sensitivity. *J Appl Physiol* 2004; 96:101–106.
11. Kay S, Fiatarone Singh M. The influence of physical activity on abdominal fat: a systematic review of the literature. *Obes Rev* 2006; 7:183–200.
12. Fagard R. Exercise characteristics and the blood pressure response to dynamic physical training. *Med Sci Sports Exerc* 2001; 33(6 suppl):S484–S492.
13. Pescatello LS, Franklin BA, Fagard R, Farquhar WB, Kelley GA, Ray CA; American College of Sports Medicine. American College of Sports Medicine position stand. Exercise and hypertension. *Med Sci Sports Exerc* 2004; 36:533–553.
14. Leon AS, Rice T, Mandel S *et al.* Blood lipid response to 20 weeks of supervised exercise in a large biracial population: the HERITAGE Family Study. *Metabolism* 2000; 49:513–520.
15. US Department of Health and Human Services. Overweight and obesity: what you can do. Being physically active can help you attain or maintain a healthy weight. http://www.surgeongeneral.gov/topics/obesity/calltoaction/fact_whatcanyoudo.htm, 2006.
16. Knowler WC, Barrett-Connor E, Fowler SE *et al.*; Diabetes Prevention Program Research Group. Reduction in the incidence of type 2 diabetes with lifestyle intervention or metformin. *N Engl J Med* 2002; 346:393–403.

17. Haskell WL, Lee IM, Pate RR *et al.*; American College of Sports Medicine; American Heart Association. Physical activity and public health: updated recommendation for adults from the American College of Sports Medicine and the American Heart Association. *Circulation* 2007; 116:1081–1093.
18. Kraus WE, Torgan CE, Duscha BD *et al.* Studies of a targeted risk reduction intervention through defined exercise (STRRIDE). *Med Sci Sports Exerc* 2001; 33:1774–1784.
19. Slentz CA, Aiken LB, Houmard JA *et al.* Inactivity, exercise, and visceral fat. STRRIDE: a randomized, controlled study of exercise intensity and amount. *J Appl Physiol* 2005; 99:1613–1618.
20. Sigal RJ, Kenny GP, Wasserman DH, Castaneda-Sceppa C, White RD. Physical activity/exercise and type 2 diabetes: a consensus statement from the American Diabetes Association. *Diabetes Care* 2006; 29:1433–1438.
21. Church TS, Earnest CP, Skinner JS, Blair SN. Effects of different doses of physical activity on cardiorespiratory fitness among sedentary, overweight or obese postmenopausal women with elevated blood pressure: a randomized controlled trial. *JAMA* 2007; 297:2081–2091.
22. Green D, Mandarino L, Pendergrass M. Exercise in Diabetes. In Fonseca VA (ed): Clinical Diabetes: Translating Research Into Practice. Philadelphia: Saunders Elsevier, 2006, pp 921–931.
23. American College of Sports Medicine position stand. Exercise for patients with coronary artery disease. *Med Sci Sports Exerc* 1994; 26:i–v.
24. American College of Sports Medicine position stand. Osteoporosis and exercise. *Med Sci Sports Exerc* 1995; 27:i–vii.
25. Fowler-Brown A, Pignone M, Pletcher M, Tice JA, Sutton SF, Lohr KN. Exercise tolerance testing to screen for coronary heart disease: a systematic review for the technical support for the US Preventive Services Task Force. *Ann Intern Med* 2004; 140:W9–W24.
26. Ogilvie D, Foster CE, Rothnie H *et al.* Interventions to promote walking: systematic review. *Br Med J* 2007; 334:1204.
27. Fogelholm M *et al.* Effects of walking training on weight maintenance after a very-low-energy diet in premenopausal obese women: a randomized controlled trial. *Arch Intern Med* 2000; 160:2177–2184.
28. Bravata DM, Smith-Spangler C, Sundaram V *et al.* Using pedometers to increase physical activity and improve health: a systematic review. *JAMA* 2007; 298:2296–2304.
29. Tudor-Locke C, Tudor-Locke BD, Jr. How many steps/day are enough? Preliminary pedometer indices for public health. *Sports Med* 2004; 34:1–8.
30. US Department of Health and Human Services. Physical Activity and Health: A Report of the Surgeon General Atlanta, GA: US Department of Health and Human Services, Centers for Disease Control and Prevention, National Center for Chronic Disease Prevention and Health Promotion, 1996.
31. Ivy J. Role of exercise training in the prevention and treatment of insulin resistance and non-insulin-dependent diabetes mellitus. *Sports Med* 1997; 24:321–336.
32. American College of Sports Medicine. Guidelines for Exercise Testing and Prescription. Philadelphia: Lippincott Williams and Wilkins, 2006.
33. American College of Sports Medicine position stand: The recommended quantity and quality of exercise for developing and maintaining cardiorespiratory and muscular fitness, and flexibility in healthy adults. *Med Sci Sports Exerc* 1998; 30:975–991.
34. Marerro D. Initiation and Maintenance in Patients With Diabetes. In Ruderman N, Schneider SH, Kriska A (eds). Handbook of Exercise in Diabetes, 2nd edition. Alexandria, VA: American Diabetes Association, 2002, pp 289–309.

4

Impact of hypoglycemic agents on the metabolic syndrome

T. K. Thethi, S. Singh, V. Fonseca

INTRODUCTION

The metabolic syndrome (MS) affects about a quarter of the population in developed countries [1]. The MS is a cluster of cardiovascular risk factors that are frequently associated with insulin resistance. MS is a major risk factor for development of type 2 diabetes mellitus (T2DM) and atherosclerosis-related cardiovascular disease (CVD) events. The prevalence of CVD is two to three times higher in individuals who have the MS than in age-matched controls [1]. They are also at five times the risk of developing T2DM. Over the years, obesity and its related disorders have reached epidemic proportions. The prevalence of obesity has increased to over 20% of the US adults and is an independent risk factor for CVD [2]. The purpose of this review is to discuss the impact of treatments commonly used in the treatment of diabetes mellitus (DM) on features of the MS as a whole, on the diagnosis and consequences of the risk factor clustering seen in the MS.

SECRETAGOGUES

Insulin secretagogues such as sulfonylureas and metiglinides reduce glucose concentrations and thereby reduce the effect of 'glucose toxicity' on insulin sensitivity. However, they do not have any direct effect on insulin sensitivity, and have very little impact on the MS [3]. Sulfonylureas cause weight gain, and although their impact on abdominal obesity has not been well studied it is unlikely that this class of drugs impacts this feature of the MS favorably. The only MS features improved are plasma glucose and occasionally triglycerides, mediated through the glucose-lowering effect.

The ongoing NAVIGATOR (Nateglinide And Valsartan in Impaired Glucose Tolerance Outcomes Research) trial is a prospective, multinational, randomized, double-blind, placebo-controlled, two-by-two factorial design trial which is being conducted in 39 countries [4]. This trial is designed to examine whether valsartan (Diovan) and/or nateglinide (Starlix) delays or prevents the progression of subjects with impaired glucose tolerance (IGT) to type 2 diabetes and/or cardiovascular events. More than 43 000 patients were screened for enrollment using a glucose tolerance test for insulin sensitivity. A multivariate analysis showed that risk factors for

Tina K. Thethi, MD, MPH, Assistant Professor of Medicine, Section of Endocrinology, Department of Internal Medicine, Tulane University Health Sciences Center, New Orleans, Louisiana, USA

Shipra Singh, MBBS, MPH, Section of Endocrinology, Department of Medicine, Tulane University, New Orleans, Louisiana, USA

Vivian Fonseca, MD, FRCP, Professor of Medicine and Pharmacology, Tullis Tulane Alumni Chair in Diabetes; Chief, Section of Endocrinology, Department of Medicine, Tulane University Health Sciences Center, New Orleans, Louisiana, USA

CVD and MS were associated with rising ALT (alanine aminotransferase). The associated risk factors included the following: increasing baseline systolic and diastolic blood pressure levels ($P = 0.03$ and $P = 0.0001$, respectively), increasing body mass index (BMI) ($P < 0.0001$), waist circumference ($P < 0.0001$), worsening glucose tolerance (both fasting and 2 hours post-challenge, $P < 0.0001$) and MS ($P < 0.0001$). Results of this study are expected to be reported in 2008.

ALPHA GLUCOSIDASE INHIBITORS (AGI)

IGT poses an increased risk for CVD, even after adjusting for the classic risk factors. [5–9]. The moderate increase in post-prandial plasma glucose levels that occurs in patients with IGT has been shown to be an independent predictor for CVD 10]. In addition to lowering glucose, alpha glucosidase inhibitors (AGIs) such as acarbose have significant lipid-lowering effects, especially on triglycerides. They therefore have the potential to favorably impact the features comprising the MS. Some small studies have also suggested that they improve insulin sensitivity.

The STOP-Non-Insulin-Dependent Diabetes Mellitus (NIDDM) [10] trial evaluated the effect of decreasing post-prandial hyperglycemia with acarbose on the risk of CVD and hypertension in patients with IGT. Study subjects had BMI between 25 and 40 mg/m^2. They were eligible for the study if they had IGT according to the World Health Organization (WHO) criteria [11], plus a fasting plasma glucose concentration of between 100 and 140 mg/dl. A cardiovascular (CV) event within the last 6 months was an exclusion criterion. Subjects that were eligible were randomized to receive either placebo or 100 mg of acarbose three times a day. All patients were instructed to go on a weight reduction or weight maintenance diet and were encouraged to exercise regularly. The STOP-NIDDM trial primarily showed a decrease in progression from IGT to T2DM.

The *post hoc* analysis of STOP-NIDDM showed that decreasing post-prandial hyperglycemia with acarbose was associated with a 49% relative risk reduction in the development of CV events (hazard ratio [HR] 0.51; 95% confidence interval [CI] 0.28–0.95; $P = 0.03$) and a 2.5% absolute risk reduction. This reduction remained significant even after adjusting for all other measured risk factors at baseline. Seventy-two percent of the patients with CV events (22, placebo group; 12, acarbose) experienced a CV event during the IGT stage before they had developed diabetes (or did not develop diabetes during the study at all). Of the patients that did experience a CV event, 28% (10, placebo; 3, acarbose) experienced an event after the onset of diabetes. Patients who developed CV events had a larger mean waist circumference (105.5 vs 102.1 cm; $P = 0.02$) and a higher mean systolic (139.5 vs 130.9 mmHg; $P < 0.001$) and diastolic blood pressure (86.3 vs 82.3 mmHg; $P = 0.004$) at baseline compared with patients who did not experience CV events. Of the total of 13 cases of clinical myocardial infarction, 12 occurred in the placebo group making the difference significant (HR 0.09; 95% CI 0.01–0.72; $P = 0.02$). The effect of acarbose on the other individual components of CVD (angina, revascularization procedures, cardiovascular death, congestive heart failure, cerebrovascular event or stroke, peripheral disease) were not significant because of the small number of events, but the trend favored the acarbose group. Acarbose was associated with a 34% relative risk reduction in the incidence of new cases of hypertension (HR 0.66; 95% CI 0.49–0.89; $P = 0.006$) and a 5.3% absolute risk reduction. Using a repeated measures analysis of variance, acarbose treatment had a significant reduction on the following parameters: weight, $P < 0.001$; BMI, $P < 0.001$; waist circumference, $P = 0.001$; systolic blood pressure, $P < 0.001$; diastolic blood pressure, $P = 0.008$; 2-h plasma glucose concentration, $P < 0.001$; and triglycerides, $P = 0.01$. The mean follow-up in the study was 3.3 years. However, 24% of the patients had discontinued their participation early, possibly due to the side-effects, which are a major limitation of the therapy.

A subgroup analysis of the STOP-NIDDM [12] study showed a significant reduction of the intima-media thickness (IMT) (mean) in the acarbose group versus placebo after an average time of 3.9 years. The annual increase of mean IMT was reduced by approximately 50% in the acarbose group vs placebo. Multiple linear regression revealed that IMT progression was related to acarbose intake in these subjects with IGT which are a high-risk population for diabetes and atherosclerosis. Acarbose inhibits carbohydrate absorption and therefore reduces post-meal hyperglycemia. Acarbose has been shown to decrease the rise in glucose, insulin and markers of coagulation activation. Ceriello *et al.*[13] studied 17 patients with diabetes that were maintained on diet therapy alone in a randomized, crossover study design comparing acarbose and placebo. Acarbose administration (100 mg orally) before a standard meal significantly reduced the rise of glucose, insulin, prothrombin fragments 1 + 2 and D-dimer from 0 to 240 min in comparison to placebo. Thus, although the AGIs do not directly impact insulin resistance by correcting post-prandial metabolic abnormalities and the associated post-prandial CV risk profile, they could possibly impact long-term events in patients with the MS.

METFORMIN

Metformin is a biguanide that has been approved for the treatment of type 2 diabetes and has also been shown to prevent diabetes in obese subjects with IGT. The primary glucose- lowering effect of metformin is due to a decrease in hepatic gluconeogenesis. There are some effects on the peripheral glucose disposal as well [14]. In the UK Prospective Diabetes Study (UKPDS) study, obese patients treated with metformin had a 36% lower risk of all-cause mortality and a 39% lower risk of myocardial infarction [15]. Patients on metformin also had less weight gain in comparison to those treated with other agents. There was no difference in glycemic control in patients treated with metformin compared to the use of other agents to achieve glycemic control. It is possible that other effects of the drug, including its effect on the insulin resistance syndrome (IRS) may have decreased CV events. Potential mechanisms by which metformin may decrease CV events, include reduced plasma triglycerides, low-density lipoprotein (LDL)-cholesterol concentration, post-prandial hyperglycemia, and plasma free fatty acid concentration [3, 16].

The Diabetes Prevention Program (DPP) randomized trial's objective was to determine the effect of metformin therapy on the incidence and resolution of the MS as compared to that of intensive lifestyle intervention and placebo [17]. Metformin was given in the dose of 850 mg twice daily. In lifetime analyses (log-rank test) [18, 19], the metformin group had a reduction in the incidence of the MS by 17% ($P = 0.03$) while the intensive lifestyle group had a reduction by 41% ($P < 0.001$) as compared with placebo. In the group of DPP participants that did not meet the criteria for MS at baseline, metformin was effective only in reducing the waist circumference and fasting glucose level. The metformin group had significantly greater reductions in weight, fasting insulin and glucose than the placebo group. In comparison to the lifestyle group, the metformin group exhibited significantly greater reduction in fibrinogen and CRP. The favorable changes in CRP were observed both in men and women. Hypertension was present in 30% of participants upon entry into the study. Participants in the placebo and metformin groups had an increase in blood pressure, which was significantly lower in the intensive lifestyle intervention group. Triglyceride levels decreased in the metformin group as well, but not to such a great extent as in the intensive lifestyle intervention group. The intensive lifestyle intervention group had a significant increase in the high-density lipoprotein (HDL)-cholesterol, but the total cholesterol and the low-density lipoprotein (LDL)-cholesterol levels were similar among all the treatment groups. Thus, metformin has been shown to have multiple effects on the various parameters of the MS. Although not approved for the treatment of the syndrome, it is likely to be used in selected patients with prediabetes in the hope of slowing the progression to overt diabetes. The ongoing follow-up of the DPP patients may tell us whether such a strategy prevents cardiovascular events.

THIAZOLIDINEDIONES

Thiazolidinediones (TZDs) are peroxisome proliferator-activated receptor (PPAR)-γ agonists that are used for the treatment of T2DM. They help elucidate the important non-hypoglycemic effects of PPAR-γ activation including modification of traditional and non-traditional markers of CVD. The non-traditional risk factors include markers of inflammation, endothelial dysfunction and abnormalities of coagulation. As stated above, the TZDs are currently indicated for the treatment of type 2 diabetes, but have potential to alter the metabolic conditions besides glycemic control. Since they target insulin resistance, they modify many of the risk factors associated with obesity and insulin resistance such as dyslipidemia, hypertension, impaired fibrinolysis and atherosclerosis [20]. Effects of several non-TZD PPAR-γ and combined PPAR-γ/α-agonists on CVD are also being evaluated. Rosiglitazone, one of the TZDs has been tested in subjects with impaired fasting glucose or IGT, or both, with the aim of assessing the drug's ability to prevent type 2 DM in these individuals, who are at high risk for developing DM, in The DREAM (Diabetes Reduction Assessment with ramipril and rosiglitazone Medication) trial [21]. Known CVD was an exclusion criterion. The primary outcome was a composite of incident diabetes or death. The primary outcome of diabetes or death was seen in significantly fewer individuals in the rosiglitazone group than in the placebo group (HR 0.40; 95% CI 0.35–0.46; P <0.0001. Rosiglitazone was also effective irrespective of baseline weight or fat distribution. While increasing baseline weight or waist-to-hip ratio (WHR) (i.e., abdominal fat distribution) predicted a higher frequency of diabetes in the placebo group, this relationship was not seen in the rosiglitazone group. Mean systolic and diastolic blood pressure were 1.7 mmHg and 1.4 mmHg lower, respectively, in the rosiglitazone group than in the placebo group (P <0.0001). There was no difference in the use of antihypertensive agents in the two groups during the trial. The mean body weight increased by 2.2 kg in the rosiglitazone group as compared to the placebo group (P < 0.0001). However, the increase in body weight observed in the rosiglitazone group was associated with a lower WHR (P <0.0001) because of an increase in hip circumference of 1.8 cm; there was no effect on waist circumference. In another study by Rennings *et al.* [22], which included obese, non-diabetic subjects with MS-treatment with rosiglitazone seemed to reduce the calculated systemic vascular resistance, but the difference failed to reach statistical significance (–3.2% [–9.6 to 3.7]; P = 0.28).

As discussed below, various groups [23, 24] have studied the effect of TZDs on endothelial function and inflammatory markers in patients with MS. In these studies, in comparison to placebo, subjects using rosiglitazone showed improvements in markers of metabolic control, inflammation and vasoreactivity. The effects of TZDs on the MS and various other markers are summarized in Table 4.1. TZDs greatly impact several features of the MS and therefore may be considered the ideal drugs for the syndrome. On the other hand, the side-effects seen in the DREAM study and recent controversies about a possible increase in risk of myocardial infarction with rosiglitazone [25] make it unlikely that the drugs will get approval outside the setting of diabetes and they are unlikely to be used purely for treatment of the MS.

INCRETINS

The incretin effect which is diminished in type 2 diabetes comprises up to 60% of the insulin secretion in the post-prandial phase [26]. One of the very important gastrointestinal hormones that promotes the incretin effect is gastric glucagon-like peptide-1 (GLP-1), discovered in 1985 [27–29]. Another important incretin hormone is glucose-dependent insulinotropic peptide (GIP), also known as gastric inhibitory polypeptide, discovered in 1971 [29, 30]. The physiological actions of GLP-1 analogs include glucose-lowering, inhibition of glucagon secretion and slowed gastric emptying besides acting as a neurotransmitter in the hypothalamus stimulating satiety. The insulinotropic effect of GLP-1 is glucose

Table 4.1 Summary of the effects of the various hypoglycemic agents on the features and sequelae of the metabolic syndrome

Drug	*Weight*	*Waist Circum.*	*WHR*	*Trig*	*HDL*	*BP*	*Microalb.*	*CRP*	*IMT*	*Vascular reactivity*
SU	↑	↔	↔	↓	↔	↔	↔	↓	↓	↔
AGIs	↓	↓	↔	↓	↔	↔	↔	↔	↔	↔
Metformin	↓	↓	↔	↓	↔	↔	↓	↓	↔	↑
TZDs	↑	↑	↑	↓	↑	↓	↓	↓	↓	↑↑
Incretin therapy	↓	↓	**	↓	↓	↔	**	↓	**	**

↑ = increase; ↓ = decrease; ↔ = no effect; ** = no data; BP = blood pressure; CRP = C-reactive protein; IMT = intima-media thickness; Microalb. = microalbuminuria; SU = sulfonylureas; TZD = thiazolidinedione; waist circum. = waist circumference; WHR = waist-to-hip ratio.

dependent, therefore having the advantage of avoiding hypoglycemia. However, GLP-1 is degraded by the enzyme dipeptidyl peptidase-IV (DPP-IV) [31, 32]. Exenatide is the synthetic form of a naturally occurring peptide, exendin-4 and is not degraded by DPP-IV. Exenatide therapy has been shown to result in moderate weight reduction [33]. In addition, it has been shown to have favorable effects on several cardiovascular risk factors, including triglyceride level, HDL-cholesterol level and diastolic blood pressure [34]. A double-blind, placebo-controlled trial by Zinman *et al.* [35] studied the effects of exenatide in patients with type 2 diabetes that was suboptimally controlled while being treated with a TZD with or without metfomin. Exenatide treatment reduced mean (±) body weight from 97.53 ± 1.73 kg to 95.38 ± 0.25 kg. Body weight did not change in the placebo group. Similar findings have been reported in other studies [36, 37]. Kendall and co-workers [34] studied patients with type 2 DM using exenatide in combination with metformin and/or sulfonylurea or metformin and/or a thizolidinedione. Their analysis revealed improvement in cardiovascular risk factors such as lipids and blood pressure when this cohort was followed for 3.5 years. Triglycerides decreased by 12% (95% CI –68.3 to –20.5, whereas total cholesterol and LDL-cholesterol decreased by 5% (95% CI –17.0 to –4.6) and 6% (95% CI –17.5 to –6.1), respectively. HDL-cholesterol increased by 24% (95% CI 7.2 to 9.7). Systolic and diastolic blood pressure decreased by 2% (95% CI –5.9 to –1.0) and –4% (95% CI –4.9 to –1.7), respectively. However, this was a cohort with type 2 DM and the drug has not been well studied in patients with obesity/MS without diabetes.

IMPACT OF DIABETES TREATMENTS ON OTHER RISK FACTORS ASSOCIATED WITH THE MS

INFLAMMATORY CYTOKINES

Adipocytes are active endocrine cells that secrete cytokines and non-cytokine active proteins termed adipokines. These include adiponectin, tumor necrosis factor alpha (TNF-α), leptin, resistin, and plasminogen-activator inhibitor type 1 (PAI-1) [38]. Adiponectin and leptin are related to increasing insulin sensitivity, while TNF-α and PAI-1 are mediators of insulin resistance [39]. Although the precise role of adipocytes in the development of the MS and atherosclerosis is unclear, cytokines and adipokines exert direct and indirect influences on the atherosclerotic process including inflammation, plaque rupture and abnormalities in coagulation and fibrinolysis.

The pro-inflammatory cytokines TNF-α, interleukin-1 (IL-1) and interleukin-6 (IL-6) may play a causal role in the development of MS and diabetes. IL-6 levels correlate with obesity and weight loss lowers the level [40]. Levels of IL-6 also correlate with increased triglycerides, free fatty acids and decreased insulin resistance [41]. IL-6 is a predictor of cardiovascular events [42]. TNF-α secretion is proportional to fat mass [43] and is involved in insulin resistance. These cytokines stimulate synthesis of acute phase proteins by the liver, such as C-reactive protein (CRP) a fibrinogen [44]. TZDs have been shown to decrease the basal levels of TNF-α and IL-6 and attenuate response to inducers of these cytokines in both obese mice [45] and in obese patients [46]. With the reduction of cytokines and subsequent inflammation, the TZD may have a positive impact on CVD.

PAI-1 is the primary inhibitor of endogenous tissue plasminogen activator (tPA). It is secreted by the adipocytes and is elevated in obesity [47]. Elevation of the plasma PAI-1 levels leads to a decrease in the fibrinolytic activity, and is associated with increased risk of atherosclerosis and CVD [48]. Increase in PAI-1 levels correlates positively with plasma insulin levels and is now recognized as an integral part of the insulin resistance syndrome. Troglitazone and pioglitazone both decrease PAI-1 expression in the human endothelial cell [49]. Raji *et al.* demonstrated that treatment with rosiglitazone significantly decreased PAI-1 levels [50]. Increased levels of PAI-1 are associated with an increased risk of myocardial infarction, but no study has been done to see the effect of decreasing PAI-1 levels on cardiovascular events.

Increases in plasma concentrations of markers of inflammation, such as CRP, are associated with insulin resistance syndrome and the development of diabetes [51] as well as CVD [52]. A significant reduction in CRP levels by TZDs has been shown in many studies [46, 50]. Mohanty *et al.* demonstrated a sustained reduction of CRP levels in obese patients treated with rosiglitazone. These effects may be related to the decrease in insulin resistance and may have beneficial consequences for long-term cardiovascular risk. In patients with coronary artery disease (CAD) without diabetes, rosiglitazone treatment reduced inflammatory markers including CRP and fibrinogen [53].

Adiponectin is an adipocyte-derived peptide from white adipose tissue. It has anti-inflammatory and insulin-sensitizing properties. Adiponectin levels are paradoxically lower in obesity, unlike most other adipokines. There is an association between low levels of adiponectin and omental obesity, insulin resistance, CAD and dyslipidemia [38]. Hypoadiponectinemia is related to the degree of insulin resistance and hyperinsulinemia [54]. Increase in the levels of adiponectin is associated with a reduced risk of type 2 diabetes [55]. Higher levels of adiponectin may positively affect the atherosclerotic process through effects on the vasculature. In the vascular endothelium, adiponectin decreases monocyte adhesion to endothelium, suppresses the transformation of macrophage to foam cell, inhibiting vascular smooth muscle cell proliferation and migration [38]. Some of the strategies to increase adiponectin levels include weight loss and TZDs. The TZDs, through PPAR-γ receptor activation, increase the levels of adiponectin in lean and obese patients, as well as those with type 2 diabetes [56].

ENDOTHELIAL FUNCTION AND VASCULAR WALL ABNORMALITIES

Obesity is associated with insulin resistance and increased plasma free fatty acids [57], which can result in impairment of endothelium-dependent vasodilatation [58]. TZDs lower plasma free fatty acid concentrations [59], which may improve insulin sensitivity [60]. Since free fatty acids are involved in lipid metabolism and have deleterious effects on the vasculature, this reduction in plasma free fatty acids may have a beneficial effect on CVD, hypertension and microvascular disease [61]. Derosa *et al.* [62] conducted a double-blind, randomized trial comparing the long-term effect of pioglitazone and rosiglitazone on blood pressure control of diabetic patients with MS treated with glimerpide. After about 9–12 months of taking these medications there was improvement in the homeostasis model assessment index (HOMA index) ($P < 0.05$ and $P < 0.01$, respectively) in both groups. Significant reduction in systolic blood pressure and diastolic blood pressure was observed in both groups at 12 months as well. However, the effect of TZDs on blood pressure has not been consistent.

Vascular endothelium plays an important role in the regulation of vascular tone, vessel permeability, and angiogenesis. Nitric oxide and endothelin-1 are both determinants of vascular tone and health. The effects of troglitazone and pioglitazone have been studied in cultured endothelial cells to assess cell growth, and secretion of endothelium-derived vasoactive substances, which affect vascular tone and remodeling in atherosclerosis [63]. Both were found to suppress endothelin, a potent vasoconstrictor, in bovine carotid artery endothelial cells.

In obesity, there is impaired endothelial function [64]. Brachial artery vasoactivity is a non-invasive method of assessing arterial endothelial function. Endothelial injury being an early event in atherogenesis, it has been suggested that impaired vasoactivity may precede the structural changes in the vessel wall. Endothelial dysfunction and inflammation is accompanied by increased reactive oxygen species (ROS) generation. The anti-inflammatory effects of TZDs have been evaluated in obese patients with and without diabetes by measuring ROS generation. Both troglitazone and rosiglitazone exert a profound anti-inflammatory effect by reducing ROS generation [46, 65]. This reduction in ROS with troglitazone use improved flow-mediated vasodilation in the brachial artery.

The MS is adversely associated with markers of early arterial dysfunction, such as common carotid arteries intimal-media thickness (CCA-IMT) [66]. Carotid intimal-medial complex thickness (CIMT) is an indicator for early atherosclerosis [67] and may serve as a surrogate marker for atherosclerotic events [68]. B-mode ultrasound is a reliable and non-invasive method for evaluating CIMT. Patients with increased CIMT have a higher rate of cardiovascular events over time. Smooth muscle proliferation is also an important feature of atherosclerotic plaques. TZDs have an antiproliferative effect on vascular smooth muscle cells [69]. Treatment with rosiglitazone decreases intimal hyperplasia after balloon catheter-induced vascular injury in Zucker rats [67, 70].

HYPERTENSION

Hypertension, a risk factor for CAD, is associated with both insulin resistance and diabetes [57]. The effects of TZDs on blood pressure have been examined in several different experimental and clinical settings. They have been found to lower blood pressure in hypertensive patients without diabetes. Raji *et al.* studied the effect of rosiglitazone on insulin resistance and blood pressure in patients with essential hypertension [50]. Patients with hypertension who were treated with rosiglitazone showed increased insulin sensitivity and reduced systolic and diastolic blood pressure. There were favorable changes in the markers of cardiovascular risk as well. Pioglitazone has also been shown to decrease diastolic blood pressure in non-diabetic patients with hypertension [71].

The mechanism of blood pressure-lowering by troglitazone was evaluated by Sung and co-workers in patients with diabetes and it has been suggested that improved insulin resistance rather than improved glycemic control was responsible for the improvement in blood pressure [72]. This decrease in blood pressure by improved insulin sensitivity promotes insulin-mediated vasodilatation. In laboratory experiments, troglitazone has been shown to lower blood pressure by blockage of the calcium channels [73].

DYSLIPIDEMIA

Insulin resistance is associated with lipid abnormalities including elevated triglycerides and decreased HDL-cholesterol, both of which are seen in the MS as well. The TZDs raise HDL-cholesterol, though only troglitazone and pioglitazone have been shown to lower triglycerides

[50, 74]. This could be due to differential effects of the various PPAR agonists on lipoproteins. PPAR-γ is a regulator of HDL and LDL, while PPAR-α regulates triglycerides.

LDL levels may not differ, but there certainly are qualitative changes in the LDL-cholesterol in patients with diabetes. The effects of TZDs on LDL are complex. In insulin resistance syndrome and diabetes, the LDL is of a small, dense particle size [75]. These particles are triglyceride rich and susceptible to oxidation, which makes them more atherogenic. This could be a key event involved in the process of atherosclerosis [76]. TZDs have been shown to increase total cholesterol and LDL-cholesterol, but the increase is primarily in larger, more buoyant LDL particles, which may be less atherogenic [48].

SUMMARY

About 47 million US residents have the MS [77]. Subjects with the MS are at an increased risk for developing diabetes and CVD. The MS also increases the mortality from CVD and all other causes. There are several modalities of treatment that are available for treatment of DM. The effect of these agents on the various metabolic and vascular parameters have been studied in patients with the MS with and without DM. Improvements in glycemic control with many agents such as insulin, insulin secretagogues and insulin sensitizers are often accompanied by weight gain, which is multifactorial. However, agents such as biguanides and alpha glucosidase inhibitors decrease or have no effect on weight. More recently, incretin therapy has been shown to result in weight loss. Various hypoglycemic agents have differing effects on features of the MS and therefore on cardiovascular risk.

ACKNOWLEDGEMENTS

Diabetes research at Tulane University Health Sciences Center is supported in part by the Susan Harling Robinson Fellowship in Diabetes Research and the Tullis-Tulane Alumni Chair in Diabetes.

REFERENCES

1. Tkáč I. Metabolic syndrome in relationship to type 2 diabetes and atherosclerosis. *Diabetes Res Clin Pract* 2005; 68(suppl 1):S2–S9.
2. Eckel RH. Obesity and heart disease: a statement for healthcare professionals from the Nutrition Committee, American Heart Association. *Circulation* 1997; 96:3248–3250.
3. Lebovitz HE. Effects of oral antihyperglycemic agents in modifying macrovascular risk factors in type 2 diabetes. *Diabetes Care* 1999; 22(suppl 3):C41–C44.
4. Nateglinide and Valsartan in Impaired Glucose Tolerance Outcomes Research (NAVIEATOR). 2007. Available at http://clinicaltrials.gov/ct/show/NCT00097786.
5. Barzilay JI, Spiekerman CF, Wahl PW *et al.* Cardiovascular disease in older adults with glucose disorders: comparison of American Diabetes Association criteria for diabetes mellitus with WHO criteria. *Lancet* 1999; 354:622–625.
6. Fontbonne A, Eschwege E, Cambien F *et al.* Hypertriglyceridaemia as a risk factor of coronary heart disease mortality in subjects with impaired glucose tolerance or diabetes. Results from the 11-year follow-up of the Paris Prospective Study. *Diabetologia* 1989; 32:300–304.
7. Fuller JH, Shipley MJ, Rose G, Jarrett RJ, Keen H. Coronary heart disease risk and impaired glucose tolerance. The Whitehall study. *Lancet* 1980; 1:1373–1376.
8. Pyörälä K. Relationship of glucose tolerance and plasma insulin to the incidence of coronary heart disease: results from two population studies in Finland. *Diabetes Care* 1979; 2:131–141.
9. Tominaga M, Eguchi H, Manaka H, Igarashi K, Kato T, Sekikawa A. Impaired glucose tolerance is a risk factor for cardiovascular disease, but not impaired fasting glucose. The Funagata Diabetes Study. *Diabetes Care* 1999; 22:920–924.
10. Chiasson JL, Josse RG, Gomis R, Hanefeld M, Karasik A, Laakso M. Acarbose treatment and the risk of cardiovascular disease and hypertension in patients with impaired glucose tolerance: the STOP-NIDDM trial. *JAMA* 2003; 290:486–494.

11. World Health Organization. Definition, diagnosis, and classification of diabetes mellitus and its complications: Report of a WHO Consultation. Part I: Diagnosis and classification of diabetes mellitus. Geneva, Switzerland: World Health Organization, 1999. Available at http://whqlibdoc.who.int/hq/1999/WHO_NCD_NCS_99.2.pdf
12. Hanefeld M, Chiasson JL, Koehler C, Henkel E, Schaper F, Temelkova-Kurktschiev T. Acarbose slows progression of intima-media thickness of the carotid arteries in subjects with impaired glucose tolerance. *Stroke* 2004; 35:1073–1078.
13. Ceriello A, Taboga C, Tonutti L *et al.* Post-meal coagulation activation in diabetes mellitus: the effect of acarbose. *Diabetologia* 1996; 39:469–473.
14. Stumvoll M, Nurjhan N, Perriello G, Dailey G, Gerich JE. Metabolic effects of metformin in non-insulin-dependent diabetes mellitus. *N Engl J Med* 1995; 333:550–554.
15. Turner RC. The U.K. Prospective Diabetes Study. A review. *Diabetes Care* 1998; 21(suppl 3):C35–C38.
16. Bailey CJ, Turner RC. Metformin. *N Engl J Med* 1996; 334:574–579.
17. Orchard TJ, Temprosa M, Goldberg R *et al.* The effect of metformin and intensive lifestyle intervention on the metabolic syndrome: the Diabetes Prevention Program randomized trial. *Ann Intern Med* 2005; 142:611–619.
18. Summary of the second report of the National Cholesterol Education Program (NCEP) Expert Panel on Detection, Evaluation, and Treatment of High Blood Cholesterol in Adults (Adult Treatment Panel II). *JAMA* 1993; 269:3015–3023.
19. Ratner R, Goldberg R, Haffner S *et al.* Impact of intensive lifestyle and metformin therapy on cardiovascular disease risk factors in the Diabetes Prevention Program. *Diabetes Care* 2005; 28:888–894.
20. Panunti B, Fonseca V. Effects of PPAR gamma agonists on cardiovascular function in obese, non-diabetic patients. *Vascul Pharmacol* 2006; 45:29–35.
21. Gerstein HC, Yusuf S, Bosch J *et al.* Effect of rosiglitazone on the frequency of diabetes in patients with impaired glucose tolerance or impaired fasting glucose: a randomised controlled trial *Lancet* 2006; 368: 1096–1105.
22. Rennings AJ, Smits P, Stewart MW, Tack CJ. Fluid retention and vascular effects of rosiglitazone in obese, insulin-resistant, nondiabetic subjects 1. *Diabetes Care* 2006; 29:581–587.
23. Esposito K, Ciotola M, Carleo D *et al.* Effect of rosiglitazone on endothelial function and inflammatory markers in patients with the metabolic syndrome. *Diabetes Care* 2006; 29:1071–1076.
24. Wang TD, Chen WJ, Cheng WC, Lin JW, Chen MF, Lee YT. Relation of improvement in endothelium-dependent flow-mediated vasodilation after rosiglitazone to changes in asymmetric dimethylarginine, endothelin-1, and C-reactive protein in nondiabetic patients with the metabolic syndrome. *Am J Cardiol* 2006; 98:1057–1062.
25. Nissen SE, Wolski K. Effect of rosiglitazone on the risk of myocardial infarction and death from cardiovascular causes 1. *N Engl J Med* 2007; 356:2457–2471.
26. Gallwitz B. New therapeutic strategies for the treatment of type 2 diabetes mellitus based on incretins. *Rev Diabet Stud* 2005; 2:61–69.
27. Holst JJ, Bersani M, Johnsen AH, Kofod H, Hartmann B, Orskov C. Proglucagon processing in porcine and human pancreas 1. *J Biol Chem* 1994; 269:18827–18833.
28. Kreymann B, Williams G, Ghatei MA, Bloom SR. Glucagon-like peptide-1 7-36: a physiological incretin in man 1. *Lancet* 1987; 2:1300–1304.
29. Meier JJ, Nauck MA, Schmidt WE, Gallwitz B. Gastric inhibitory polypeptide: the neglected incretin revisited 1. *Regul Pept* 2002; 107:1–13.
30. Brown JC, Dryburgh JR. A gastric inhibitory polypeptide. II. The complete amino acid sequence 1. *Can J Biochem* 1971; 49:867–872.
31. Mentlein R, Gallwitz B, Schmidt WE. Dipeptidyl-peptidase IV hydrolyses gastric inhibitory polypeptide, glucagon-like peptide-1(7–36)amide, peptide histidine methionine and is responsible for their degradation in human serum. *Eur J Biochem* 1993; 214:829–835.
32. Deacon CF, Johnsen AH, Holst JJ. Degradation of glucagon-like peptide-1 by human plasma in vitro yields an N-terminally truncated peptide that is a major endogenous metabolite in vivo. *J Clin Endocrinol Metab* 1995; 80:952–957.
33. Poon T, Nelson P, Shen L *et al.* Exenatide improves glycemic control and reduces body weight in subjects with type 2 diabetes: a dose-ranging study. *Diabetes Technol Ther* 2005; 7:467–477.
34. Blonde L, Klein EJ, Han J *et al.* Interim analysis of the effects of exenatide treatment on A1C, weight and cardiovascular risk factors over 82 weeks in 314 overweight patients with type 2 diabetes. *Diabetes Obes Metab* 2006; 8:436–447.

35. Zinman B, Hoogwerf BJ, Duran GS *et al*. The effect of adding exenatide to a thiazolidinedione in suboptimally controlled type 2 diabetes: a randomized trial. *Ann Intern Med* 2007; 146:477–485.
36. Amori RE, Lau J, Pittas AG. Efficacy and safety of incretin therapy in type 2 diabetes: systematic review and meta-analysis. *JAMA* 2007; 298:194–206.
37. Buse JB, Henry RR, Han J, Kim DD, Fineman MS, Baron AD. Effects of exenatide (exendin-4) on glycemic control over 30 weeks in sulfonylurea-treated patients with type 2 diabetes. *Diabetes Care* 2004; 27:2628–2635.
38. Chandran M, Phillips SA, Ciaraldi T, Henry RR. Adiponectin: more than just another fat cell hormone? *Diabetes Care* 2003; 26:2442–2450.
39. Bloomgarden ZT. Adiposity and diabetes. *Diabetes Care* 2002; 25:2342–2349.
40. Bastard JP, Jardel C, Bruckert E *et al*. Elevated levels of interleukin 6 are reduced in serum and subcutaneous adipose tissue of obese women after weight loss. *J Clin Endocrinol Metab* 2000; 85: 3338–3342.
41. Trujillo ME, Sullivan S, Harten I, Schneider SH, Greenberg AS, Fried SK. Interleukin-6 regulates human adipose tissue lipid metabolism and leptin production in vitro. *J Clin Endocrinol Metab* 2004; 89:5577–5582.
42. Ridker PM, Rifai N, Pfeffer M, Sacks F, Lepage S, Braunwald E. Elevation of tumor necrosis factor-alpha and increased risk of recurrent coronary events after myocardial infarction. *Circulation* 2000; 101:2149–2153.
43. Corica F, Allegra A, Corsonello A *et al*. Relationship between plasma leptin levels and the tumor necrosis factor-alpha system in obese subjects. *Int J Obes Relat Metab Disord* 1999; 23:355–360.
44. Pickup JC. Inflammation and activated innate immunity in the pathogenesis of type 2 diabetes. *Diabetes Care* 2004; 27:813–823.
45. Sigrist S, Bedoucha M, Boelsterli UA. Down-regulation by troglitazone of hepatic tumor necrosis factor-alpha and interleukin-6 mRNA expression in a murine model of non-insulin-dependent diabetes. *Biochem Pharmacol* 2000; 60:67–75.
46. Mohanty P, Aljada A, Ghanim H *et al*. Evidence for a potent antiinflammatory effect of rosiglitazone. *J Clin Endocrinol Metab* 2004; 89:2728–2735.
47. Juhan-Vague I, Vague P, Alessi MC *et al*. Relationships between plasma insulin triglyceride, body mass index, and plasminogen activator inhibitor 1. *Diabete Metab* 1987; 13:331–336.
48. Huber K, Christ G, Wojta J, Gulba D. Plasminogen activator inhibitor type-1 in cardiovascular disease. Status report 2001. *Thromb Res* 2001; 103(suppl 1):S7–19.
49. Kato K, Satoh H, Endo Y *et al*. Thiazolidinediones down-regulate plasminogen activator inhibitor type 1 expression in human vascular endothelial cells: A possible role for PPARgamma in endothelial function. *Biochem Biophys Res Commun* 1999; 258:431–435.
50. Raji A, Seely EW, Bekins SA, Williams GH, Simonson DC. Rosiglitazone improves insulin sensitivity and lowers blood pressure in hypertensive patients. *Diabetes Care* 2003; 26:172–178.
51. Pradhan AD, Manson JE, Rifai N, Buring JE, Ridker PM. C-reactive protein, interleukin 6, and risk of developing type 2 diabetes mellitus. *JAMA* 2001; 286:327–334.
52. Ridker PM, Rifai N, Rose L, Buring JE, Cook NR. Comparison of C-reactive protein and low-density lipoprotein cholesterol levels in the prediction of first cardiovascular events. *N Engl J Med* 2002; 347:1557–1565.
53. Sidhu JS, Cowan D, Kaski JC. The effects of rosiglitazone, a peroxisome proliferator-activated receptor-gamma agonist, on markers of endothelial cell activation, C-reactive protein, and fibrinogen levels in non-diabetic coronary artery disease patients. *J Am Coll Cardiol* 2003; 42:1757–1763.
54. Weyer C, Funahashi T, Tanaka S *et al*. Hypoadiponectinemia in obesity and type 2 diabetes: close association with insulin resistance and hyperinsulinemia. *J Clin Endocrinol Metab* 2001; 86:1930–1935.
55. Spranger J, Kroke A, Mohlig M *et al*. Adiponectin and protection against type 2 diabetes mellitus. *Lancet* 2003; 361:226–228.
56. Yu JG, Javorschi S, Hevener AL *et al*. The effect of thiazolidinediones on plasma adiponectin levels in normal, obese, and type 2 diabetic subjects. *Diabetes* 2002; 51:2968–2974.
57. DeFronzo RA, Ferrannini E. Insulin resistance. A multifaceted syndrome responsible for NIDDM, obesity, hypertension, dyslipidemia, and atherosclerotic cardiovascular disease. *Diabetes Care* 1991; 14:173–194.
58. Steinberg HO, Tarshoby M, Monestel R *et al*. Elevated circulating free fatty acid levels impair endothelium-dependent vasodilation. *J Clin Invest* 1997; 100:1230–1239.
59. Kersten S, Desvergne B, Wahli W. Roles of PPARs in health and disease. *Nature* 2000; 405:421–424.

60. Santomauro AT, Boden G, Silva ME *et al.* Overnight lowering of free fatty acids with Acipimox improves insulin resistance and glucose tolerance in obese diabetic and nondiabetic subjects. *Diabetes* 1999; 48:1836–1841.
61. de Jongh RT, Serné EH, Ijzerman RG, de Vries G, Stehouwer CD. Impaired microvascular function in obesity: implications for obesity-associated microangiopathy, hypertension, and insulin resistance. *Circulation* 2004; 109:2529–2535.
62. Derosa G, Cicero AF, Dangelo A *et al.* Thiazolidinedione effects on blood pressure in diabetic patients with metabolic syndrome treated with glimepiride. *Hypertens Res* 2005; 28:917–924.
63. Fukunaga Y, Itoh H, Doi K *et al.* Thiazolidinediones, peroxisome proliferator-activated receptor gamma agonists, regulate endothelial cell growth and secretion of vasoactive peptides. *Atherosclerosis* 2001; 158:113–119.
64. Oflaz H, Ozbey N, Mantar F *et al.* Determination of endothelial function and early atherosclerotic changes in healthy obese women. *Diabetes Nutr Metab* 2003; 16:176–181.
65. Garg R, Kumbkarni Y, Aljada A *et al.* Troglitazone reduces reactive oxygen species generation by leukocytes and lipid peroxidation and improves flow-mediated vasodilatation in obese subjects. *Hypertension* 2000; 36:430–435.
66. Czernichow S, Bertrais S, Blacher J *et al.* Metabolic syndrome in relation to structure and function of large arteries: a predominant effect of blood pressure. A report from the SU.VI.MAX. Vascular Study. *Am J Hypertens* 2005; 18:1154–1160.
67. Salonen JT, Salonen R. Ultrasound B-mode imaging in observational studies of atherosclerotic progression. *Circulation* 1993; 87:II56–II65.
68. Burke GL, Evans GW, Riley WA *et al.* Arterial wall thickness is associated with prevalent cardiovascular disease in middle-aged adults. The Atherosclerosis Risk in Communities (ARIC) Study. *Stroke* 1995; 26:386–391.
69. Marx N, Schonbeck U, Lazar MA, Libby P, Plutzky J. Peroxisome proliferator-activated receptor gamma activators inhibit gene expression and migration in human vascular smooth muscle cells. *Circ Res* 1998; 83:1097–1103.
70. Desouza CV, Murthy SN, Diez J *et al.* Differential effects of peroxisome proliferator activator receptor-alpha and gamma ligands on intimal hyperplasia after balloon catheter-induced vascular injury in Zucker rats. *J Cardiovasc Pharmacol Ther* 2003; 8:297–305.
71. Fullert S, Schneider F, Haak E *et al.* Effects of pioglitazone in nondiabetic patients with arterial hypertension: a double-blind, placebo-controlled study. *J Clin Endocrinol Metab* 2002; 87:5503–5506.
72. Sung BH, Izzo JL, Jr, Dandona P, Wilson MF. Vasodilatory effects of troglitazone improve blood pressure at rest and during mental stress in type 2 diabetes mellitus. *Hypertension* 1999; 34:83–88.
73. Ali SS, Igwe RC, Walsh MF, Sowers JR. Troglitazone and vascular reactivity: role of glucose and calcium. *Metabolism* 1999; 48:125–130.
74. Chiquette E, Ramirez G, Defronzo R. A meta-analysis comparing the effect of thiazolidinediones on cardiovascular risk factors. *Arch Intern Med* 2004; 164:2097–2104.
75. Friedlander Y, Kidron M, Caslake M, Lamb T, McConnell M, Bar-On H. Low density lipoprotein particle size and risk factors of insulin resistance syndrome. *Atherosclerosis* 2000; 148:141–149.
76. Steinberg D, Parthasarathy S, Carew TE, Khoo JC, Witztum JL. Beyond cholesterol. Modifications of low-density lipoprotein that increase its atherogenicity. *N Engl J Med* 1989; 320:915–924.
77. Ford ES, Giles WH, Dietz WH. Prevalence of the metabolic syndrome among US adults: findings from the third National Health and Nutrition Examination Survey. *JAMA* 2002; 287:356–359.

5

Weight loss agents and the metabolic syndrome

W. T. Cefalu, C. Champagne, F. Greenway

INTRODUCTION

The prevalence of metabolic syndrome continues to reach epidemic proportions around the world. As outlined in this book, one of the major contributors to the increase in the prevalence of metabolic syndrome is the growing obesity problem. While it is recognized that there have been many changes in our environment that promote obesity, it is also clear that many individuals manage to resist obesity. Thus, there appears to be evidence that the variable susceptibility to obesity in response to environmental factors is undoubtedly modulated by specific genes [1, 2]. As well-established, those individuals considered obese, i.e. body mass index (BMI) $\geq$30 mg/m^2, are at much higher risk for cardiovascular mortality than those considered overweight, i.e. BMI between 25 and 29.9 mg/m^2 [3–6].

It is estimated that over one billion adults worldwide are overweight and at least 300 million are considered obese. Major contributors to this epidemic across the world are sedentary lifestyles, consumption of high-fat, caloric-dense diets and increased urbanization. Data from the National Health and Nutrition Examination Surveys (NHANES) in the United States find that 64% of the US adult population is classified as either overweight or obese (defined as BMI >25 mg/m^2). The prevalence of overweight adults increased slightly from data collected in 1960, from approximately 30.5% to 34.0% whereas the prevalence of obesity (defined as a BMI $\geq$30 mg/m^2) has more than doubled (13% in 1960 to over 30% in the year 2000) [6]. The prevalence of individuals with extreme obesity as defined by a BMI $\geq$40 mg/m^2 has increased even more dramatically as it has increased over 6-fold in the 40-year period (0.8% vs 4.7%).

Clinically, the concerns associated with the obesity epidemic are the dramatic increase in prevalence of the associated comorbidities that define the metabolic syndrome. Specifically, obesity is significantly associated with both the traditional risk factors, i.e. hypertension, dyslipidemia, diabetes and the non-traditional risk factors, i.e. fibrinogen and inflammatory markers, of cardiovascular disease (CVD). In addition, if one considers the presence of insulin resistance as the hallmark for the presence of metabolic syndrome, it is clear that obesity is the major contributor for the development of metabolic syndrome.

In general, every major organ system may be affected by the development of obesity (Table 5.1). In addition to cardiovascular diseases and diabetes, obesity has been suggested to increase an individual's risk for cancer, gastrointestinal diseases and arthritis.

William T. Cefalu, MD, Douglas L. Manship Senior Professor of Diabetes; Chief, Division of Nutrition and Chronic Diseases, Pennington Biomedical Research Center, Louisiana State University System, Baton Rouge, Louisiana, USA

Catherine M. Champagne, PhD, RD, Professor and Chief, Nutritional Epidemiology, Pennington Biomedical Research Center, Louisiana State University System, Baton Rouge, Louisiana, USA

Frank L. Greenway, MD, Professor and Director of Outpatient Clinical Research, Pennington Biomedical Research Center, Louisiana State University System, Baton Rouge, Louisiana, USA

Table 5.1 Medical complications associated with obesity (with permission from [3])

Gastrointestinal	Gallstones, pancreatitis, abdominal hernia, NAFLD (steatosis, steatohepatitis, and cirrhosis), and possibly GERD
Endocrine/metabolic	Metabolic syndrome, insulin resistance, impaired glucose tolerance, type 2 diabetes mellitus, dyslipidemia, polycystic ovary syndrome
Cardiovascular	Hypertension, coronary heart disease, congestive heart failure, dysrhythmias, pulmonary hypertension, ischemic stroke, venous stasis, deep vein thrombosis, pulmonary embolus
Respiratory	Abnormal pulmonary function, obstructive sleep apnea, obesity hypoventilation syndrome
Musculoskeletal	Osteoarthritis, gout, low back pain
Gyneocologic	Abnormal menses, infertility
Genitourinary	Urinary stress incontinence
Ophthalmologic	Cataracts
Neurologic	Idiopathic intracranial hypertension (pseudotumor cerebri)
Cancer	Esophagus, colon, gallbladder, prostate, breast, uterus, cervix, kidney
Post-operative events	Atelectasis, pneumonia, deep vein thrombosis, pulmonary embolus

GERD = gastro-esophageal reflux disease; NAFLD = non-alcoholic fatty liver disease

Table 5.2 BMI-associated disease risk

	Obesity class	*BMI (kg/m²)*	*Risk*
Underweight		<18.5	Increased
Normal		18.5–24.9	Normal
Overweight		25.0–29.9	Increased
Obesity	I	30.0–34.9	High
	II	35.0–39.9	Very high
Extreme obesity	III	≥40	Extremely high

Additional risks: (1) waist circumference >40 inches in men and >35 inches in woman; (2) weight gain of ≥5 kg since age 18–20 years; (3) poor aerobic fitness; and (4) Southeast Asian descent

DEFINITION AND NEW CONCEPTS OF OBESITY

The simplest and most useful clinical assessments to define obesity consist of body weight and BMI. Classification of obesity into specific risk categories is based on the BMI from data collected from large population-based studies that assessed the relationship between body weight and mortality (Table 5.2) [4, 5]. The BMI represents the relationship between weight and height and is derived by:

- Calculating either the weight (in kg) and dividing by the height (in meters) squared; or
- Calculating weight (in pounds) times 704 divided by height in inches squared [3].

In addition to weight and BMI, there has been great interest in assessing the specific distribution of the body fat, e.g. central or abdominal obesity, in an effort to help define cardiovascular risk. Body fat distribution, in the past, has been assessed by anthropometric measurements, i.e. waist circumference, the waist-to-hip ratio (WHR) or skinfold thicknesses,

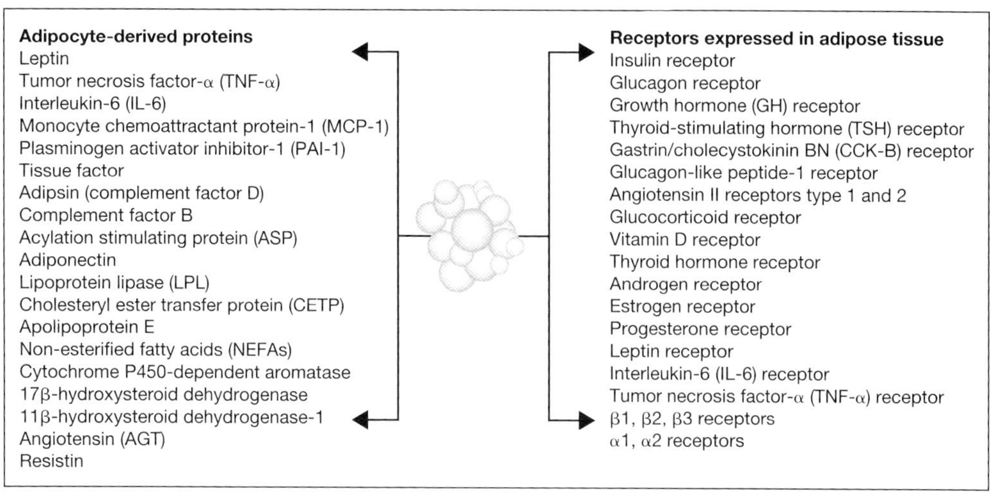

Figure 5.1 Adipocyte-derived proteins and receptor (with permission from [7]).

but more sophisticated techniques such as computed tomography (CT) scans or magnetic resonance imaging (MRI) scans more precisely quantify abdominal fat depots. Using these techniques, the relationship between specific adipose tissue depots, e.g. visceral fat depots, to peripheral muscle insulin sensitivity and other metabolic risk factors can be assessed.

When one considers the importance of treating obesity, it is important to note that adipose tissue does not just serve as a passive reservoir for energy storage, but has an equally important role as an active endocrine organ. Specifically, adipose tissue contributes greatly to biological processes that include energy metabolism, neuroendocrine and immune function, via secretion of a number of bioactive proteins, e.g. adipocytokines. In addition, it expresses numerous receptors that allow it to respond to different hormonal signals (Figure 5.1) [7].

STRATEGIES FOR WEIGHT LOSS

By definition, obesity is defined as an excessive amount of body fat, which increases the risk of medical illness and premature death. Obesity develops over time when an individual consumes more calories than he/she burns and, as such, can be viewed as developing secondary to an imbalance in energy balance. Energy balance is required to maintain a stable body weight and is achieved when food consumption, i.e. '*energy intake*', matches energy output, i.e. '*energy expenditure*'. The major determinants of energy expenditure are:

- The thermogenic effect of food (TEF) which represents the amount of energy utilized by ingestion and digestion of food we consume.
- Physical activity.
- Resting metabolic rate (RMR), determined in large measure by the amount of lean body mass.

Thus, in very simple terms, weight loss should be directed toward either reducing food intake and/or increasing expenditure as the basic rationale for weight loss and such a concept is the cornerstone of treatment. However, as is well recognized, obesity is not such a simple process. The mechanisms responsible for its development are complex and highly integrated. It has also been determined that there is a dynamic interplay between the adipose tissue and other key tissues in the body, such as the liver, muscle and regulatory centers of the brain. Altered regulation of this integrated and coordinated system inevitably leads to accumulation of body fat, insulin resistance and the development of associated risk factors contributing to the metabolic syndrome. But, on clinical grounds, it is clear that altering energy balance to achieve an overall deficit in energy intake either with nutritional or pharmacologic approaches is the goal of treatment for obesity.

SPECIFIC TREATMENT OPTIONS

The options available for treatment of obesity associated with metabolic syndrome will consist of a lifestyle program as a cornerstone in management to be optimally effective. In addition, pharmacologic agents and surgery may be required. Regardless of what treatment options are used, a team approach involving medical and surgical disciplines to deliver treatment with optimal safety is required.

BEHAVIOR MODIFICATION AND LIFESTYLE CHANGE

The first option available for any weight loss program should be one that strives for lifestyle modification. Unfortunately, there are considerable hurdles in this regard as it relates to patient compliance and time available for the primary care physician to adequately instruct the patient. Specifically, most physicians in primary care may lack the necessary preparation required to deliver such a program. In addition, based on the current medical practice paradigm, the physician may not have the time for this activity. Thus, a specific referral for behavior modification and lifestyle counseling may be required. This also raises additional hurdles relating to reimbursement of services. So, even this simple non-pharmacologic step has hurdles that may limit its success.

Lifestyle modification may result in a weight loss of approximately 10% of initial body weight over 16–26 weeks [8]. A 5–10% loss of initial body weight has been demonstrated to produce clinically important benefits as discussed in the section outlined below for the Diabetes Prevention Program (DPP) [9]. Continued contact with the therapist can help maintain the major proportion of that weight loss. In the Diabetes Prevention Program, subjects in the lifestyle change program lost an initial 7% of body weight and at 3 years maintained a 4% body weight loss accompanied by a 58% reduction in the conversion from impaired glucose tolerance to diabetes [10].

Calorie-controlled portions

Calorie-controlled portions using commercially available products, e.g. SlimFast®, Glucerna®, once or twice a day, have been compared to diets of comparable caloric content that use an exchange system. A 1-year long study compared a group taking two meal replacements a day for 3 months followed by 1 meal replacement a day to a group following an exchange diet of similar calories for 3 months followed by one meal replacement a day. The group starting on meal replacements lost 11.3 ± 6.8% of initial body weight at 1 year compared to the group starting on an exchange diet which lost 5.9 ± 5.0% [11]. Thus, calorie-controlled portions can be a powerful tool in delivering a weight loss program.

Commercial weight loss programs

Weight Watchers is a commercial program that delivers a lifestyle change program using counselors that are successful graduates of the program. The program uses a balanced diet constructed from food lists, is conducted in a group context and is relatively inexpensive. A 6-month controlled trial comparing Weight Watchers to a self-help weight loss group gave a 4.8 ± 5.6 kg weight loss in the Weight Watchers group compared to a 1.4 ± 4.7 kg weight loss in the self-help group [12]. This weight loss was greater than 5% of initial body weight and clinically significant. At 2 years, subjects in the Weight Watchers group maintained more than a 3% weight loss while weight in the self-help group returned to baseline [13].

A recent review of commercial weight loss programs concluded that the only well controlled trial was the study of the Weight Watchers program, but called for 'naturalistic studies' of program results [14]. The Jenny Craig program, which combines calorie-controlled portions with individual behavior and lifestyle counseling, recently published such a study of their program [15]. Those subjects who remained in the program for a year lost 15.6 ± 7.5% of their initial body weight. Rock *et al.* published a one-year study comparing the Jenny Craig program with a self-help control group [16]. At six months, the Jenny Craig group lost 7.8 + 7.2% of initial body weight compared to 0.4 + 4.5% in the control group. The Jenny Craig program is more expensive than the Weight Watchers program, in addition to being more effective; however, any program which is associated with high adherence would be effective. These studies give the physician some basis upon which to make a referral to a commercial weight loss program.

Diabetes Prevention Program meal plan

The participants in the lifestyle intervention group of the Diabetes Prevention Program received intensive training in diet, exercise, and behavior modification. By eating less fat and fewer calories and exercising for a total of 150 min a week, they aimed to lose 7% of their body weight and maintain that loss.

They were not given specific meal plans, but rather were taught strategies to adhere to a low-fat diet with fewer calories. They were taught how to figure out the fat content of foods using labels and given other resources needed to self-monitor their dietary intake. That was necessary to figure out what they were currently eating and in order to change their behavior to decrease all fat intake. Counting fat grams was essential. Weighing and measuring foods was also critical and most people are surprised when they weigh and measure foods since it heightens awareness of exactly what they are eating. The DPP focused on three ways to eat less fat: eating high-fat foods less often, eating smaller amounts of high-fat foods, and just eating lower-fat foods.

Of course, just telling people to eat less fat needs to be accompanied by making changes in all food groups to be successful. DPP used the Food Guide Pyramid as a key concept in making wise choices towards a healthy diet. Strategies like 'rating your plate' helped participants determine whether or not they were eating a healthy diet with variety. The lifestyle interventionists also addressed cooking techniques to help achieve a healthy diet. The issues of building healthy dietary habits in shopping and focusing on cues that make someone want to eat were also discussed with participants. There were a myriad of lifestyle changes that were addressed in 16 sessions with participants.

However, increasing physical activity was also an essential component of the DPP lifestyle program, and while not discussed in this section, it is important to realize that this was all part of the participants' learning. Behavioral strategies to achieve lifestyle changes were critically important and an essential part of the training from the lifestyle interventionists. Without addressing life problems, work issues, family support, motivation and adherence, the success in the DPP undoubtedly would have not been as high.

PHARMACOLOGIC TREATMENT

While lifestyle modification remains the cornerstone of treatment, there are two medications presently approved for the long-term treatment of obesity, sibutramine and orlistat. Medications approved before 1985, the year the National Institutes of Health (NIH) conference declared obesity to be a chronic disease, were approved and tested for up to 12 weeks as an adjunct to diet and lifestyle change [17]. We will review drugs approved for the treatment of obesity.

Obesity medication approved for short-term use

Drugs approved before 1985 for the treatment of obesity are chemically related to amphetamine, and are all associated with some degree of central nervous system (CNS) stimulation. Phentermine and diethylpropion are in Drug Enforcement Administration (DEA) class IV and are felt to have a lower abuse potential than phendimetrazine and benzphetamine that are in DEA class III or phenmetrazine that is in DEA class II. One might logically ask if these drugs can be useful in a chronic disease when they are all approved for up to 12 weeks of use. There is a study comparing phentermine given continuously to phentermine given every other month and to a placebo in a 36-week trial [18]. The intermittent use of phentermine gave equivalent weight loss to continuous use. The intermittent regimen gave lower drug exposure, was less expensive and allowed phentermine to be used in a way that is consistent with its package insert. Although the long-term studies of these drugs are limited, phentermine gave a 7.9 kg greater weight loss than placebo in a 1-year trial [19].

Sibutramine

Sibutramine is a reuptake inhibitor of norepinephrine and serotonin. It gives 2.8 kg more weight loss than a placebo at 3 months and 4.5 kg more weight loss than placebo at 1 year [20]. Adverse events associated with the use of sibutramine are associated with its adrenergic mechanism of action and include dry mouth, insomnia and nausea. Sibutramine gives the improvement in glucose and lipids expected with weight loss. Sibutramine is associated with an average increase in pulse rate of four beats per minute and the expected improvement in blood pressure is not seen, probably due to noradrenergic stimulation.

A clear dose response was seen in a 6-month dose-ranging study of 1047 patients. However, patients regained weight when the drug was stopped [21]. In a trial in patients who initially lost weight eating a very low-calorie diet before being randomized to sibutramine (10 mg per day) or placebo, sibutramine produced additional weight loss, while the placebo-treated patients regained weight [22]. The Sibutramine Trial of Obesity Reduction and Maintenance (STORM) lasted 2 years and provided evidence for weight maintenance [23]. Patients were initially enrolled in an open-label phase and treated with 10 mg per day of sibutramine for 6 months. Of the patients who lost more than 8 kg, two-thirds were then randomized to sibutramine and one-third to placebo. During the 18-month double-blind phase of this trial, the placebo-treated patients steadily regained weight, maintaining only 20% of their initial weight loss at the end of the trial. In contrast, the subjects treated with sibutramine maintained their weight for 12 months and then regained an average of only 2 kg, thus maintaining 80% of their initial weight loss after 2 years [23]. Despite the higher weight loss with sibutramine at the end of the 18 months of controlled observation, the blood pressure levels of the sibutramine-treated patients were still higher than in the patients treated with placebo.

The recommended starting level of sibutramine is 10 mg per day and it is available in 5-, 10-, and 15-mg doses. Titration can be up or down depending on the response, but doses higher than 15 mg/day are not recommended. Of the patients who lost 2 kg (4 lb) in the first 4 weeks of treatment, 60% achieved a weight loss of more than 5%, compared with less than 10% of those who did not lose 2 kg (4 lb) in 4 weeks. Combining data from eleven studies on sibutramine showed a reduction in triglyceride, total cholesterol, LDL-cholesterol levels and an increase in HDL-cholesterol levels that were related to the magnitude of the weight loss.

Orlistat

Orlistat is an inhibitor of pancreatic lipase and causes dietary fat, up to one-third, to be lost in the stool [24]. Orlistat is designed for use with a 30% fat diet. It gives approximately 3.2 kg more weight loss than placebo at 6 months and 3.2 kg more weight loss than placebo at 1 year [25]. Adverse events associated with the use of orlistat are an increased incidence of diarrhea, flatulence and dyspepsia. Orlistat gives the expected decrease in blood glucose and blood pressure with weight loss, but gives a reduction in lipids in excess of that expected for the degree of weight loss, probably because it enforces a low-fat diet. Orlistat is recommended at a dose of 120 mg three times per day with meals. An over-the-counter dose of 60 mg three times is now available.

In a one-year study of 391 diabetic subjects taking sulfonylurea medication, the orlistat group lost 6.2 ± 0.45% of initial body weight compared to 4.3 + 0.49% in the placebo group, and diabetic control improved to a greater degree in the orlistat group commensurate with the weight loss [26]. A 4-year trial randomized 3305 subjects, 79% with normal glucose tolerance and 21% with impaired glucose tolerance to orlistat 120 mg three times a day or a placebo. At the end of 4 years, 52% remained in the orlistat group compared to 34% in the placebo group. The orlistat group not only lost more weight, 3.6 kg vs 1.4 kg, but the orlistat group also reduced the conversion to diabetes by one-third, 6.2% in the orlistat group and 9% in the placebo group [27].

Comparing and combining orlistat and sibutramine

Orlistat and sibutramine were compared in a double-blind, randomized clinical trial of 113 subjects over 1 year. Both medications gave significant weight loss but there was no statistically significant difference between them [28]. A similar trial in 144 type 2 diabetic subjects confirmed these results [29].

Since orlistat and sibutramine work by different mechanisms, it is logical to ask whether using them in combination might give additive weight loss. The first trial addressing this question treated subjects with sibutramine for 1 year and added orlistat during weight maintenance. No further weight was lost by the addition of orlistat [30]. Three studies compared sibutamine, orlistat and the combination. The first trial of 80 subjects showed more weight loss in the combination and sibutramine 10 mg/day groups than either the orlistat 120 mg three times a day or the diet alone groups, but the sibutramine group and the combination group did not differ from each other [31]. This finding was confirmed by a second study using a similar design [32]. The third trial compared orlistat 120 mg three times a day to sibutramine 10 mg/day and the combination in 89 obese subjects. The sibutramine and the combination groups lost 10.2% and 10.6% of initial body weight, respectively, which was not different but was greater than the 5.5% weight loss in the orlistat group [33]. A trial in obese type 2 diabetic subjects compared metformin 850 mg twice a day to sibutramine 10 mg twice a day and orlistat 120 mg three times a day. The sibutramine group lost more weight (10.4%) than the orlistat group (6.6%) or the metformin group (8.1%) [34]. In summary, sibutramine appears to give superior weight loss and is better tolerated than orlistat, but orlistat gave the expected decrease in blood pressure not seen with sibutramine.

Rimonabant

Rimonabant is not yet approved for the treatment of obesity in the USA. The mechanism by which rimonabant causes weight loss is thought to be through inhibition of the cannabinoid-1 receptor. There are two cannabinoid receptors, CB-1 (470 amino acids in length) and CB-2 (360 amino acids in length). The CB-1 receptor has almost all the amino acids that comprise the CB-2 receptor and additional amino acids at both ends. CB-1 receptors are distributed throughout the brain in the areas related to feeding, on fat cells, in the gastrointestinal tract and on immune cells. Marijuana and tetrahydrocannabinol stimulate the CB-1 receptor, increase high-fat and high-sweet food intake, and increase fasting levels of endocannabinoids such as anandamide and 2-arachidonyl-glycerol. The rewarding properties of cannabinoid agonists are mediated through the meso-limbic dopaminergic system. Rimonabant, being a specific antagonist of the CB-1 receptor, inhibits sweet food intake in marmosets as well as high-fat food intake in rats, but not food intake in rats fed standard chow. In addition to being specific in inhibiting highly palatable food intake, pair feeding experiments in diet-induced obese rats show that the rimonabant-treated animals lost 21% of their body weight compared to 14% in the pair-fed controls. This suggests, at least in rodents, that rimonabant increases energy expenditure in addition to reducing food intake. CB-1 knockout mice are lean and resistant to diet-induced obesity, but have an accelerated cognitive decline with aging [35]. CB-1 receptors are upregulated on adipocytes in diet-induced obese mice, and rimonabant increases adiponectin, a fat cell hormone associated with insulin sensitivity [36].

The results of three phase III trials of rimonabant for the treatment of obesity have been published. The first trial to be announced was called the Rio-Lipids trial. This was a 1-year trial that randomized 1018 obese subjects equally to placebo, rimonabant 5 mg/day or rimonabant 20 mg/day. The subjects in this trial had untreated dyslipidemia, a BMI between 27 and 40 kg/m^2 and a mean weight of 96 kg. Weight loss was 2% in the placebo group and 8.5% in the 20 mg rimonabant group. In the 20 mg/day rimonabant group, waist circumference was reduced 9 cm, triglycerides were reduced by 15% and HDL-cholesterol was increased by 23%, compared to 3.5 cm, 3% and 12%, respectively, in the placebo group. In the 20 mg/day group, the LDL particle size increased, adiponectin increased, glucose decreased, insulin decreased, C-reactive protein decreased and the metabolic syndrome prevalence was cut in half. Although blood pressure did not increase, the expected improvement with weight loss was not seen. Fifteen percent of subjects in the rimonabant 20 mg/day group dropped from the trial for adverse events. The most common reasons for discontinuation were anxiety, depression and nausea, as one might expect from the location of the CB-1 receptors [37].

In the second 1-year study called Rio-Europe, 305 subjects were randomized to placebo, 603 subjects to rimonabant 5 mg/day and 599 subjects to rimonabant 20 mg/day. Weight loss at 1 year in the placebo group was 1.8 kg compared to 7.2 kg in the 20 mg rimonabant group, and triglycerides, HDL-cholesterol, waist circumference, insulin resistance and the metabolic syndrome all improved [38]. The third study, Rio-North America, was a 2-year study that randomized 3045 obese subjects without diabetes to placebo, 5 mg rimonabant or 20 mg rimonabant. At 1 year, half the rimonabant groups were re-randomized to placebo. At 1 year, only 55% of the rimonabant 20 mg group remained in the trial. Weight loss was 1.6 kg in the placebo group and 6.3 kg in the 20 mg rimonabant group. At 2 years, there was weight regain in those re-randomized to placebo and weight maintenance in those re-randomized to continued rimonabant [39].

DIABETES MEDICATIONS

Although not specifically indicated for obesity, there are a number of diabetes medications which may have a favorable effect on weight which include metformin, pramlintide and exenatide. The specific role of these agents in the treatment of obesity and metabolic syndrome has not been firmly established.

Metformin

Metformin is a biguanide that reduces hepatic glucose production, decreases intestinal glucose absorption and enhances insulin sensitivity. In clinical trials where metformin was compared with sulfonylureas, it produced weight loss [40]. In one French trial, BIGPRO, metformin was compared to placebo in a 1-year multicenter study of 324 middle-aged subjects with upper body obesity and the insulin resistance syndrome (metabolic syndrome). Subjects on metformin lost significantly more weight (1–2 kg) than the placebo group, and the study concluded that metformin may have a role in the primary prevention of type 2 diabetes [41].

The best trial of metformin, however, is the Diabetes Prevention Program enrolling individuals with impaired glucose tolerance. Subjects were over 25 years of age and overweight with impaired glucose tolerance. They were randomized to lifestyle change ($n = 1079$), metformin ($n = 1073$) or usual care ($n = 1082$). At the end of 2.8 years, on average, the trial was terminated because lifestyle change and metformin were clearly superior to usual care. During this time, the metformin-treated group lost 2.5% of their body weight ($P < 0.001$ compared to usual care), and the conversion to diabetes was reduced by 31% compared to placebo. Metformin was most effective in reducing conversion to diabetes in those who were younger and more overweight [10]. Although metformin does not produce enough weight loss (5%) to qualify as a 'weight-loss drug' using the Food and Drug Administration (FDA) criteria, it would appear to be a very useful choice for overweight individuals with diabetes or those at high risk for diabetes.

Pramlintide

Amylin is secreted from the β cell along with insulin, and amylin is deficient in type 1 diabetes where β cells are immunologically destroyed. Pramlintide, a synthetic amylin analog, is approved by the FDA for the treatment of diabetes. Unlike insulin, pramlintide is associated with weight loss. Maggs and colleagues analyzed the data from two 1-year studies in insulin-treated type 2 diabetic subjects randomized to pramlintide 120 μg twice a day or 150 μg three times a day [42]. Weight decreased by 2.6 kg and hemoglobin A1c (HbA1c) decreased 0.5%. When weight loss was analyzed by ethnic group, African-Americans lost 4 kg, Caucasians lost 2.4 kg, Hispanics lost 2.3 kg, and the improvement in diabetes correlated with the weight loss, suggesting that pramlintide is more effective in an ethnic group with the greatest obesity burden. The most common adverse event was nausea, which was usually mild and confined to the first 4 weeks of therapy. Thus, pramlintide should be considered in insulin-treated patients with obesity and type 2 diabetes.

Exenatide

Exendin-4 (exenatide) is a 39 amino acid peptide that is produced in the salivary gland of the Gila monster lizard and has been approved for the treatment of type 2 diabetes. It has 53% homology with GLP-1 but has a much longer half-life. Exenatide decreases food intake and body weight gain in Zucker rats while lowering HbA1c [43]. Exenatide increases β-cell mass to a greater extent than would be expected for the degree of insulin resistance [44]. Exenatide induces satiety and weight loss in Zucker rats with peripheral administration and crosses the blood–brain barrier to act in the central nervous system [45, 46]. In humans, exenatide reduces fasting and post-prandial glucose levels, slows gastric emptying and decreases food intake by 19%. The side-effects of exenatide in humans are headache, nausea and vomiting that are lessened by gradual dose escalation [47]. Exenatide at 10 μg subcutaneously per day or a placebo was given to 377 type 2 diabetic subjects for 30 weeks who were failing maximal sulfonylurea therapy. The HbA1c fell 0.74% more than placebo, fasting glucose decreased and there was a progressive weight loss of 1.6 kg [48]. In ongoing open-label clinical trials, the weight loss at 18 months is –4.5 kg without using behavior therapy or diet.

Acarbose

Acarbose, an alpha glucosidase inhibitor that is approved for the treatment of diabetes, has been evaluated for weight loss in a 9-month trial randomizing 354 obese type 2 diabetic subjects to acarbose or placebo. The placebo group gained 0.3 kg while the acarbose group lost 0.5 kg [49]. Although this is a small weight loss, it was statistically significant, and even a lack of weight gain can be a victory in treating the obese type 2 diabetic individual.

OBESITY SURGERY

As reviewed earlier in this chapter, behavior modification gives an approximate 10% weight loss, and obesity drugs give about the same. Medical weight loss programs rarely last more than 2 years and weight maintenance has been disappointing. The prevalence of class III obesity, a BMI >40 kg/m^2 and the degree of obesity that would qualify for obesity surgery, increased from 0.5% in 1995 to 7.5% in 2002 in African-American women alone [50]. Individuals with class III obesity cannot, with rare exceptions, lose and keep off the weight needed to achieve a healthy body weight with medical interventions. It is in that context that those with class III obesity are turning in greater numbers to obesity surgery.

Surgical procedures have evolved since the 1950s when the first operative attempts to treat obesity were made. The present surgical procedures in common use can be divided into those that restrict the stomach, represented most commonly by the lap-band, and those that both restrict the stomach and have a malabsorptive component, represented most commonly by the gastric bypass. Although there are other restrictive procedures such as vertical gastric banding and other restrictive-malabsorptive procedures such as biliopancreatic bypass with and without a duodenal switch, one can generalize the discussion to these two classes of surgical procedures.

Restrictive procedures

The lap-band, a restrictive procedure, is the preferred operation in most of Europe due to its minimal distortion of the normal gastrointestinal anatomy and its ease of reversal. Despite these advantages, the weight loss with this procedure is less (20–25% vs 30–35% of initial body weight) and the need for surgical revision is higher (10% vs 5%) than restrictive-malabsorptive procedures like the gastric bypass [51]. The improvement in diabetes and other obesity-associated diseases following restrictive procedures is proportional to the weight loss. The Swedish Obese Study consisted mostly of restrictive procedures. Weight loss in the lap-band group was 20–25% at 1 year post-operatively but only 10–15% at 10 years. Only 9 (47%) of the 19 subjects with diabetes had resolution of their diabetes following the lap-band placement. The incidence of developing diabetes at 10 years was 7% in the surgical group and 24% in the medically treated control group [52]. These incidence rate reductions appear to be related to the weight loss in contradistinction to the restrictive-malabsorbtive procedures where the reduction in diabetes is greater than can be attributed to weight loss alone [53].

Restrictive-malabsorptive procedures

Surgeries in this group cause food to bypass the upper gastrointestinal tract reaching the distal small intestine earlier and in a less digested state. This causes a decrease of hormones from the upper gastrointestinal tract like ghrelin, a hormone that initiates meals. This decrease in upper gastrointestinal hormones is not associated with medical weight loss [54]. Hormones like PYY-3-36 from the distal gut are increased after gastric bypass, and PYY-3-36 has been shown to decrease food intake by 30–35% after intravenous infusion [55, 56]. Thus, PYY-3-36 may be partly responsible for the more efficient weight loss seen after bypass operations compared to purely restrictive procedures. Glucagon-like peptide-1, another distal gut hormone that increases after gastric bypass, along with a decreased food intake, may be partly responsible for the enhanced effect that bypass operations have on reducing the prevalence of diabetes [57]. GLP-1 inhibits pancreatic glucagon secretion, a hormone that increases glucose levels in the blood, and GLP-1 also stimulates insulin secretion, a hormone that lowers blood glucose [58]. GLP-1 only stimulates insulin secretion at high glucose levels, so it is not associated with hypoglycemia, and GLP-1 is known to increase β-cell mass [59]. Exenitide stimulates the GLP-1 receptor and is a treatment for diabetes that causes weight loss as described earlier in this chapter.

Possibly due, in part, to the effects of gastric bypass on gut hormones, the gastric bypass is much more efficient in reversing diabetes. Pories and colleagues, and Hickey and his co-workers reported a 14-year experience of the gastric bypass with an extraordinary 97%

follow-up in which 121 (82.9%) of the 146 patients with type 2 diabetes and 150 (99%) of the 152 patients with IGT returned to euglycemia with complete normalization of their glucose metabolism [60, 61]. In a comparison study of morbidly obese patients undergoing gastric bypass and morbidly obese controls, Long and colleagues showed the gastric bypass imparted a greater than 30-fold decrease in the risk of developing type 2 diabetes after weight loss [62].

SUMMARY

Treatment of metabolic syndrome will involve treatment of multiple risk factors and includes addressing the associated obesity. Lifestyle modification is the cornerstone of treatment, but is difficult to sustain over time and physicians are not prepared or generally interested in administering the essential lifestyle program. Pharmaceutical treatment, combined with lifestyle, may result in a 5–10% weight loss that is clinically significant. More aggressive therapy will involve surgery. The surgical treatment of obesity is complex and requires interaction with dietitians and other healthcare professionals in addition to the surgeon. Thus, the optimal treatment of obesity is a team discipline, whether the treatment is surgical or medical.

REFERENCES

1. Bouchard C. Genetics and the metabolic syndrome. *Int J Obes Relat Metab Disord* 1995; 19(suppl 1): S52–S59.
2. Liese AD, Mayer-Davis EJ, Haffner SM. Development of the multiple metabolic syndrome: an epidemiologic perspective. *Epidemiol Rev* 1998; 20:157–172.
3. Klein S, Wadden T, Sugerman HJ. AGA technical review on obesity. *Gastroenterology* 2002; 123:882–932.
4. Troiano RP, Frongillo EA, Jr, Sobal J, Levitsky DA. The relationship between body weight and mortality: a quantitative analysis of combined information from existing studies. *Int J Obes Relat Metab Disord* 1996; 20:63–75.
5. Calle EE, Thun MJ, Petrelli JM, Rodriguez C, Heath CW, Jr. Body-mass index and mortality in a prospective cohort of U.S. adults. *N Engl J Med* 1999; 341:1097–1105.
6. Flegal KM, Carroll MD, Kuczmarski RJ, Johnson CL. Overweight and obesity in the United States: prevalence and trends, 1960–1994. *Int J Obes Relat Metab Disord* 1998; 22:39–47.
7. Kershaw EE, Flier JS. Adipose tissue as an endocrine organ. *J Clin Endocrinol Metab* 2004; 89:2548–2556.
8. Wadden TA, Butryn ML, Byrne KJ. Efficacy of lifestyle modification for long-term weight control. *Obes Res* 2004; 12(suppl):151S–162S.
9. Blackburn G. Effect of degree of weight loss on health benefits. *Obes Res* 1995; 2(suppl 3):211s–216s.
10. Knowler WC, Barrett-Connor E, Fowler SE *et al.* Reduction in the incidence of type 2 diabetes with lifestyle intervention or metformin. *N Engl J Med* 2002; 346:393–403.
11. Ditschuneit HH, Flechtner-Mors M, Johnson TD, Adler G. Metabolic and weight-loss effects of a long-term dietary intervention in obese patients. *Am J Clin Nutr* 1999; 69:198–204.
12. Heshka S, Greenway F, Anderson JW *et al.* Self-help weight loss versus a structured commercial program after 26 weeks: a randomized controlled study. *Am J Med* 2000; 109:282–287.
13. Heshka S, Anderson JW, Atkinson RL *et al.* Weight loss with self-help compared with a structured commercial program: a randomized trial. *JAMA* 2003; 289:1792–1798.
14. Tsai AG, Wadden TA. Systematic review: an evaluation of major commercial weight loss programs in the United States. *Ann Intern Med* 2005; 142:56–66.
15. Finley CE, Barlow CE, Greenway FL, Rock CL, Rolls BJ, Blair SN. Retention rates and weight loss in a commercial weight loss program. *Int J Obes* 2007; 31:292–298.
16. Rock CL, Pakiz B, Flatt SW, Quintane EL. Randomized trial of a multifaceted commercial weight loss program. *Obesity* 2007; 15:939–949.
17. NIH Consensus Development Conference Statement. Health implications of obesity. *Ann Intern Med* 1985; 103:1973–1977.
18. Munro JF, MacCuish AC, Wilson EM, Duncan LJ. Comparison of continuous and intermittent anorectic therapy in obesity. *Br Med J* 1968; 1:352–354.

19. Glazer G. Long-term pharmacotherapy of obesity 2000: a review of efficacy and safety. *Arch Intern Med* 2001; 161:1814–1824.
20. Arterburn DE, Crane PK, Veenstra DL. The efficacy and safety of sibutramine for weight loss: a systematic review. *Arch Intern Med* 2004; 164:994–1003.
21. Bray GA, Blackburn GL, Ferguson JM *et al.* Sibutramine produces dose-related weight loss. *Obes Res* 1999; 7:189–198.
22. Apfelbaum M, Vague P, Ziegler O, Hanotin C, Thomas F, Leutenegger E. Long-term maintenance of weight loss after a very-low-calorie diet: a randomized blinded trial of the efficacy and tolerability of sibutramine. *Am J Med* 1999; 106:179–184.
23. James WP, Astrup A, Finer N *et al.* Effect of sibutramine on weight maintenance after weight loss: a randomised trial. STORM Study Group. Sibutramine Trial of Obesity Reduction and Maintenance. *Lancet* 2000; 356:2119–2125.
24. Zhi J, Melia AT, Guerciolini R *et al.* Retrospective population-based analysis of the dose-response (fecal fat excretion) relationship of orlistat in normal and obese volunteers. *Clin Pharmacol Ther* 1994; 56:82–85.
25. O'Meara S, Riemsma R, Shirran L, Mather L, ter Riet G. A systematic review of the clinical effectiveness of orlistat used for the management of obesity. *Obes Rev* 2004; 5:51–68.
26. Hollander PA, Elbein SC, Hirsch IB *et al.* Role of orlistat in the treatment of obese patients with type 2 diabetes. A 1-year randomized double-blind study. *Diabetes Care* 1998; 21:1288–1294.
27. Torgerson JS, Hauptman J, Boldrin MN, Sjostrom L. XENical in the prevention of diabetes in obese subjects (XENDOS) study: a randomized study of orlistat as an adjunct to lifestyle changes for the prevention of type 2 diabetes in obese patients. *Diabetes Care* 2004; 27:155–161.
28. Derosa G, Cicero AF, Murdolo G *et al.* Efficacy and safety comparative evaluation of orlistat and sibutramine treatment in hypertensive obese patients. *Diabetes Obes Metab* 2005; 7:47–55.
29. Derosa G, Cicero AF, Murdolo G, Ciccarelli L, Fogari R. Comparison of metabolic effects of orlistat and sibutramine treatment in Type 2 diabetic obese patients. *Diabetes Nutr Metab* 2004; 17:222–229.
30. Wadden TA, Berkowitz RI, Womble LG, Sarwer DB, Arnold ME, Steinberg CM. Effects of sibutramine plus orlistat in obese women following 1 year of treatment by sibutramine alone: a placebo-controlled trial. *Obes Res* 2000; 8:431–437.
31. Aydin N, Topsever P, Kaya A, Karasakal M, Duman C, Dagar A. Orlistat, sibutramine, or combination therapy: which performs better on waist circumference in relation with body mass index in obese patients? *Tohoku J Exp Med* 2004; 202:173–180.
32. Kaya A, Aydin N, Topsever P *et al.* Efficacy of sibutramine, orlistat and combination therapy on short-term weight management in obese patients. *Biomed Pharmacother* 2004; 58:582–587.
33. Sari R, Balci MK, Cakir M, Altunbas H, Karayalcin U. Comparison of efficacy of sibutramine or orlistat versus their combination in obese women. *Endocr Res* 2004; 30:159–167.
34. Gokcel A, Gumurdulu Y, Karakose H *et al.* Evaluation of the safety and efficacy of sibutramine, orlistat and metformin in the treatment of obesity. *Diabetes Obes Metab* 2002; 4:49–55.
35. Bilkei-Gorzo A, Racz I, Valverde O *et al.* Early age-related cognitive impairment in mice lacking cannabinoid CB1 receptors. *Proc Natl Acad Sci USA* 2005; 102:15670–15675.
36. Bensaid M, Gary-Bobo M, Esclangon A *et al.* The cannabinoid CB1 receptor antagonist SR141716 increases Acrp30 mRNA expression in adipose tissue of obese fa/fa rats and in cultured adipocyte cells. *Mol Pharmacol* 2003; 63:908–914.
37. Despres JP, Golay A, Sjostrom L. Effects of rimonabant on metabolic risk factors in overweight patients with dyslipidemia. *N Engl J Med* 2005; 353:2121–2134.
38. Van Gaal LF, Rissanen AM, Scheen AJ, Ziegler O, Rossner S. Effects of the cannabinoid-1 receptor blocker rimonabant on weight reduction and cardiovascular risk factors in overweight patients: 1-year experience from the RIO-Europe study. *Lancet* 2005; 365:1389–1397.
39. Pi-Sunyer FX, Aronne LJ, Heshmati HM, Devin J, Rosenstock J. Effect of rimonabant, a cannabinoid-1 receptor blocker, on weight and cardiometabolic risk factors in overweight or obese patients: RIO-North America: a randomized controlled trial. *JAMA* 2006; 295:761–775.
40. Bray GA, Greenway FL. Current and potential drugs for treatment of obesity. *Endocr Rev* 1999; 20:805–875.
41. Fontbonne A, Charles MA, Juhan-Vague I *et al.* The effect of metformin on the metabolic abnormalities associated with upper-body fat distribution. BIGPRO Study Group. *Diabetes Care* 1996; 19:920–926.
42. Maggs D, Shen L, Strobel S, Brown D, Kolterman O, Weyer C. Effect of pramlintide on A1C and body weight in insulin-treated African Americans and Hispanics with type 2 diabetes: a pooled post hoc analysis. *Metabolism* 2003; 52:1638–1642.

43. Szayna M, Doyle ME, Betkey JA *et al.* Exendin-4 decelerates food intake, weight gain, and fat deposition in Zucker rats. *Endocrinology* 2000; 141:1936–1941.
44. Gedulin BR, Nikoulina SE, Smith PA *et al.* Exenatide (exendin-4) improves insulin sensitivity and beta-cell mass in insulin-resistant obese fa/fa Zucker rats independent of glycemia and body weight. *Endocrinology* 2005; 146:2069–2076.
45. Rodriquez de Fonseca F, Navarro M, Alvarez E *et al.* Peripheral versus central effects of glucagon-like peptide-1 receptor agonists on satiety and body weight loss in Zucker obese rats. *Metabolism* 2000; 49:709–717.
46. Kastin AJ, Akerstrom V. Entry of exendin-4 into brain is rapid but may be limited at high doses. *Int J Obes Relat Metab Disord* 2003; 27:313–318.
47. Fineman MS, Shen LZ, Taylor K, Kim DD, Baron AD. Effectiveness of progressive dose-escalation of exenatide (exendin-4) in reducing dose-limiting side effects in subjects with type 2 diabetes. *Diabetes Metab Res Rev* 2004; 20:411–417.
48. Buse JB, Henry RR, Han J, Kim DD, Fineman MS, Baron AD. Effects of exenatide (exendin-4) on glycemic control over 30 weeks in sulfonylurea-treated patients with type 2 diabetes. *Diabetes Care* 2004; 27:2628–2635.
49. Wolever TM, Chiasson JL, Josse RG *et al.* Small weight loss on long-term acarbose therapy with no change in dietary pattern or nutrient intake of individuals with non-insulin-dependent diabetes. *Int J Obes Relat Metab Disord* 1997; 21:756–763.
50. Roberts A, King J, Greenway F. Class III obesity continues to rise in African-American women. *Obes Surg* 2004; 14:533–535.
51. Greenway FL. Surgery for obesity. *Endocrinol Metab Clin North Am* 1996; 25:1005–1027.
52. Sjostrom L, Lindroos AK, Peltonen M *et al.* Lifestyle, diabetes, and cardiovascular risk factors 10 years after bariatric surgery. *N Engl J Med* 2004; 351:2683–2693.
53. Greenway SE, Greenway FL, 3rd, Klein S. Effects of obesity surgery on non-insulin-dependent diabetes mellitus. *Arch Surg* 2002; 137:1109–1117.
54. Cummings DE, Weigle DS, Frayo RS *et al.* Plasma ghrelin levels after diet-induced weight loss or gastric bypass surgery. *N Engl J Med* 2002; 346:1623–1630.
55. Korner J, Bessler M, Cirilo LJ *et al.* Effects of Roux-en-Y gastric bypass surgery on fasting and postprandial concentrations of plasma ghrelin, peptide YY, and insulin. *J Clin Endocrinol Metab* 2005; 90:359–365.
56. Batterham RL, Cohen MA, Ellis SM *et al.* Inhibition of food intake in obese subjects by peptide YY3-36. *N Engl J Med* 2003; 349:941–948.
57. le Roux CW, Aylwin SJ, Batterham RL *et al.* Gut hormone profiles following bariatric surgery favor an anorectic state, facilitate weight loss, and improve metabolic parameters. *Ann Surg* 2006; 243:108–114.
58. Mason EE. Ileal [correction of ilial] transposition and enteroglucagon/GLP-1 in obesity (and diabetic?) surgery. *Obes Surg* 1999; 9:223–228.
59. Gallwitz B. Glucagon-like peptide-1-based therapies for the treatment of type 2 diabetes mellitus. *Treat Endocrinol* 2005; 4:361–370.
60. Pories WJ, Swanson MS, MacDonald KG *et al.* Who would have thought it? An operation proves to be the most effective therapy for adult-onset diabetes mellitus. *Ann Surg* 1995; 222:339–350; discussion 350–352.
61. Hickey MS, Pories WJ, MacDonald KG, Jr. *et al.* A new paradigm for type 2 diabetes mellitus: could it be a disease of the foregut? *Ann Surg* 1998; 227:637–643; discussion 643–644.
62. Long SD, O'Brien K, MacDonald KG, Jr. *et al.* Weight loss in severely obese subjects prevents the progression of impaired glucose tolerance to type II diabetes. A longitudinal interventional study. *Diabetes Care* 1994; 17:372–375.

6

Blockage of the renin–angiotensin system in metabolic syndrome: implications for the prevention of diabetes

K. Vijayaraghavan, P. C. Deedwania

INTRODUCTION

The epidemics of obesity, metabolic syndrome and increasing age are playing an important role in the increased prevalence of diabetes. In addition, the changes in diagnostic criteria have allowed us to predict the exponential rise from 171 million subjects in year 2000 to a staggering 366 million by year 2030 [1, 2]. The prevalence of diabetes has increased by 61% from 1990 to 2001 with type 2 diabetes mellitus (T2DM) accounting for 95% of this increase [3]. The annual cost of the disease is estimated at $132 billion, accounting for more than 10% of US healthcare expenditure. Moreover, the lifetime risk for developing diabetes among Americans born in year 2000 is 32.8% for men and 38.5% for women [4]. The increase in prevalence of T2DM is paralleled by the rising rate of obesity and metabolic syndrome (MS). As body mass index (BMI) increases, the risk of developing type 2 diabetes increases in a dose-dependent manner [5, 6]. The prevalence of T2DM is 3–7 times higher in obese subjects and 20 times higher if BMI $>35\,kg/m^2$ than those with a BMI between 18.5 and $24.9\,kg/m^2$. This, however, may be different in other ethnic groups [7–9]. Obesity is a component of metabolic syndrome. According to the National Cholesterol Education Program Adult Treatment Panel (NECP ATP III), MS is defined by objective clinical criteria [10]. Any three of the components of risk factors will qualify as MS. Clustering of risk factors associated with this syndrome predicts development of manifest diabetes and cardiovascular disease (CVD). Other risk factors for T2DM include age ≥45 years, family history of diabetes (parent or siblings), physical inactivity, race (ethnicity such as Afro-American, Hispanic, Native American, Asian-American, and Pacific Islanders), impaired glucose tolerance (IGT), history of gestational diabetes or delivery of a baby weighing >9 lbs, hypertension (blood pressure [BP] ≥140/90 mmHg in adults), high-density lipoprotein (HDL)-cholesterol <35 mg/dl and triglyceride >250 mg/dl, polycystic ovary syndrome and history of vascular disease [10]. The increased prevalence along with the complications of micro- and macrovascular disease will impose a significant public health and economic burden. Even though a number of efficacious treatments are available, suboptimal applications of these in clinical practice has led

Krishnaswami Vijayaraghavan, MD, FACP, FACC, Director of Cardiovascular Research, Scottsdale Healthcare, Scottsdale, Arizona; Consultant Cardiologist, Scottsdale Cardiovascular Center; Clinical Professor of Medicine, Midwestern University School of Medicine, Glendale, Arizona, USA

Prakash C. Deedwania, MD, FACC, FAHA, Chief, Cardiology Division, Veterans Administration Central California Health Care System, Fresno; Professor of Medicine, UCSF School of Medicine, San Francisco, California, USA

to gaps in diabetes prevention and management. Impediments include paucity of healthcare provider and patient education of outcomes from clinical trials, inadequate comprehension of the gravity of the disease, little motivation towards prevention of diabetes and its complications, insufficient time and lack of socioeconomic resources and support [6, 11]. Hence, there is an urgent need to prevent the onset of diabetes in the high-risk population and prevention of T2DM should aim to treat and prevent components of MS. This review addresses the role of the renin–angiotensin–aldosterone system (RAAS) activation, evidence of prevention of diabetes through pharmacological interventions specifically targeting the RAAS from recent clinical studies, the potential mechanisms of RAAS inhibition and future directions that may reduce the overall public health and economic burden.

MS AND ITS EFFECTS

MS carries with it the underlying pathophysiologic feature of insulin resistance with tissue resistance to insulin action, compensatory hyperinsulinemia and excessive circulating free fatty acids [12–14]. In addition, cardiovascular risk factors of low HDL, high triglycerides, hypertension and lack of physical activity have all been shown to be predictors of non-insulin dependent diabetes [15]. The relationships between MS and cardiovascular mortality as well as chronic complication of T2DM have been well described [16, 17]. Several studies have shown impaired glucose tolerance to be a predictor of progression to T2DM [18–21]. It follows, then, that aggressive intervention in subjects with IGT or MS would translate to diabetes prevention.

PREVENTION OF DIABETES BY LIFESTYLE MODIFICATIONS

Multiple clinical trials have been performed that tested lifestyle modification to prevent T2DM. The inclusion criteria for all trials were IGT based on two blood glucose measurements, a fasting value of <126 mg/dl and a glucose value of 140–200 mg/dl 2 h after 75 g consumption of glucose. In the United Kingdom, Jarrett and colleagues in the 'Borderline Diabetes' study [22], and Keen *et al.* in the Bedford Survey [23] found no effect of diet or oral modification on preventing diabetes. However, the Swedish study found that diabetes counseling and tolbutamide reduced incidence of diabetes, albeit, intention to treat analysis was not performed [24]. More recently, three studies of primary prevention that utilized lifestyle intervention have shown significant results. The Finnish Diabetes Prevention Study, the Da Qing IGT and Diabetes study and the Diabetes Prevention Program (DPP) revealed that aggressive dietary intervention and exercise program reduced the incidence of diabetes by 58%, 42% and 58% respectively compared to controls [25–28]. In addition to the Da Qing study, Finnish Diabetes Prevention Study and DPP, there have been several smaller studies reflecting the benefit of lifestyle modifications [29–32]. However, a weight loss program, dietary modification and aggressive exercise regimen are fraught with challenges [33–35]. As urbanization becomes more and more widespread, exercise as a modality for losing weight will become increasingly difficult and possibly destined to failure. A group of Hawaiians, who were obese, changed their diet to *ad libitum* feeding of their traditional diet, which provided only 7% of energy as fat. They lost 7.8 kg in 3 weeks [36]. This was accomplished without increasing exercise activity, questioning the validity and need for exercise. Lack of motivation, transient loss of weight with rebound increase, socioeconomic status and different priorities in life with multiple other stressful issues taking precedence over preventing diabetes in the long run are all factors that impede the success of such programs. Many studies have assessed delivery of multifaceted, system-oriented and integrated approaches aimed at primary prevention of T2DM. Unfortunately, the long-term success of these programs has been disappointing. Suboptimal reductions in cardiovascular (CV) risk were noticed without any overall reduction in mortality [29, 37–38]. Weight loss itself is difficult to accomplish and maintain and one cannot assume that such strategies are inexpensive. Analysis from the DPP showed that in clinical practice, cost per case of diabetes delayed or

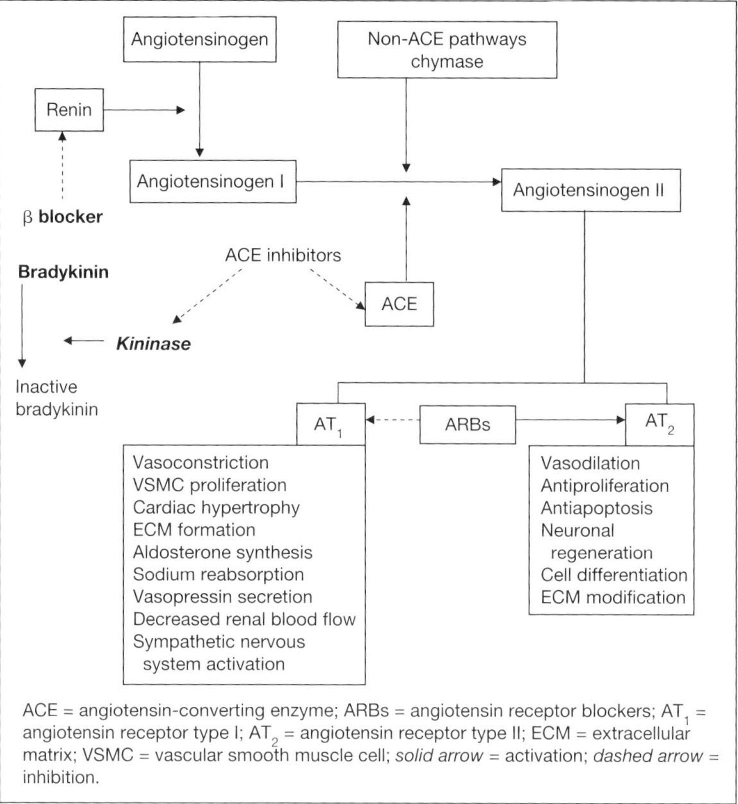

Figure 6.1 RAAS pathway.

prevented was similar for metformin ($14 300) and lifestyle interventions ($13 200) [39]. Pharmacologic interventions that may delay the onset of diabetes should be taken into account concurrently in the context of lifestyle modifications. Hence, it is imperative for us to consider all means available for preventing development of diabetes including pharmacological interventions such as RAAS inhibition.

ROLE OF RAAS ACTIVATION

Angiotensin II (Ang II) formation occurs from the substrate angiotensinogen through a series of steps. Renin catalyzes the conversion of angiotensinogen to angiotensin I which is subsequently hydrolyzed by angiotensin-converting enzymes (ACE) to form Ang II. Alternate pathways exist that convert angiotensinogen directly to Ang II, such as tissue plasminogen activator, cathepsin G and tonin; whereas angiotensin I is also catalyzed to Ang II by chymase and cathepsin G [40, 41]. Ang II mediates deleterious effects by binding specific receptors located on the cell membrane. Ang II receptor type I mediates the biological activities that are harmful to the tissues. Ang II receptor type II expression is less well studied, but appears to mediate beneficial effects that include vasodilation, inhibition of cell growth and proliferation as well as cell differentiation [42, 43]. The differential effects are shown in Figure 6.1. The sequential progression of CV disease begins with the risk factors of hypertension, diabetes, smoking, MS and dyslipidemia. These risk factors are independently

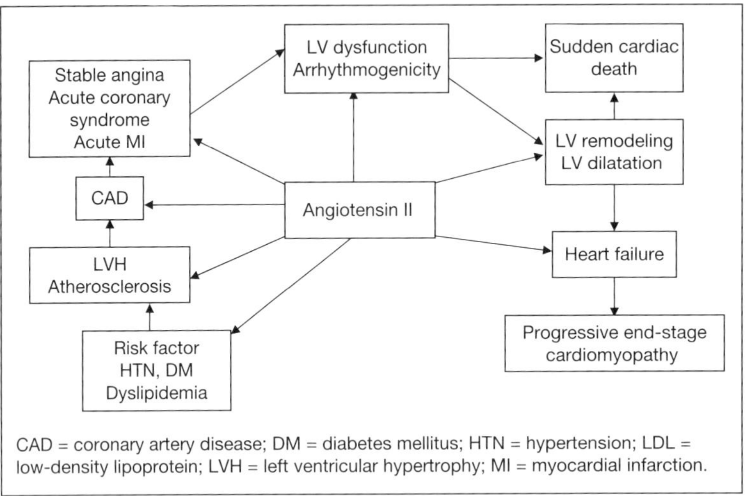

CAD = coronary artery disease; DM = diabetes mellitus; HTN = hypertension; LDL = low-density lipoprotein; LVH = left ventricular hypertrophy; MI = myocardial infarction.

Figure 6.2 Ang II and the sequential progression of CV disease.

associated with levels of Ang II, which in turn triggers the cascade of events. Progression to atherosclerotic disease and left ventricular hypertrophy leads to plaque destabilization in the face of uncontrolled risk factors with acute coronary syndrome and myocardial infarction as the sequelae [44]. Loss of cardiac muscle, while potentially increasing sudden cardiac death, will eventually lead to remodeling of left ventricle progressing relentlessly to heart failure and end-stage cardiomyopathy (Figure 6.2).

RAAS AND VASCULAR ENDOTHELIAL FUNCTION

Endothelium has five functions. First, it acts as a permeability barrier blocking exocytosis of macrophage and small dense low-density lipoproteins (LDL) entering the subendothelial layer to initiate genesis of the fatty streak, an initial step in atheroformation. Second, it plays an important role in maintaining vascular tone by releasing Ang II and endothelin, powerful vasoconstrictors, and balancing it by release of nitric oxide for vasodilator effect. Third, it balances hemostasis by mediating coagulation by inhibiting platelet aggregation and expressing adhesion molecules as well as by releasing von Willebrand factor, tissue plasminogen activator and plasminogen-activator inhibitor type 1 (PAI-1), all of which maintains a balance between bleeding and clotting. Fourth, it releases inflammatory cytokines such as IL-6, tumor necrosis factor alpha (TNF-α) and others that are involved in compensatory mechanisms in atherogenesis. Finally, it acts as a transducer of biomechanical forces and prevents sheer stress from denudation of the endothelial layer to allow plaque accumulation [45, 46] (Figure 6.3). Ang II contributes to endothelial dysfunction by increasing oxidative stress, attenuating chemoattractants, and adhesion molecule expression leading to inflammation [47]. In addition, Ang II can also exert proliferative and prothrombotic actions, produce superoxide radicals scavenging nitric oxide and reduce vasodilation [48]. There is evidence that an increased expression of ACE is present in endothelial growth arrest. ACE is induced by glucocorticoids in vascular smooth muscle [49] while activation of ACE induces PAI-1 levels, which are contributors to atherothrombosis [50]. Bradykinin, which is unopposed with blockade of ACE, has significant beneficial effects on endothelium, primarily due to its powerful vasodilating properties [51, 52]. Thus, there is evidence that Ang II accumulation impairs endothelial function and enhances atherogenic process.

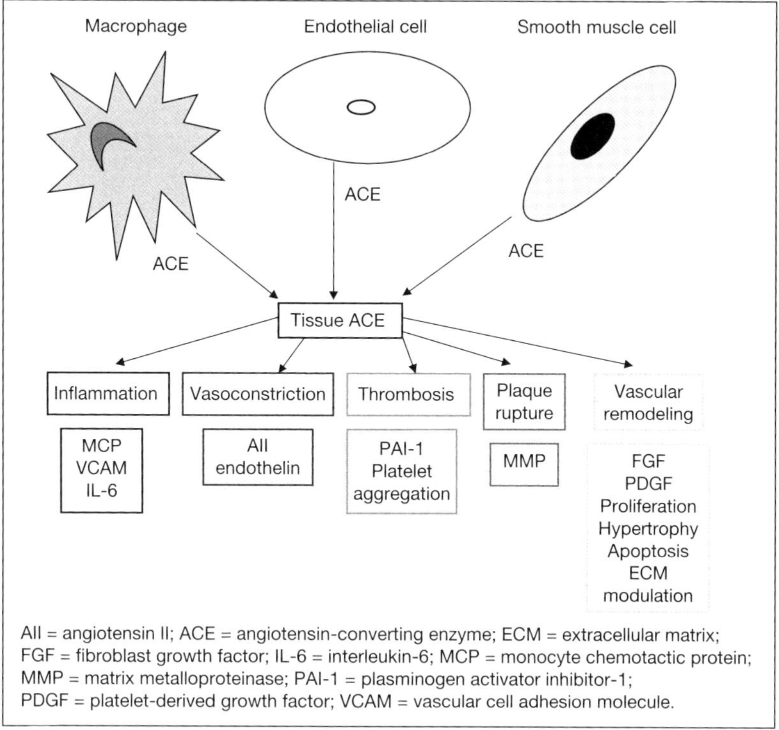

Figure 6.3 Role of ACE in vascular function.

CROSSTALK BETWEEN ANGIOTENSIN, ENDOTHELIUM, AND INSULIN RESISTANCE

Insulin resistance is associated with MS, which in turn increases risk of adverse cardiovascular outcomes. There is definitive evidence of a parallel progression between insulin resistance and endothelial dysfunction. As insulin resistance progresses to clinical MS, IGT and development of diabetes, there is a parallel track that leads from endothelial dysfunction to inflammation, thrombosis and oxidation to overt atherosclerotic disease. Insulin resistance has been shown to interact with this parallel track of endothelial dysfunction by accumulation of free fatty acids, pro-inflammatory adipokines and TNF-α [53]. In addition, increased oxidative stress and oxidized LDL with reduction of HDL, development of hypertension, hyperuricemia and hyperglycemia contribute to the underlying mechanisms of endothelial dysfunction in insulin resistance [45].

As Ang II plays a significant role in endothelial dysfunction, interplay of Ang II in glucose homeostasis has been of significant interest to biochemical and molecular biologists. The relationship between Ang II and insulin signaling pathways is becoming evident in preclinical studies. Insulin binds to the cell surface receptor, tyrosine kinase, which leads to autophosphorylation of tyrosine residue turning on the insulin signaling pathways. The initial step is activation of the phosphotidyl inositol kinase pathway (PI-3K), which is important for glucose transport in skeletal muscle. In addition, this pathway enhances nitric oxide production and insulin-induced vasodilatory response [54, 55]. The second pathway that is activated is the mitogen activated protein kinase (MAPK). This pathway promotes vascular smooth muscle cell proliferation and migration induced by insulin, thrombin and

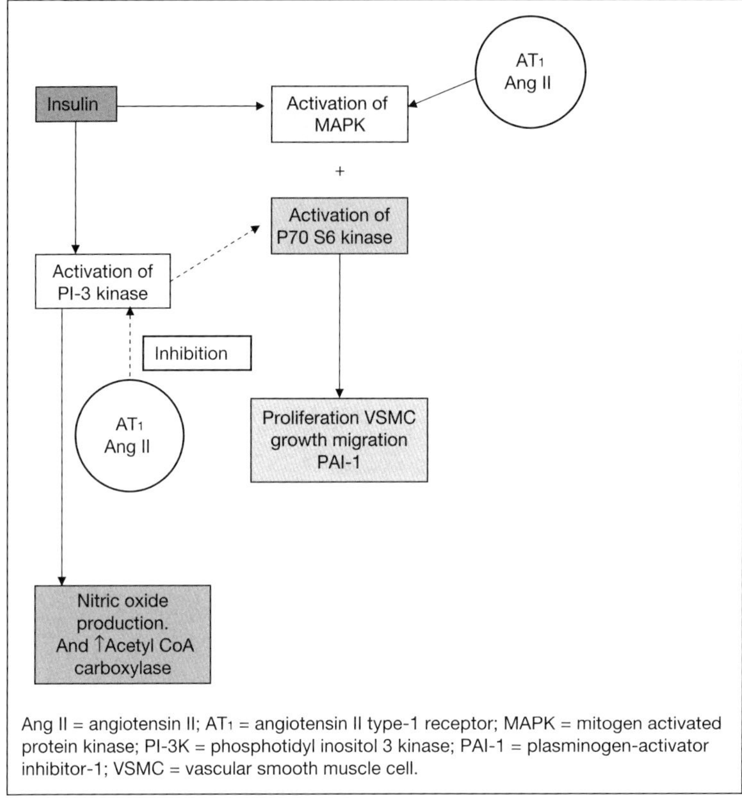

Ang II = angiotensin II; AT1 = angiotensin II type-1 receptor; MAPK = mitogen activated protein kinase; PI-3K = phosphotidyl inositol 3 kinase; PAI-1 = plasminogen-activator inhibitor-1; VSMC = vascular smooth muscle cell.

Figure 6.4 Ang II, insulin signaling and crosstalk.

platelet- derived growth factors (Figure 6.4). In addition, a third pathway is triggered that leads to activation of P70 S6 kinase, a regulator of protein synthesis [56–58].

Ang II plays an important role in signaling pathways for maintaining structure and function of the heart. Angiotension II type-1 (AT_1) stimulation results in activation of the MAPK, PI-3K and tyrosine phosphorylation both *in vivo* and *in vitro*. In the heart, Ang II blocks the insulin-induced PI-3K but stimulates MAPK, thus inhibiting the metabolic effects of insulin, but not the proliferative ones [59]. This crosstalk between the two signaling pathways may play a pivotal role in understanding how cardiovascular and neuroendocrine physiologies relate to each other and thus explain the role of Ang II blockade in insulin resistance and prevention of diabetes.

RAAS AS A THERAPEUTIC TARGET

ACE inhibitors were initially developed in the late 1970s for treatment of hypertension. Their utilization has since been expanded to heart failure, post-myocardial infarction (MI) and renal disease. ACE inhibitors, by blocking the conversion of angiotensin I to Ang II, as well as by catalyzing the breakdown of bradykinin, exert numerous beneficial effects that maintain blood pressure, and salt and water homeostasis. In addition, salutary effects are seen with ACE inhibitors due to its vasodilating, anti-inflammatory, plaque stabilizing, antithrombotic and antiproliferative properties. Numerous studies in literature have demonstrated a significant benefit with use of ACE inhibition. Enalapril in CONSENSUS, SOLVD treatment

Table 6.1 ACE inhibitor clinical trials summary

Trial	*ACE inhibitor*	*Patient group*	*Outcome*
CONSENSUS (*n* = 253)	Enalapril vs placebo	NYHA IV, CHF	↓ Overall mortality
SOLVD, treatment arm (*n* = 2569)	Enalapril vs placebo	NYHA II & III, CHF	↓ Overall mortality
V-HeFT II (*n* = 804)	Enalapril vs hydralazine-isosorbide	NYHA II & III, CHF	↓ Overall mortality
SAVE (*n* = 2231)	Captopril vs placebo	Recent MI with asymptomatic LVD	↓ Overall mortality
SOLVD, prevention arm (*n* = 4228)	Enalapril vs placebo	Asymptomatic LVD	↓ Death and hospitalization due to CHF
AIRE (*n* = 2006)	Ramipril vs placebo	Recent MI with overt CHF	↓ Overall mortality
ISIS-4 (*n* >50 000)	Captopril vs placebo	Acute MI	↓ Overall mortality
GISSI-3 (*n* = 19 394)	Lisinopril vs open control	Acute MI	↓Overall mortality
TRACE (*n* = 1749)	Trandolapril vs placebo	Recent MI with LVD	↓ Overall mortality
SMILE (*n* = 1556)	Zofenopril vs placebo	Acute MI	↓ Overall mortality

AIRE = Acute Infarction Ramipril Efficacy trial; CHF = congestive heart failure; CONSENSUS = Cooperative New Scandinavian Enalapril Survival Study; GISSI-3 = Gruppo Italiano per lo Studio della Sopravivenza nell'Infarto Miocardica III; ISIS-4 = International Study of Infarct Survival 4; LVD = left ventricular dysfunction; MI = myocardial infarction; NYHA = New York Heart Association; SAVE = Survival and Ventricular Enlargement trial; SOLVD = Studies on Left Ventricular Dysfunction; SMILE = Survival of Myocardial Infarction Long-Term Evaluation trial; TRACE = Trandolapril Cardiac Evaluation trial; V-HeFTII = Vasodilator-Heart Failure Trial II.

and prevention, and V-HeFT II demonstrated significant overall mortality reduction in patients with congestive heart failure (CHF). Captopril in the SAVE study and ISIS-4 also revealed a survival benefit in post-myocardial infarction patients. Ramipril showed a reduction in mortality in the AIRE study in patients with recent MI and overt CHF. In addition, ramipril showed a significant benefit in cardiovascular outcomes and mortality in patients with CV disease or diabetes and one other risk factor in the Heart Outcomes Prevention Evaluation (HOPE) study Lisinopril, trandolapril and zofenopril revealed improved survival in patients with acute MI, recent MI with left ventricular dysfunction and acute MI respectively (Table 6.1) [60–69]. Angiotensin receptor blockers (ARBs) have also shown significant benefit in both cardiovascular and renal outcomes (Table 6.2) [70–82]. Losartan compared to atenolol in patients with hypertension and left ventricular hypertrophy, showed reduction in composite cardiovascular mortality, MI and stroke in the LIFE study (relative risk [RR] = 0.13; $P = 0.021$) [70, 83]; however, losartan showed no difference in all-cause mortality compared to captopril in the OPTIMAAL study in subjects with acute MI [73]. Also, no difference in mortality was noted with losartan compared to captopril in CHF in the ELITE II study [77]. But, in the RENAAL study, there was a significant reduction of serum creatinine, end-stage renal disease and death using losartan compared to placebo in patients with diabetic nephropathy (RR = 0.16; $P = 0.02$) [74]. Valsartan compared to placebo for heart failure revealed no difference in mortality in the V-HeFT study, but there was a reduction in hospitalization [78]. When valsartan was added to captopril in subjects following acute MI, there was no difference in mortality or composite endpoints compared to either one of the

Table 6.2 ARBs in clinical trials

Condition	*Trial*	*Drugs*	*n*	*Duration*	*Outcome*	*Result*
LVH and hypertension	LIFE	Losartan 50–100 mg vs atenolol 50–100 mg	9193	5 years	Composite CV mortality, MI, stroke	13% RR ($P = 0.021$)
HTN	VALUE	Valsartan up to 160 mg vs amlodipine up to 10 mg	15 245	4.2 years	Composite endpoint of mortality and morbidity	No difference between valsartan and amlodipine
Diabetic nephropathy	IDNT	Irbesartan up to 300 mg vs amlodipine up to 10 mg vs placebo	1715	2.6 years	Doubling of SCr, ESRD or death	20% lower than placebo ($P = 0.02$); 23% lower than amlodipine ($P = 0.006$)
	IRMA	Irbesartan 150 mg or 300 mg vs placebo	590	3 months	Albuminuria, overt proteinuria	24% lower albumin excretion with 150 mg irbesartan ($P < 0.001$); 38% lower albumin excretion with 300 mg irbesartan ($P < 0.001$); 70% reduction of overt proteinuria ($P < 0.001$)
	RENAAL	Losartan 50–100 mg vs placebo	1513	3.4 years	Doubling of SCr, ESRD or death	16% reduction of composite ($P = 0.02$); 25% reduction in doubling of SCr; 28% reduction in ESRD; no change in deaths
Acute MI	OPTIMAAL	Losartan 50 mg/day or captopril 50 mg tid	5477	6 months	All-cause mortality, SCD and total and NFMI	No difference between captopril and losartan; 13.3% death captopril vs. 15.3% death losartan ($P = 0.03$)

	VALIANT	Valsartan 160 mg bid, captopril 50 mg tid or combinations of valsartan 30 mg bid and captopril 50 mg tid	14 703	2.1 years	All-cause mortality, CV death, MI, hospitalization to CHF	No difference between groups
CHF	ELITE II	Losartan 50 mg/day, captopril 50 mg tid	3152	555 days	All-cause mortality	No difference
	ValHeft	Valsartan 160 mg, placebo	5010		Mortality and composite endpoint of mortality and morbidity	No difference in mortality; improvement in hospitalization with valsartan
	CHARM, overall	Candesartan 32 mg/day, placebo	7601	2 years	All-cause mortality	17% reduction, statistically significant
	CHARM, alternate	Candesartan 32 mg/day, placebo	2028	33.7 months	Composite of CV death at hospital	23% reduction, statistically significant
	CHARM, added	Candesartan 32 mg/day, placebo	2548	41 months	Composite	15% reduction, statistically significant
	CHARM, preserved	Candsesartan 32 mg/day, placebo	3023	36.6 months	CV death or hospitalization	11% reduction, statistically significant

CHF = congestive heart failure; CV = cardiovascular; ESRD = end-stage renal disease; LVD = left ventricular dysfunction; MI = myocardial infarction; NFMI = non-fatal myocardial infarction; RR = relative risk; SCD = sudden cardiovascular death; SCr = serum creatinine

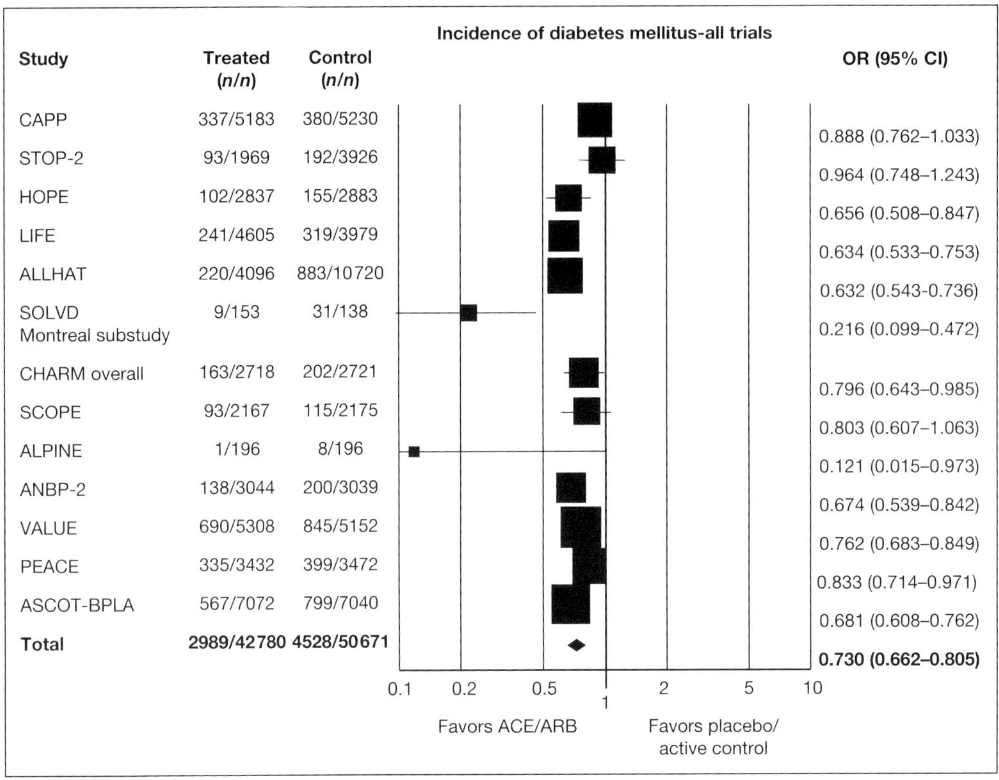

Figure 6.5 Meta-analysis of randomized trials with use of ACE inhibitors/ARBs on development of diabetes (with permission from [92] and [95]).

medications (VALIANT study) [76]. In the VALUE trial, there was no difference in composite endpoints of mortality and morbidity between valsartan and amlodipine [71]. Irbesartan was studied in patients with diabetic nephropathy. When compared to amlodipine (IDNT study) [35] and placebo (IRMA study) [71], irbesartan showed significant reduction of overt proteinuria, end-stage renal disease and doubling of serum creatinine. In the CHARM study, candesartan also showed reduction in composite endpoints of mortality and morbidity in heart failure patients with LV dysfunction compared to placebo (Table 6.2) [79–81]. As evidenced in these clinical trials, there appears to be reasonable justification for considering RAAS inhibition to prevent adverse cardiovascular and renal outcomes. In addition, as we examine the role of the renin–angiotensin axis and its interaction with endothelium and the insulin signaling pathways, there appears to be potential in the prevention of diabetes using agents that block the renin–angiotensin–aldosterone system.

Clinical studies on RAAS inhibition and outcomes of new-onset diabetes as a secondary endpoint

ACE inhibition and angiotensin receptor blockers have been studied extensively in hypertension, congestive heart failure, coronary artery disease and renal disease. Both drugs consistently prevent CAD (particularly ACE inhibition), stroke, and diabetic complications of microvascular disease. In addition, secondary endpoints of some of these studies have suggested reduced incidence of new-onset diabetes (Figure 6.5). In the HOPE study, the incidence of diabetes was 34% lower in the ramipril-treated group compared to the placebo group [66, 84]. In the LIFE

Table 6.3 Prevention of type II DM by RAAS inhibition

Study	*Treatment arm: Number of patients with new T2DM*	*Treatment arm: Total number of subjects without DM*	*Control arm: Total number of patients with new DM*	*Control arm: Total number of patients without DM*	*Relative risk (RR)*	*Confidence interval (CI)*	*P-value favoring Treatment arm*
CAPP (1999)	337	5184	380	5229	0.86	0.70–1.03	NS
STOP-HTN-2 (1999)	93	1969	97	1961	0.95	0.72–1.26	NS
LIFE (2002)	241	4006	319	3592	0.75	0.63–0.88	$P = 0.001$
HOPE (2001)	102	2837	155	2883	0.66	0.51–0.85	$P < 0.001$
ALLHAT (2002)	473	5840	1129	9733	0.70	0.53–0.81	$P < 0.001$
SOLVD (2003)	9	153	31	138	0.26	0.13–0.53	$P < 0.001$
ALPINE (2003)	1	196	8	196	0.13	0.02–0.97	$P = 0.03$
SCOPE (2003)	93	2160	115	2170	0.75	0.62–1.06	NS
CHARM (2003)	163	2715	202	2721	0.81	0.66–0.97	$P < 0.001$
VALUE (2004)	690	5267	845	5152	0.77	0.69–0.86	$P < 0.0001$
PEACE (2004)	335	3432	399	3472	0.83	0.72–0.96	$P < 0.01$
ANBP-2	138	3044	200	3039	0.674	0.539–0.842	$P < 0.001$
ASCOT-BPLA	567	7072	799	7040	0.681	0.608–0.762	$P < 0.001$

ALLHAT = Antihypertensive and Lipid Lowering treatment to prevent Heart Attack Trial; ALPINE = Antihypertensive treatment and Lipid Profile In a North of Sweden Efficacy; ANBP-2 = Second Australian National Blood Pressure Study; ASCOT-BPLA = Anglo Scandinavian Cardiac Outcomes Trial Blood Pressure Lowering Arm; CAPP = Captopril Prevention Project; PEACE = Prevention of Events with Angiotensin Converting Enzyme inhibition; SCOPE = Study of Cognition and Prognosis in the Elderly; STOP-HTN-2 = Cardiovascular events in elderly patients with isolated systolic hypertension.

study, where losartan was compared to atenolol while treating hypertension with left ventricular hypertrophy, losartan was associated with a 25% reduction in new onset of diabetes compared to atenolol [70, 83]. Even in the more recent ALLHAT study, the lisinopril arm had significantly lower events of new-onset diabetes compared to chlorthalidone [85]. The chlorthalidone arm had 302 cases of new-onset diabetes out of 9733 subjects while the lisinopril arm had only 119 patients with new-onset diabetes out of 5840 participants providing a relative risk of 0.66 (confidence interval [CI] 0.53–0.81). In the CHARM study, candesartan reduced onset of diabetes by 19% (RR 0.81; CI 0.66–0.97) compared to placebo when used in patients with chronic heart failure [79–82]. The SOLVD study recently analyzed data on new-onset diabetes in an enalapril group compared to placebo treatment for chronic heart failure. There was a significant reduction (RR 0.26; CI 0.13–0.53) of new onset of diabetes with use of enalapril [86]. In addition, in the ALPINE study, compared to hydrochlorothiazide, candesartan decreased new onset of diabetes significantly (RR 0.13; CI 0.02–0.97; $P = 0.03$) [87]. More recently, VALUE trial results suggested that when treating hypertensive patients with valsartan, there was a 23% reduction (RR 0.77; CI 0.69–0.86; $P < 0.001$) in new onset of diabetes compared to amlodipine [71]. The CAPP study, SCOPE study and STOP-HTN study on the other hand showed no difference between use of ACE inhibitor or ARB and control in new onset of diabetes (Table 6.3) [88–90]. In the PEACE trial, even though there was no difference in the primary endpoint of cardiovascular outcomes between trandolapril and placebo, trandolapril reduced the risk of development of diabetes by 17% compared to placebo

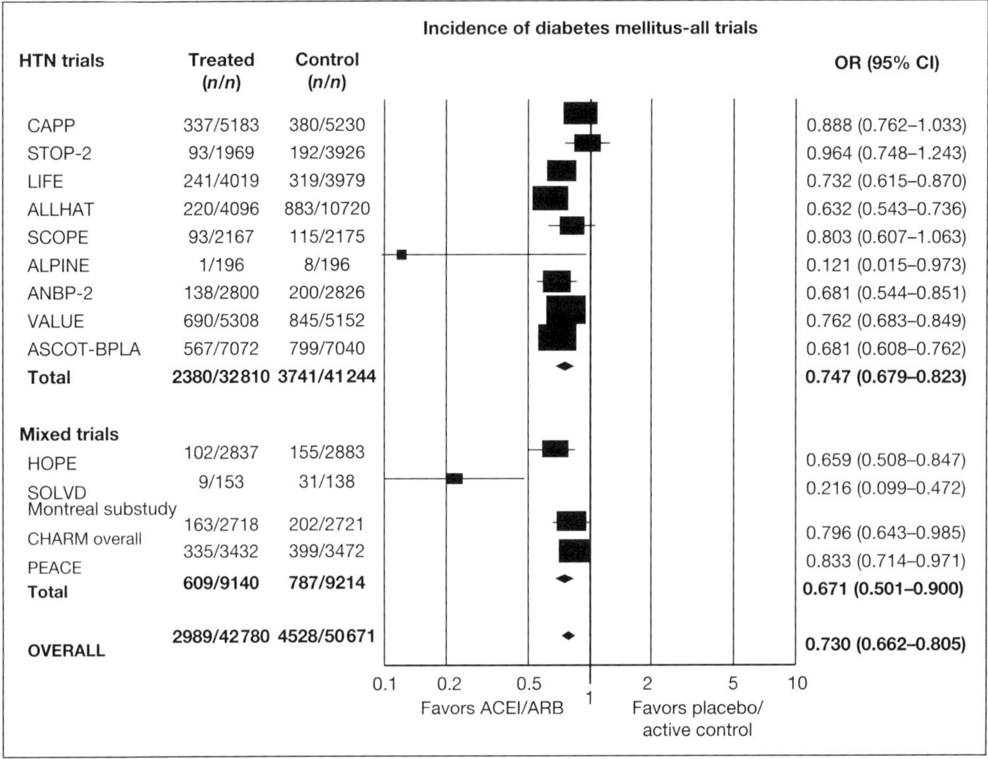

Figure 6.6 Effect of RAAS inhibition between hypertensives and non-hypertensives (with permission from [92] and [95]). ACEI = ACE inhibitor; ARB = angiotensin receptor blocker; HTN = hypertension

(RR 0.83; CI 0.72–0.96; $P = 0.01$) [91]. A comprehensive meta-analysis was recently performed to assess new onset of diabetes in patients treated with ACE inhibitor or ARB [92]. Thirteen randomized trials were included that had enrolled 93 451 patients without diabetes, of whom 42 780 patients received an ACE inhibitor or an ARB. Overall, 2989 new cases of type 2 diabetes were observed in 42 780 patients treated with the RAAS blocking agent (7.12%) compared to 4528 events in 50 671 patients in the control group (8.95%). An absolute risk reduction of 1.85% ($P < 0.001$) was observed with RAAS inhibitors. This was also significant regardless of the comparator, suggesting a positive beneficial effect of RAAS blockade rather than a negative deleterious effect of the control group agent. The number needed to treat to prevent one new case of diabetes averaged 46 over a 4–5-year period.

Exclusion of any single trial from the meta-analysis did not alter the findings. Nine trials randomized hypertensive patients and four trials randomized patients with left ventricular dysfunction or vascular disease. In hypertensive subjects, there was a 27% reduction in new onset of diabetes, and in the non-hypertensive trials, there was a 33% reduction in new-onset diabetes with use of ACE inhibitors or ARBs. In addition, when separating the effects of ACE inhibitors and ARBs, diabetes developed in 6.5% of patients randomized to ACE inhibitors compared to 8.4% in placebo (odds ratio [OR] 0.73; $P < 0.001$) and 8.2% in ARBs compared to 10.5% in placebo (OR 0.73; $P < 0.001$). There were no gender differences or effect of age noted in any of the studies for new-onset diabetes (mean age 65 years) [92–95]. There was no significant difference in effect size of diabetes prevention between hypertensives and

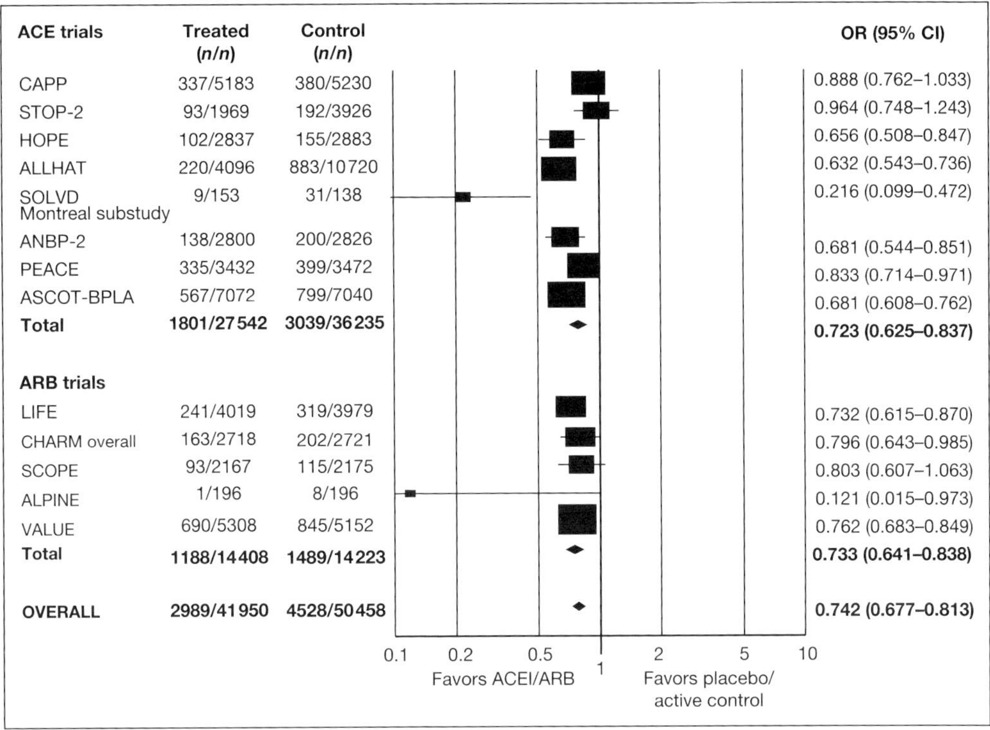

Figure 6.7 Effect of RAAS inhibition on development of diabetes between ACE inhibitors and ARBs (with permission from [92] and [95]. ACEI = ACE inhibitor; ARB = angiotensin receptor blocker

non-hypertensives (Figure 6.6). Furthermore, there were no differences in effect size between ACE inhibitors and ARBs (Figure 6.7).

However, there are multiple limitations in recommending RAAS blockers for prevention of diabetes. First, many of the above-mentioned studies recruited populations that differed widely. For instance, in the HOPE study, there were significant differences in baseline characteristics of the utilization of β-blockers and thiazide diuretic, both of which affect insulin sensitivity adversely. It is not clear if the benefit seen with lisinopril in ALLHAT is due to a positive effect of the RAAS blocker or a negative effect of chlorthalidone, a thiazide diuretic. In addition, in the LIFE study, the question whether losartan had a favorable effect on insulin sensitivity by its peripheral vascular dilating mechanism or atenelol had a deleterious effect by its negative effect on insulin sensitivity remains unanswered. Second, none of the studies described in the meta-analysis were designed to address 'new onset of diabetes' as a primary endpoint. Third, the definition of development of diabetes varied significantly and did not use glucose tolerance tests before the onset of the study or as an endpoint to define new onset of diabetes, raising the possibility of ascertainment or classification bias. While attempts to decrease insulin resistance and inhibit the renin–angiotensin system may reduce the risk of cardiovascular disease, lessons learned from these trials should facilitate adoption of different strategies in future clinical trials [96–98].

Studies addressing prevention of diabetes with RAAS inhibition as a primary endpoint

The DREAM (Diabetes Reduction Assessment with Ramipril and Rosaglitazone Medication) trial was designed to address whether ramipril or rosaglitazone could prevent new onset of diabetes as a primary endpoint [99–101]. The investigators randomized 5269 patients with impaired fasting glucose (fasting plasma glucose >6.1 mmol/l or >110 mg/dl but <7 mmol/l or <126 mg/dl), IGT (plasma glucose level more than or equal to 7.8 mmol/l or 140 mg/dl but less than or equal to 11.1mmol/l or 200 mg/dl two h after a glucose load), or both, to receive ramipril (5 mg daily, increased to 10 mg after 2 months and to 15 mg after 1 year), rosiglitazone (4 mg daily, increased to 8 mg daily after 2 months), both or placebo. The subjects were assessed at 2 months, 6 months, 12 months and once a year thereafter, for the composite primary outcome of death or diabetes and secondary outcomes of regression to normoglycemia. Mean age was 54.7 and mean BMI was 31 kg/m^2. At 3-year follow-up, a significant reduction in the primary endpoint was noted with rosiglitazone (11.6% vs 26% in placebo with a hazard ratio (HR) of 0.40 and P <0.001). There was no difference in the primary endpoint with ramipril compared to placebo (17.1% ramipril and 18.5% placebo; HR 0.91; P = 0.15). Regression to normoglycemia was significantly more frequent in the ramipril group than in the placebo group (42.5% vs 38.2%; HR 1.16; P <0.001) and with rosiglitazone compared to placebo (38.6% vs 20.5%; HR 1.83; P <0.001).

The implications of these results are multifaceted. The DREAM investigators point out some of these. First, the aforementioned studies not only looked at diabetes as secondary endpoints, but also included patients who were older, and had hypertension and/or cardiovascular disease. This confluence of *a priori* risk, possibly increases the magnitude of RAAS activation in these subjects, allowing for a better response with ACE inhibitors or ARBs. Second, the observed reduction in onset of diabetes in other trials may be due to an improvement in unrecognized hyperglycemia at baseline or reduced detection of diabetes in the RAAS blockade arm due to reduced hospitalization for their primary endpoint of cardiovascular events. Third, the effect on regression to normoglycemia with ramipril is intriguing despite no reduction in development of diabetes. Several arguments were raised that could have contributed to this phenomenon. Blood pressure was reduced significantly in the ramipril arm at 2 months compared to placebo (4.3 mmHg vs 1.6 mmHg). Whether this had an effect on the secondary endpoint was clarified by further analysis with adjustment for blood pressure reduction. There was still a consistent effect on regression to normoglycemia with ramipril compared to placebo (HR 1.12; P = 0.008). Adjustment of use of ARBs at baseline had no effect on the primary or secondary endpoints. Whether maintaining potassium homeostasis with RAAS blockers has a protective effect on development of diabetes (compared to the potassium depleting effect of thiazide diuretics and its propensity to increase development of diabetes) is still unclear as potassium levels were not tested following randomization in the DREAM trial.

In contrast to ramipril, there was a significant benefit noted with use of rosiglitazone in preventing onset of diabetes (60% reduction) compared to placebo. The peroxisome proliferator activator receptor-gamma (PPAR-γ) agonists have been shown to prevent diabetes in high-risk Hispanic women as noted by Buchanan and colleagues in previous studies [102–104]. Troglitazone, used in the TRIPOD study [102], was unfortunately taken off the market due to its side-effect profile of hepatotoxicity. It is, however, not surprising that an agent having similar mechanism of action, such as rosiglitazone, would have a favorable effect on new-onset diabetes [105]. Although this medication was generally safe, the adverse events noted in the trial should be viewed in the context of risk versus benefit. The prevalence of side-effects was higher with use of rosiglitazone compared to placebo (peripheral edema: 6.8% vs 4.9%; heart failure: 0.5% vs 0.1% and a weight gain of 2.2 kg in rosiglitazone compared to placebo).

The authors of the DREAM trial argue that, although the side-effects of rosiglitazone were slightly higher compared to placebo, the incidence of heart failure with rosiglitazone was about ten times lower in participants at low risk of cardiovascular events in the DREAM trial than in the PROACTIV trial [106], a cardiovascular prevention trial of participants at high risk. This, according to them, could be explained by a reduced susceptibility of lower-risk people to heart failure. Nevertheless, there were 16 cases of heart failure in this study, which needs to be addressed by identifying individuals who may be at risk for heart failure.

Table 6.4 Mechanisms of RAAS inhibition in diabetes prevention

- Improves β-cell function of pancreas
- Prevents fibrosis and apoptosis of β cells of the pancreas
- Activation of bradykinin and nitric oxide pathways
- Enhances insulin sensitivity by augmenting skeletal muscle blood flow
- Promotes insulin signaling of the beneficial PI-3 kinase pathway and attenuates MAPK pathway in vascular wall
- Increases GLUT 4 expression
- Inhibits differentiation of pre-adipocytes to mature adipocytes
- Activates PPAR-γ nuclear receptor expression
- Direct benefit in improvement of endothelial function

GLUT 4 = glucose transporter 4; MAPK = mitogen activated protein kinase; PI-3 kinase = phosphotidyl inositol kinase; PPAR = peroxisome proliferator activator receptor; RAAS = renin–angiotensin–aldosterone system.

There was a difference in the absolute risk between the treatment groups of 14.4%. This suggests that for every seven people with impaired fasting glucose or IGT, rosiglitazone given over a 3-year period will prevent one individual from developing diabetes. Moreover, rosiglitazone significantly increased the likelihood of regression to normoglycemia by about 70–80% compared with placebo. The reduction achieved with lifestyle approaches was similar to that achieved in the DREAM trial and greater reductions were achieved with rosiglitazone compared to metformin or acarbose. The effect on regression is much the same or larger than that of lifestyle approaches or acarbose, and larger than that with metformin, which did not promote more regression than placebo.

POTENTIAL MECHANISM OF RAAS BLOCKADE IN DIABETES PREVENTION

The precise mechanism of action of RAAS blockade in prevention of diabetes is unclear. Potential mechanisms responsible for reduced incidence of diabetes in these trials include improvement in insulin-mediated glucose uptake, enhanced endothelial function, increased nitric oxide activation, reduced inflammatory response and increased bradykinin levels [107–109].

Other possibilities include multifactorial beneficial effects on β-cell function, skeletal muscle blood flow and its effects on adipocyte and insulin signaling pathways. (Table 6.4). Significant vasoconstrictive effects of Ang II on pancreatic vasculature lead to disruption of islet cell structure, fibrosis and apoptosis. RAAS inhibition attenuates this negative response in the islet cells [110–113]. It is known that increased Ang II activity leads to increased oxidative stress, which in turn can lead to islet cell apoptosis, and RAAS blockade will attenuate this process as well. Furthermore, bradykinin and nitric oxide production from ACE inhibition improves blood flow to the skeletal muscle leading to enhanced insulin-mediated glucose disposal [114, 115]. In addition, glucose utilization is increased by amplified expression of GLUT 4, a glucose transporter protein, in skeletal muscle and myocardium. Insulin sensitivity is also augmented by preferential stimulation of phosphoinositol signaling pathway in the vascular wall [116]. Ang II inhibits differentiation of preadipocytes to mature adipocytes leading to deposition of lipids in muscle, liver and pancreas. Insulin resistance resulting from this process can be attenuated by blockade of the renin–angiotensin pathway [117, 118]. In a recent study, low levels of adiponectin were found to be an independent predictor of type 2 diabetes [119]. There are multiple studies addressing the mechanistic ways ACE inhibitors and ARBs affect insulin sensitivity and insulin action [120–128]. The ACE inhibitors quinapril significantly improved endothelial function in multiple studies, both in normotensive volunteers and subjects with CAD [121–124, 127]. In addition, ACE inhibitors and ARBs have been shown to increase adiponectin levels and insulin sensitivity. This may explain another mechanism of prevention of diabetes with RAAS inhibition [129–144]. Recent work has revealed a new mechanism of an ARB, telmisartan. It appears to activate PPAR-γ, a nuclear receptor expressed in adipocytes, macrophages and muscle that functions as a transcription factor controlling carbohydrate and lipid metabolism [142]. PPAR agonists and thiazolidinediones have been effective in the treatment of diabetes and prevention of diabetes in insulin resistant women. Hence, activation of this nuclear receptor may have a significant role in diabetes prevention. In addition, improvement in endothelial function may have a direct benefit. Endothelial dysfunction leads to defects in insulin-mediated glucose uptake. Blockade of vascular nitric oxide synthesis with L-arginine analog also impairs endothelial-dependent vasodilation. Improvement of endothelial function occurs with exercise, low-fat and low-carbohydrate diets as well as with statins and ACE inhibitors [121–126, 143].

PREVENTING VERSUS DELAYING THE ONSET OF DIABETES

Type 2 diabetes may be prevented or delayed by three types of interventions: those that limit fat accumulation in the body; those that uncouple obesity from insulin resistance; and those that directly preserve β-cell mass and/or function, despite the high secretory demands imposed by insulin. Prevention of type 2 diabetes requires cessation of the progressive β-cell dysfunction and stabilization of glucose concentrations to normoglycemia. Allowing even a partial β-cell dysfunction will only delay the onset of diabetes, not prevent it.

Current efforts to prevent type 2 diabetes have utilized interventions that modify body weight and/or insulin resistance or that change glucose levels directly. The studies have not paid careful attention to the endpoints of stable glycemia and β-cell function. Rather, they have focused on reducing a proportion of patients with slightly elevated glucose levels, as in IGT, who convert to diabetes, at which point the risk of microvascular complications begins. The duration of the studies have been short relative to the years required for the development of diabetes. Studies of such short duration will reveal a reduction in the incidence of diabetes if active interventions stabilize glucose at non-diabetic levels in some or all individuals. Interventions that lower glucose levels acutely without changing the rate of increase, and interventions that slow rather than arrest increasing glucose levels, will also cause an apparent reduction in the incidence of diabetes. However, these types of interventions delay rather than prevent diabetes. Eventually, these individuals will develop diabetes because their glucose levels continue to rise. Outcomes should ideally include measures of β-cell function in relation to insulin resistance, and stabilization of β cells over time. In the absence of such measures, stability of glycemia should be assessed to determine whether diabetes is prevented or only delayed in groups that receive active treatment. Diagnostic testing for diabetes after a relevant post-drug washout period should be included if the intervention has an antidiabetic effect. Finally, prolonged follow-up to look for an impact on chronic diabetes complications, both microvascular and cardiovascular, should be included as endpoints [145].

The survival curve in the DREAM trial for ramipril seems to diverge starting at 3.5 years. Whether this is truly representative of the effect of ramipril or purely a chance effect will only be evident if further follow-up is performed on these subjects. The ONTARGET, a simple randomized trial evaluating telmisartan, ramipril and their combination, in high-risk patients with cardiovascular disease has recently been completed and preliminary results presented at the annual convention of the American College of Cardiology. These revealed that telmisartan was not inferior to ramipril in reducing the incidence of major adverse cardiovascular events in high-risk patients with cardiovascular disease or diabetes, but that combination therapy with both agents was not superior to either agent alone. Moreover, the incidence of side-effects including hypotension, syncope, and renal dysfunction was higher with the combination therapy compared with ramipril alone. Telmisartan was associated with a lower incidence of cough and angioedema, but a higher incidence of hypotension compared with ramipril. A 4000 patient substudy of Telmisartan Randomized Assessment Study in ACE Intolerant Subjects with Cardiovascular Disease (TRANSCEND) will investigate whether chronic AT_1 blockade with telmisartan can improve glucose metabolism and prevent onset of diabetes as detected by an oral glucose tolerance test [146]. Baseline data from 2837 patients in TRANSCEND reveal that at least 59.9% have dysglycemia. A third of them have diabetes and an additional 8% were diagnosed with diabetes, 13.9% with IGT and 8.7% with impaired fasting glucose during their glucose tolerance test.

Further follow-up in the DREAM trial and data from the ONTARGET–TRANSCEND trial will provide new insights into the role of RAAS blockade in the prevention of diabetes.

SUMMARY

The role of the renin–angiotensin–aldosterone system in development and maintenance of blood pressure is well established. In addition, the deleterious effects of Ang II on the heart, vasculature and kidneys have been clearly defined. There appears to be a close relationship between endothelial dysfunction, insulin resistance (a precursor to diabetes and CAD) and Ang II. The signaling pathways for insulin in the vascular wall interact with angiotensin signaling giving rise to potential mechanisms for the development of diabetes and resultant harmful effects. A large number of clinical trials using ACE inhibitors or ARBs have shown significant reductions in the secondary endpoint of development of new onset of diabetes. Meta-analysis has methodological limitations due to the combination of different trial designs, therapies with different properties and heterogeneous patient populations. In addition, there may be variations in study level characteristics, risk factors in the population studied, diagnostics for diabetes, and cutpoints used for diagnosis of new onset of diabetes. Also, it is not clear from the meta-analysis if RAAS inhibition prevented new onset of diabetes or just prolonged the overt manifestation of the disease state. The DREAM trial showed benefit in reduction of incidence of diabetes with rosiglitazone, but not with ramipril. A prospective study involving an antidiabetic agent and an ARB is being studied in the Nateglinide and Valsartan Impaired Glucose Tolerance Outcomes Research (NAVIGATOR) trial that is ongoing and being tested for their ability to prevent type 2 diabetes. The ONTARGET–TRANSCEND study will also address the primary endpoint of new-onset diabetes [137]. In the meantime, it is important to recognize insulin resistance and MS as entities with increased risk for CV disease; in addition to lifestyle modifications, management of endothelial dysfunction and protecting the vasculature will blaze the trail towards preventing diabetes and cardiovascular disease.

REFERENCES

1. American Heart Association. Heart Disease and stroke statistics – 2005 Update. Dallas, TX: American Heart Association, 2004.
2. Zimmer P, Alberti KGMM, Shaw J. Global and societal implications of the diabetes epidemic. *Nature* 2001; 414:782–787.
3. Centers for Disease Control and Prevention. National diabetes fact sheet: general information and national estimates on diabetes in the United States, 2003. Atlanta, GA: US Department of Human Services, Centers for Disease Control and Prevention, 2003. Accessed at www.cdc.gov/diabetes/pubs/factsheet.htm on 24 February 2004.
4. Narayan KM, Boyle JP, Thompson TJ, Sorensen SW, Williamson DF. Lifetime risk for diabetes mellitus in the United States. *JAMA* 2003; 290:1884–1890.
5. Eyre H, Kahn R, Robertson RM; the ACS/ADA/AHA Collaborative Writing Committee. Preventing cancer, cardiovascular disease, and diabetes: a common agenda for the American Cancer Society, the American Diabetes Association, and the American Heart Association. *Stroke* 2004; 35:1999–2010.

6. Chin MH, Zhang JX, Merrell K. Diabetes in the African-American Medicare population. Morbidity, quality of care, and resource utilization. *Diabetes Care* 1998; 21:1090–1095.
7. Steinberger J, Daniels SR. Obesity, insulin resistance, diabetes, and cardiovascular risk in children: an American Heart Association scientific statement from the Atherosclerosis, Hypertension, and Obesity in the Young Committee (Council on Cardiovascular Disease in the Young) and the Diabetes Committee (Council on Nutrition, Physical Activity, and Metabolism). *Circulation* 2003; 107:1448–1453.
8. Sowers JR. Obesity as a cardiovascular risk factor. *Am J Med* 2003; 115(suppl 8A):37S–41S.
9. McFarlane SI, Jacober SJ, Winer N *et al.* Control of cardiovascular risk factors in patients with diabetes and hypertension at urban academic medical centers. *Diabetes Care* 2002; 25:718–723.
10. Executive Summary of the Third Report of the National Cholesterol Education Program (NCEP) Expert Panel on Detection, Evaluation and Treatment of High Blood Cholesterol in Adults (Adult Treatment Panel III). *JAMA* 2001; 285:2486–2497.
11. Harris MI, Flegal KM, Cowie CC *et al.* Prevalence of diabetes, impaired fasting glucose, and impaired glucose tolerance in U.S. adults. The Third National Health and Nutrition Examination Survey, 1988–1994. *Diabetes Care* 1998; 21:518–524.
12. McVea K, Crabtree BF, Medder JD *et al.* An ounce of prevention? Evaluation of the "Put Prevention into Practice" program. *J Fam Pract* 1996; 43:361–369.
13. Deedwania PC, Fonseca VA. Diabetes, prediabetes and cardiovascular risk: shifting the paradigm. *Am J Med* 2005; 118:939–947.
14. Reaven GM. Syndrome X. *Clinical Diabetes* 1994; 12:32–36.
15. Haffner SM, Valdez RA, Hazuda HP, Mitchell BD, Morales PA, Stern MP. Prospective analysis of the insulin-resistance syndrome (syndrome X). *Diabetes* 1992; 41:715–722.
16. Mykkanen L, Kuusisto J, Pyörälä K, Laakso M. Cardiovascular disease risk factors as predictors of type 2 (non-insulin-dependent) diabetes mellitus in elderly subjects. *Diabetologia* 1993; 36:553–559.
17. Lakka HM, Laaksonen D, Lakka T *et al.* The MetS and total cardiovascular mortality in middle-aged men. *JAMA* 2002; 228:2709–2716.
18. Isomaa B, Henricsson M, Almgren P, Tuomi T, Taskinen M-R, Groop L. The MetS influences the risk of chronic complications in patients with type II diabetes. *Diabetologia* 2001; 44:1148–1154.
19. Alberti KG. The clinical implications of impaired glucose tolerance. *Diabet Med* 1996; 13:927–937.
20. Edelstein SL, Knowler WC, Bain RP *et al.* Predictors of progression from impaired glucose tolerance to NIDDM: an analysis of six prospective studies. *Diabetes* 1997; 46:701–710.
21. Lorenzo C, Okoloise M, Williams K, Stern MP, Haffner SM. The MetS as predictor of type 2 diabetes. *Diabetes Care* 2003; 26:3153–3159.
22. Jarrett RJ, Keen H, Fuller JH, McCartney M. Worsening to diabetes in men with impaired glucose tolerance ("borderline diabetes"). *Diabetologia* 1979; 16:25–30.
23. Keen H, Jarrett RJ, McCartney P. The ten-year follow-up of the Bedford survey (1962–1972): glucose tolerance and diabetes. *Diabetologia* 1982; 22:73–78.
24. Sartor G, Schersten B, Carlstrom S, Melander A, Norden A, Persson G. Ten-year follow-up of subjects with impaired glucose tolerance: prevention of diabetes by tolbutamide and diet regulation. *Diabetes* 1980; 29:41–49.
25. Pan XR, Li GW, Hu YH *et al.* Effects of diet and exercise in preventing NIDDM in people with impaired glucose tolerance. The Da Qing IGT and Diabetes Study. *Diabetes Care* 1997; 20:537–544.
26. Tuomilehto J, Geboers J, Salonen JT, Nissinen A, Kuulasmaa K, Puska P. Decline in cardiovascular mortality in North Karelia and other parts of Finland. *Br Med J* 1986; 293:1068–1071.
27. Knowler WC, Barrett-Connor E, Fowler SE *et al.* Reduction in the incidence of type 2 diabetes with lifestyle intervention or Metformin. *N Engl J Med* 2002; 346:393–403.
28. Lindstrom J, Louheranta A, Mannelin M *et al.* Natl Publ Hlth Inst, Diabetes & Genet Epidemiol Unit, FI-00300 Helsinki, Finland. The Finnish Diabetes Prevention Study (DPS). *Diabetes Care* 2003; 26:3230–3236.
29. Klein S, Sheard NF, Pi-Sunyer X *et al.* Weight management through lifestyle modification for the prevention and management of type 2 diabetes: rationale and strategies. *Diabetes Care* 2004; 27:2067–2073.
30. Farquhar JW, Fortmann SP, Flora JA *et al.* Effects of communitywide education on cardiovascular disease risk factors. The Stanford Five-City Project. *JAMA* 1990; 264:359–365.
31. Luepker RV, Murray DM, Jacobs DR Jr. *et al.* Community education for cardiovascular disease prevention: risk factor changes in the Minnesota Heart Health Program. *Am J Public Health* 1994; 84:1383–1393.
32. Younis N, Soran H, Farook S. The prevention of type 2 diabetes mellitus: recent advances. *Q J Med* 2004; 97:451–455.

33. Watanabe M, Yamaoka K, Yokotsuka M, Tango T. Randomized controlled trial of a new dietary education program to prevent type 2 diabetes in a high-risk group of Japanese male workers. *Diabetes Care* 2003; 26:3209–3214.
34. Tuomilehto J, Lindstrom J, Eriksson JG *et al.* Prevention of type 2 diabetes mellitus by changes in lifestyle among subjects with impaired glucose tolerance. *N Engl J Med* 2001; 344:1343–1350.
35. Jacques CH, Jones RL. Problems encountered by primary care physicians in the care of patients with diabetes. *Arch Fam Med* 1993; 2:739–741.
36. Shintani TT, Hughes CK, Beckham S, O'Connor HK. Obesity and cardiovascular risk intervention through the ad libitum feeding of traditional Hawaiian diet. *Am J Clin Nutr* 1991; 53:1647S–1651S.
37. Rosenson RS, Reasner CA. Therapeutic approaches in the prevention of cardiovascular disease in metabolic syndrome and in patients with type 2 diabetes. *Curr Opin Cardiol* 2004; 19:480–487.
38. Wing R, Venditti E, Jakcic J, Polley B, Lang W. Lifestyle intervention in overweight individuals with a family history of diabetes. *Diabetes Care* 1998; 21:350–359.
39. Zimmet P, Shaw J, Alberti KGMM. Preventing type 2 diabetes and the dysmetabolic syndrome in the real world: a realistic view. *Diabet Med* 2003; 20:693–702.
40. Lucius R, Gallinat S, Busche S, Rosenstiel P, Unger T. Beyond blood pressure: new roles for angiotensin II. *Cell Mol Life Sci* 1999; 56:1008–1019.
41. Johnston CI, Risvanis J. Preclinical pharmacology of angiotensin II receptor antagonists: update and outstanding issues. *Am J Hypertens* 1997; 10:306S–310S.
42. Chung O, Stoll M, Unger T. Physiologic and pharmacologic implications of AT_1 versus AT_2 receptors. *Blood Press* 1996; 5(suppl 2):47–52.
43. Timmermans PB, Wong PC, Chiu AT *et al.* Angiotensin II receptors and angiotensin II receptor antagonists. *Pharmacol Rev* 1993; 45:205–251.
44. Unger T, Culman J, Gohlke P. Angiotensin II receptor blockade and end-organ protection: pharmacological rationale and evidence. *J Hypertens* 1998; 16(suppl 7):S3–S9.
45. Drexler H, Hornig B. Endothelial dysfunction in human disease. *J Mol Cell Cardiol* 1999; 31:51–60.
46. Britten MB, Zeiher AM, Schachinger V. Clinical importance of coronary endothelial vasodilator dysfunction and therapeutic options. *J Intern Med* 1999; 245:315–327.
47. Diet F, Pratt RE, Berry GJ, Momose N, Gibbons GH, Dzau VJ. Increased accumulation of tissue ACE in human atherosclerotic coronary artery disease. *Circulation* 1996; 94:2756–2767.
48. Shai SY, Fishel RS, Martin BM, Berk BC, Bernstein KE. Bovine angiotensin converting enzyme cDNA cloning and regulation. Increased expression during endothelial cell growth arrest. *Circ Res* 1992; 70:1274–1281.
49. Fishel RS, Eisenberg S, Shai SY, Redden RA, Bernstein KE, Berk BC. Glucocorticoids induce angiotensin-converting enzyme expression in vascular smooth muscle. *Hypertension* 1995; 25:343–349.
50. Brown NJ, Agirbasli MA, Williams GH, Litchfield WR, Vaughan DE. Effect of activation and inhibition of the renin-angiotensin system on plasma PAI-1. *Hypertension* 1998; 32:965–971.
51. Gainer JV, Morrow JD, Loveland A, King DJ, Brown NJ. Effect of bradykinin-receptor blockade on the response to angiotensin-converting enzyme inhibitor in normotensive and hypertensive subjects. *N Engl J Med* 1998; 339:1285–1292.
52. Hornig B, Kohler C, Drexler H. Role of bradykinin in mediating vascular effects of angiotensin-converting enzyme inhibitors in humans. *Circulation* 1997; 95:1115–1118.
53. Lyon CJ, Law RE, Hsueh WA. Minireview: adiposity, inflammation, and atherogenesis. *Endocrinology* 2003; 144:2195–2200.
54. Moule KS, Denton RM. Multiple signaling pathways involved in the metabolic effects of insulin. *Am J Cardiol* 1997; 80:41A–49A.
55. Nascimben L, Bothwell JH, Dominguez DY *et al.* Angiotensin II stimulates insulin-independent glucose uptake in hypertrophied rat hearts [abstract]. *J Hypertens* 1997; 15(suppl 4):S84.
56. Schorb W, Peeler TC, Madigan NN *et al.* Angiotensin II-induced protein tyrosine phosphorylation in neonatal rat. *J Biol Chem* 1994; 269:19626–19632.
57. Wan J, Kurosaki T, Huant XY *et al.* Tyrosine kinases in activation of the MAP-kinase cascade by G protein-coupled receptors. *Nature* 1996; 380:541–544.
58. Saad MJA, Velloso LA, Carvalho CRO. Angiotensin II induces tyrosine phosphorylation of insulin receptor substrate 1 and its association with phosphatidylinositol 3-kinase in rat heart. *Biochem J* 1995; 310:741–744.
59. Bernobich E, de Angelis L, Lerin C, Bellini G. The role of the angiotensin system in cardiac glucose homeostasis: therapeutic implications. *Drugs* 2002; 62:1295–1314.

60. The CONSENSUS Trial Study Group. Effects of enalapril on mortality in severe congestive heart failure. Results of the Cooperative North Scandinavian Enalapril Survival Study (CONSENSUS). *N Engl J Med* 1987; 316:1429–1435.
61. Garg R, Yusuf S. Overview of randomized trials of angiotensin-converting enzyme inhibitors on mortality and morbidity in patients with heart failure. Collaborative Group on ACE Inhibitor Trials. *JAMA* 1995; 273:1450–1456.
62. Flather MD, Yusuf S, Kober L *et al.* Long-Term ACE-inhibitor therapy in patients with heart failure or left-ventricular dysfunction: a systematic overview of data from individual patients. ACE-Inhibitor Myocardial Infarction Collaborative Group. *Lancet* 2000; 355:1575–1581.
63. The Acute Infarction Ramipril Efficacy (AIRE) Study Investigators. Effect of ramipril on mortality and morbidity of survivors of acute myocardial infarction with clinical evidence of heart failure. *Lancet* 1993; 342:821–828.
64. ACE Inhibitor Myocardial Infarction Collaborative Group. Indications for ACE inhibitors in the early treatment of acute myocardial infarction: systematic overview of individual data from 100,000 patients in randomized trials. *Circulation* 1998; 97:2202–2212.
65. Honan MB, Harrell FE, Jr, Reimer KA *et al.* Cardiac rupture, mortality and the timing of thrombolytic therapy: a meta-analysis. *J Am Coll Cardiol* 1990; 16:359–367.
66. Yusuf S, Sleight P, Pogue J, Bosch J, Davies R, Dagenais G. Effects of an angiotensin-converting-enzyme inhibitor, ramipril, on cardiovascular events in high-risk patients. The Heart Outcomes Prevention Evaluation Study Investigators. *N Engl J Med* 2000; 342:145–153.
67. Lonn E, Yusuf S, Dzavik V, Doris I, Yi Q, Smith S, Moore-Cox A. Effects of ramipril and vitamin E on atherosclerosis: the Study to Evaluate Carotid Ultrasound Changes in Patients Treated with Ramipril and Vitamin E (SECURE). *Circulation* 2001; 103:919–925.
68. Lonn EM, Shaishkoleslami R, Yi Q, Bosch J, Magi A, Yusuf S. Effects of rampiril on left ventricular mass and function in normotensive, high-risk patients with normal ejection fraction. A substudy of HOPE. *J Am Coll Cardiol* 2001; 37(suppl 2A):165A.
69. Yusuf S. From the Heart Outcomes Prevention Evaluation Study to Ongoing Telmisartan Alone and in Combination with Ramipril Global Endpoint Trial and the Telmisartan Randomized Assessment Study in Angiotensin-Converting Enzyme Inhibitor Intolerant Patients with Cardiovascular Disease: challenges in improving prognosis. *Am J Cardiol* 2002; 89(suppl):18A–26A.
70. Dahlof B, Devereux RB, Kjeldsen SE *et al.* Cardiovascular morbidity and mortality in the Losartan Intervention for Endpoint reduction in hypertension study (LIFE): a randomized trial against atenolol. *Lancet* 2002; 359:995–1003.
71. Julius S, Kjeldsen SE, Weber M *et al.*, for the VALUE trial group. Outcomes in hypertensive patients at high cardiovascular risk treated with regimens based on Valsartan or Amlodipine: the VALUE randomized trial. *Lancet* 2004; 363:2022–2031.
72. Lewis EJ, Hunsicker LG, Clarke WR *et al.* Renoprotective effect of the angiotensin-receptor antagonist irbesartan in patients with nephropathy due to type 2 diabetes. *N Engl J Med* 2001; 345:851–860.
73. Parving HH, Lehnert H, Brochner-Mortensen J *et al.* The effect of irbesartan on the development of diabetic nephropathy in patients with type 2 diabetes. *N Engl J Med* 2001; 345:870–878.
74. Brenner BM, Cooper ME, de Zeeuw D *et al.* Effects of losartan on renal and cardiovascular outcomes in patients with type 2 diabetes and nephropathy. *N Engl J Med* 2001; 345:861–869.
75. Dickstein K, Kjekshus J, OPTIMAAL Steering Committee of the OPTIMAAL Study Group. Effects of losartan and captopril on mortality and morbidity in high-risk patients after acute myocardial infarction: the OPTIMAAL randomized trial. Optimal Trial in myocardial infarction with angiotensin II antagonist Losartan. *Lancet* 2002; 360:752–760.
76. Pfeffer MA, McMurray JJV, Velazquez EJ *et al.*, for the Valsartan in Acute Myocardial Infarction Trial Investigators. Valsartan, captopril, or both in myocardial infarction complicated by heart failure, left ventricular dysfunction, or both. *N Engl J Med* 2003; 349:1893–1906.
77. Pitt B, Poole-Wilson PA, Segal R *et al.* Effect of losartan compared with captopril on mortality in patients with symptomatic heart failure: randomized trial – the Losartan Heart Failure Survival Study ELITE II. *Lancet* 2000; 355:1582–1587.
78. Cohn JN, Tognoni G, Valsartan Heart Failure Trial Investigators. A randomized trial of the angiotensin-receptor blocker valsartan in chronic heart failure. *N Engl J Med* 2001; 345:1667–1675.
79. Pfeffer MA, Swedberg K, Granger CB *et al.;* CHARM Investigators and Committees. Effects of candesartan on mortality and morbidity in patients with chronic heart failure: the CHARM-Overall programme. *Lancet* 2003; 362:759–766.

80. Granger CB, McMurray JJ, Yusuf S *et al.*; CHARM Investigators and Committees. Effects of candesartan in patients with chronic heart failure and reduced left-ventricular systolic function intolerant to angiotensin-converting-enzyme inhibitors: the CHARM-Alternative Trial. *Lancet* 2003; 362:772–776.
81. McMurray JJ, Ostergren J, Swedberg K *et al.*; CHARM Investigators and Committees. Effects of candesartan in patients with chronic heart failure and reduced left ventricular systolic function taking angiotensin-converting-enzyme inhibitors: the CHARM-Added trial. *Lancet* 2003; 362:767–771.
82. Yusuf S, Pfeffer MA, Swedberg K *et al.*; CHARM Investigators and Committees. Effects of candesartan in patients with chronic heart failure and preserved left-ventricular ejection fraction: the CHARM-Preserved trial. *Lancet* 2003; 362:777–781.
83. Lindholm LH, Ibsen H, Dahlof B *et al.* Cardiovascular morbidity and mortality in patients with diabetes in the Losartan Intervention for Endpoint reduction in hypertension study (LIFE): a randomized trial against Atenolol. *Lancet* 2002; 359:1004–1010.
84. Yusuf S, Gerstein H, Hoogwerf B *et al.* for the HOPE Study Investigators. Ramipril and the development of diabetes. *JAMA* 2001; 286:1882–1885.
85. The ALLHAT Officers and Coordinators for the ALLHAT Collaborative Research Group. Major outcomes in high-risk hypertensive patients randomized to angiotensin-converting enzyme inhibitor or calcium channel blocker vs diuretic: The Antihypertensive and Lipid-Lowering Treatment to Prevent Heart Attack Trial (ALLHAT). *JAMA* 2002; 288:2981–2997.
86. Vermes E, Ducharme A, Bourassa MG, Lessard M, White M, Tardiff JC. Enalapril reduces the incidence of diabetes in patients with chronic heart failure : insight from the Studies Of Left Ventricular Dysfunction (SOLVD). *Circulation* 2003; 107:1291–1296.
87. Lindholm LH, Persson M, Alaupovic P, Carlberg B, Svensson A, Samuelsson O. Metabolic outcome during 1 year in newly detected hypertensives: results of the Antihypertensive Treatment and Lipid Profile in a North of Sweden Efficacy Evaluation (ALPINE study). *J Hypertens* 2003; 21:1563–1574.
88. Papademetriou V, Farsang C, Elmfeldt D *et al.* Study on cognition and prognosis in the elderly study group. Stroke prevention with the angiotensin II type 1-receptor blocker candesartan in elderly patients with isolated systolic hypertension: the Study on Cognition and Prognosis in the Elderly (SCOPE). *J Am Coll Cardiol* 2004; 44:1175–1180.
89. Ekbom T, Linjer E, Hedner T *et al.* Cardiovascular events in elderly patients with isolated systolic hypertension. A subgroup analysis of treatment strategies in STOP-Hypertension-2. *Blood Press* 2004; 13:137–141.
90. The Captopril Prevention Project (CAPP) Study Group. Effect of angiotensin-converting enzyme inhibition compared with conventional therapy on cardiovascular morbidity and mortality in hypertension: the Captopril Prevention Project (CAPP) randomized trial. *Curr Hypertens Rep* 1999; 1:466–467.
91. The PEACE Trial Investigators. Angiotensin converting enzyme inhibitors in stable coronary disease. *N Eng J Med* 2004; 350:2058–2068.
92. Andraws R, Brown DL. Effect of inhibition of the renin–angiotensin system on development of type 2 diabetes mellitus (meta-analysis of randomized trials). *Am J Cardiol* 2007; 99:1006–1012.
93. Yusuf S, Ostergren JB, Hertzel C *et al* on behalf of the Candesartan in Heart Failure – Assessment of Reduction in Mortality and Morbidity Program (CHARM) Investigators. Effects of candesartan on the development of a new diagnosis of diabetes mellitus in patients with heart failure. *Circ* 2005; 112:48–53.
94. Kurtz TW, Pravenec M. Antidiabetic mechanisms of angiotensin-converting enzyme inhibitors and angiotensin II receptor antagonists: beyond the renin-angiotensin system. *J Hypertens* 2004; 22:2253–2261.
95. Scheen AJ. Renin-angiotensin system inhibition prevents type 2 diabetes mellitus. Part 1. A meta-analysis of randomised clinical trials. *Diabetes Metab* 2004; 30:487–496.
96. Fonseca VA. Insulin resistance, diabetes, hypertension, and renin-angiotensin system inhibition: reducing risk for cardiovascular disease. *J Clin Hypertens* (*Greenwich*) 2006; 8:713–720.
97. Mazzone T. Strategies in ongoing clinical trials to reduce cardiovascular disease in patients with diabetic mellitus and insulin resistance. *Am J Cardiol* 2004; 93:27C–31C.
98. Drexler AJ. Lessons learned from landmark trials of type 2 diabetes mellitus and potential applications to clinical practice. *Postgrad Med* 2003; Spec. no.:15–26.
99. DREAM Trial Investigators. Rationale, design and recruitment characteristics of a large, simple international trial of diabetes prevention: the DREAM trial. *Diabetologia* 2004; 47:1519–1527.

100. DREAM Trial Investigators. Ramipril's effect on incident diabetes in impaired glucose regulation. *N Engl J Med* 2006; 355:1551–1562.
101. The DREAM (Diabetes REduction Assessment with ramipril and rosiglitazone Medication) Trial Investigators. Effect of rosiglitazone on the frequency of diabetes in patients with impaired glucose tolerance or impaired fasting glucose: a randomised controlled trial. *Lancet* 2006; 368:1096–1105.
102. Buchanan TA, Xiang AH, Peters RK *et al.* Preservation of pancreatic beta-cell function and prevention of type 2 diabetes by pharmacological treatment of insulin resistance in high-risk hispanic women. *Diabetes* 2002; 51:2796–2803.
103. Buchanan TA, Xiang AH, Peters RK *et al.* Response of pancreatic beta-cells to improved insulin sensitivity in women at high risk for type 2 diabetes. *Diabetes* 2000; 49:782–728.
104. Diabetes Prevention Program Research Group. Prevention of type 2 diabetes with troglitazone in the Diabetes Prevention Program. *Diabetes* 2005; 54:1150–1156.
105. Leiter LA. Beta-cell preservation: a potential role for thiazolidinediones to improve clinical care in type 2 diabetes. *Diabet Med* 2005; 22:963–972.
106. Dormandy J, Charbonnel B, Eckland DJ *et al.* Secondary prevention of macrovascular events in patients with type 2 diabetes in the PROactive Study (PROspective pioglitAzone Clinical Trial In macroVascular Events): a randomised controlled trial. *Lancet* 2005; 366:1279–1289.
107. Aranda JM, Jr, Conti R. Angiotensin II blockade: A therapeutic strategy with wide applications. *Clin Cardiol* 2003; 26:500–502.
108. Hsueh WA, Quinones MJ. Role of endothelial dysfunction in insulin resistance. *Am J Cardiol* 2003; 92:10J–17J.
109. Savoia C, Schiffrin EL. Inhibition of the renin angiotensin system: implications for the endothelium. *Curr Diab Rep* 2006; 6:274–278.
110. Kingston R. Blockade of the renin-angiotensin system decreases adipocyte size with improvement in insulin sensitivity. *J Hypertens* 2004; 22:1867–1868.
111. Carlsson PO, Bernie C, Jansson, L. Angiotensin II and the endocrine pancreas; effects on islet blood flow and insulin secretion in rats. *Diabetologia* 1998; 41:127–133.
112. Sharma AM, Janke J, Gorzelniak K *et al.* Angiotensin blockade prevents type 2 diabetes by formation of fat cells. *Hypertension* 2002; 40:609–611.
113. Furuhashi M, Ura N, Takizawa H *et al.* Blockade of the renin-angiotensin system decreases adipocyte size with improvement in insulin sensitivity. *J Hypertens* 2004; 22:1977–1982.
114. Henriksen EJ, Jacob S. Angiotensin converting enzyme inhibitors and modulation of skeletal muscle insulin resistance. *Diabetes Obes Metab* 2003; 5:214–222.
115. Henriksen EJ, Jacob S, Kinnick TR *et al.* ACE inhibition and glucose transport in insulin resistant muscle: roles of bradykinin and nitric oxide. *Am J Physiol* 1999; 277:R332–R336.
116. Folli F, Saad MJ, Velloso L *et al.* Crosstalk between insulin and angiotensin II signaling systems. *Exp Clin Endocrinol Diabetes* 1999; 196:171–179.
117. Sharma AM, Janke J. Gorzelniak K, Engeli S, Luft SC. Angiotensin blockade prevents type 2 diabetes by formation of fat cells. *Hypertension* 2002; 40:609–611
118. Furuhashi M, Ura N, Higashiura K *et al.* Blockade of the renin-angiotensin system increases adiponectin concentrations in patients with essential hypertension. *Hypertension* 2003; 42:76–81.
119. Snehalatha C, Mukesh B, Simon M, Viswanathan V, Haffner SM, Ramachandran A. Plasma adiponectin is an independent predictor of type 2 diabetes in Asian indians. *Diabetes Care* 2003; 26:3226–3229.
120. Saris JJ, van Dijk MA, Kroon I, Schalekamp MA, Danser AH. Functional importance of angiotensin-converting enzyme-dependent in situ angiotensin II generation in the human forearm. *Hypertension* 2000; 35:764–768.
121. Lyons D, Webster J, Benjamin N. Effect of enalapril and quinapril on forearm vascular ACE in man. *Eur J Clin Pharmacol* 1997; 51:373–378.
122. Padmanabhan N, Jardine AG, McGrath JC, Connell JM. Angiotensin-converting enzyme-independent contraction to angiotensin I in human resistance arteries. *Circulation* 1999; 99:2914–2920.
123. Hornig B, Arakawa N, Haussmann D, Drexler H. Differential effects of quinaprilat and Enalapril on endothelial function of conduit arteries in patients with chronic heart failure. *Circulation* 1998; 98:2842–2848.
124. Prasad A, Husain S, Quyyumi AA. Effect of enalapril on nitric oxide activity in coronary artery disease. *Am J Cardiol* 1999; 84:1–6.
125. Anderson TJ, Elstein E, Haber H, Charbonneau F. Comparative study of ACE-inhibition, angiotensin II antagonism, and calcium channel blockade on flow-mediated vasodilation in patients with coronary disease (BANFF study). *J Am Coll Cardiol* 2000; 35:60–66.

126. Scheen AJ. Part 2. Overview to physiological and biochemical mechanisms. Renin-angiotensin system inhibition prevents type 2 diabetes mellitus. *Diabetes* 2004; 30:498–505.
127. Scheen AJ. Pathophysiology of insulin secretion. *Ann Endocrinol* 2004; 65:29–36
128. White M, Racine N, Ducharme A, de Champlain J. Therapeutic potential of angiotensin II receptor antagonists. *Expert Opin Investig Drugs* 2001; 10:1687–1701.
129. Bak JF, Gerdes LU, Sorenson NS *et al.* Effects of perindopril on insulin sensitivity and plasma lipid profile in hypertensive non-insulin-dependent diabetic patients. *Am J Med* 1992; 92:69S–72S.
130. Paolisso G, Balbi V, Gambardella A *et al.* Lisinopril administration improves insulin action in aged patients with hypertension. *J Hum Hypertens* 1995; 9:541–546.
131. Thurig C, Bohlen L, Schneider M *et al.* Lisinopril is neutral to insulin sensitivity and serum lipoproteins in essential hypertensive patients. *Eur J Clin Pharmacol* 1995; 49:21–26.
132. Vuorinen-Markolla H, Yki-Jarvinen H. Antihypertensive therapy with enalapril improves glucose storage and insulin sensitivity in hypertensive patients with non-insulin-dependent diabetes mellitus. *Metabolism* 1995; 44:85–89.
133. Falkner B, Canessa M, Anzalone D. Effect of angiotensin converting enzyme inhibitor (lisinopril) on insulin sensitivity and sodium transport in mild hypertension. *Am J Hypertens* 1995; 8:454–460.
134. Bohlen L, Bienz R, Doser M *et al.* Metabolic neutrality of perindopril: focus on insulin sensitivity in overweight patients with essential hypertension. *J Cardiovasc Pharmacol* 1996; 27:770–776.
135. Petrie JR, Morris AD, Ueda S *et al.* Trandopril does not improve insulin sensitivity in patients with hypertension and type 2 diabetes: a double-blind, placebo-controlled crossover trial. *J Clin Endocrinol Metab* 2000; 85:1882–1889.
136. Laasko M, Karjalainen L, Lempiainen-Kuosa P. Effects of losartan on insulin sensitivity in hypertensive subjects. *Hypertension* 1996; 28:392–396.
137. Paolisso G, Tagliamonte MR, Gambardella A *et al.* losartan mediated improvement in insulin action is mainly due to a non-oxidative glucose metabolism and blood flow in insulin-resistant hypertensive patients. *J Hum Hypertens* 1997; 11:307–312.
138. Fogari R, Zoppi A, Lazzari P *et al.* ACE-inhibition but not angiotensin II antagonism reduces plasma fibrinogen and insulin resistance in overweight hypertensive patients. *J Cardiovasc Pharmacol* 1998; 32:616–620.
139. Fogari R, Zoppi A, Corradi L *et al.* Comparative effects of lisinopril and losartan on insulin sensitivity in the treatment of non-diabetic hypertensive patients. *Br J Clin Pharmacol* 1998; 46:467–471.
140. Trenkwalder P, Dahl K, Lehtovirta M *et al.* Antihypertensive treatment with candesartan cilexitil does not affect glucose homeostasis or serum lipid profile in patients with mild hypertension and type II diabetes. *Blood Press* 1998; 7:170–175.
141. Higashiura K, Ura N, Miyazaki Y *et al.* Effects of angiotensin II receptor antagonist, candesartan cilexitil, on insulin resistance and pressor mechanisms in essential hypertension. *J Hum Hypertens* 1999; 13(suppl 1):S71–S74.
142. Schupp M, Janke J, Clasen R *et al.* Angiotensin type I receptor blockers induce peroxisome proliferator activated receptor gamma activity. *Circulation* 2004; 109:2054–2057.
143. Shepherd J, Cobbe SM, Ford I *et al.* Prevention of coronary heart disease with pravastatin in men with hypercholesterolemia. West of Scotland Coronary Prevention Study Group. *N Engl J Med* 1995; 333:1301–1307.
144. Hennes MMI, O'Shaughnessy IM, Kelly TM, LaBelle P, Egan BM, Kissebah AH. Insulin-resistant lipolysis in abdominally obese hypertensive individuals. Role of the renin-angiotensin system. *Hypertension* 1996; 28:120–126.
145. Buchanan TA. Prevention of type 2 diabetes: What is it really? *Diabetes Care* 2003; 26:1306–1308.
146. The ONTARGET/TRANSCEND Investigators. Rationale, design, and baseline characteristics of 2 large, simple randomized trials evaluating telmisartan, ramipril, and their combination in high-risk patients; the ongoing Telmisartan alone and in combination with Ramipril Global Endpoint Trial/Telmisartan Randomized Assessment Study in ACE Intolerant Subjects with Cardiovascular Disease (ONTARGET/TRANSCEND) trials. *Am Heart J* 2004; 148:52–61.

7

Lipid management in the metabolic syndrome

O. P. Ganda

INTRODUCTION

The metabolic syndrome is a strong predictor of diabetes as well as cardiovascular disease as shown in many long-term studies. In one of the longest prospective studies, the Nurses Health Study, approximately 6000 of the 117 000 women developed diabetes during 20 years of follow-up. During the prediabetes period, the risk of myocardial infarction (MI) or stroke was 2.8-fold greater in those who subsequently developed diabetes compared to those who remained non-diabetic [1]. There is evidence from multiple studies in men and women that lipid abnormalities, along with other features of metabolic syndrome, namely abdominal obesity, hypertension and glucose intolerance predominate in a vast majority of individuals in the prediabetic phase. Moreover, multiple features of metabolic syndrome contributed to the progressive increase in the risk of coronary heart disease (CHD) events in >4400 subjects followed over 10 years in the Strong Heart Study of Native Americans (Figure 7.1) [2].

LIPOPROTEIN ABNORMALITIES ASSOCIATED WITH METABOLIC SYNDROME

The dyslipidemia of type 2 diabetes, metabolic syndrome and insulin resistance is characterized by a number of interrelated atherogenic abnormalities consisting of increased levels of triglyceride-rich lipoproteins (very low-density lipoprotein [VLDL], intermediate-density lipoprotein [IDL], and remnant particles), low levels of high-density lipoprotein (HDL)-cholesterol, as well as increased levels of small, dense low-density lipoprotein (LDL) particles (Figure 7.2) [3, 4].

There is an increase in the lipid-rich, large VLDL (VLDL-1) upregulation of hepatic sterol regulatory element binding protein (SREBP-1), which stimulates *de novo* lipid synthesis; and increased availability of free fatty acids (FFA). All of these effects are probably linked with insulin resistance [3]. The activity of lipoprotein lipase (LPL) is suppressed leading to reduced catabolism of triglyceride-rich particles, while hepatic lipase (HL) activity is increased, facilitating the compositional changes in LDL and HDL particles.

In addition, there is enhanced activity of cholesteryl ester transfer protein (CETP), which mediates the transfer of triglyceride to LDL and HDL while cholesteryl esters from HDL are shunted to the larger triglyceride-rich particles. Thus, hypertriglyceridemia is indirectly linked with changes in the HDL and LDL composition and associated with increased atherogenesis. The small, dense LDL particles bind to intimal proteoglycans more avidly, are more susceptible to oxidation and glycation, and have impaired binding to LDL receptors. All of these factors contribute to enhanced atherosclerosis in patients with metabolic syndrome.

Om P. Ganda, MD, Director, Lipid Clinic, Joslin Diabetes Center; Associate Clinical Professor of Medicine, Harvard Medical School, Boston, Massachusetts, USA

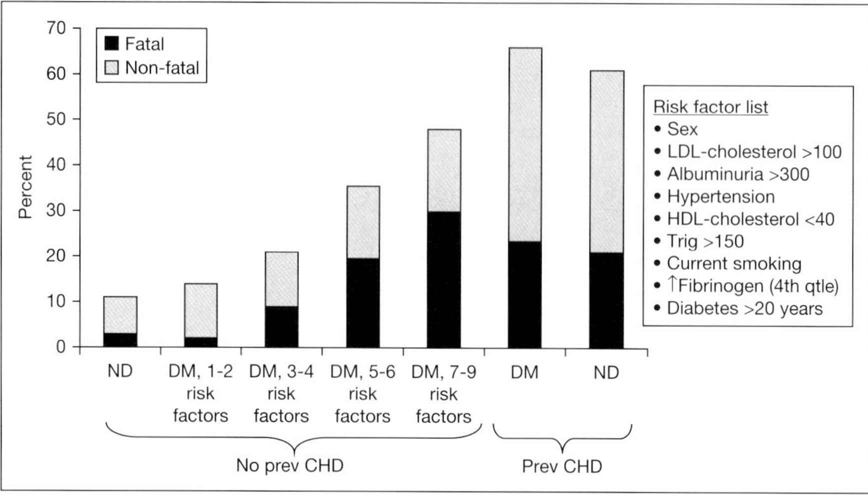

Figure 7.1 The 10-year cumulative incidence of CHD by numbers of baseline risk factors. With permission from [2]. DM = diabetes mellitus; ND = non-diabetic

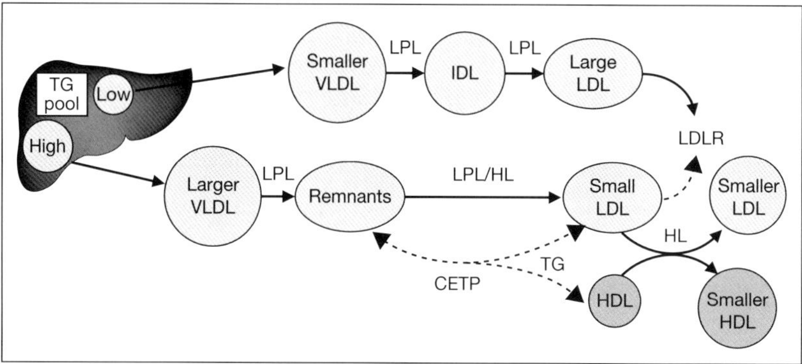

Figure 7.2 Pathophysiology of dislipidemia in type 2 diabetes. With permission from [3]. CETP = cholesteryl ester transfer protein; HDL = high-density lipoprotein; HL = hepatic lipase; IDL = intermediate-density lipoprotein; LDL = low-density lipoprotein; TG = triglyceride; VLDL = very low-density lipoprotein.

Lipoprotein particle size and concentrations have been characterized by nuclear magnetic resonance (NMR) in subjects with type 2 diabetes, and normal or impaired insulin sensitivity characterized by euglycemic, hyperinsulinemic clamp technique [5]. There was a progressive increase in the size of VLDL particles in insulin-sensitive, insulin-resistant, and type 2 diabetes subjects respectively, as well as a reciprocal decrease in the size of LDL and HDL particles. On the other hand, the cholesterol content in large LDL was increased and that in small LDL was decreased in those with insulin resistance and type 2 diabetes, whereas the calculated LDL-cholesterol was relatively unchanged despite increased LDL particle number.

In view of the compositional changes in lipoproteins, the LDL-cholesterol determined in routine assays tends to underestimate the LDL particle number, particularly in patients with hypertriglyceridemia. It has therefore been proposed that direct measurement of apoliprotein B (apoB) might provide a better estimate of risk in such patients [6, 7]. However, the assays for

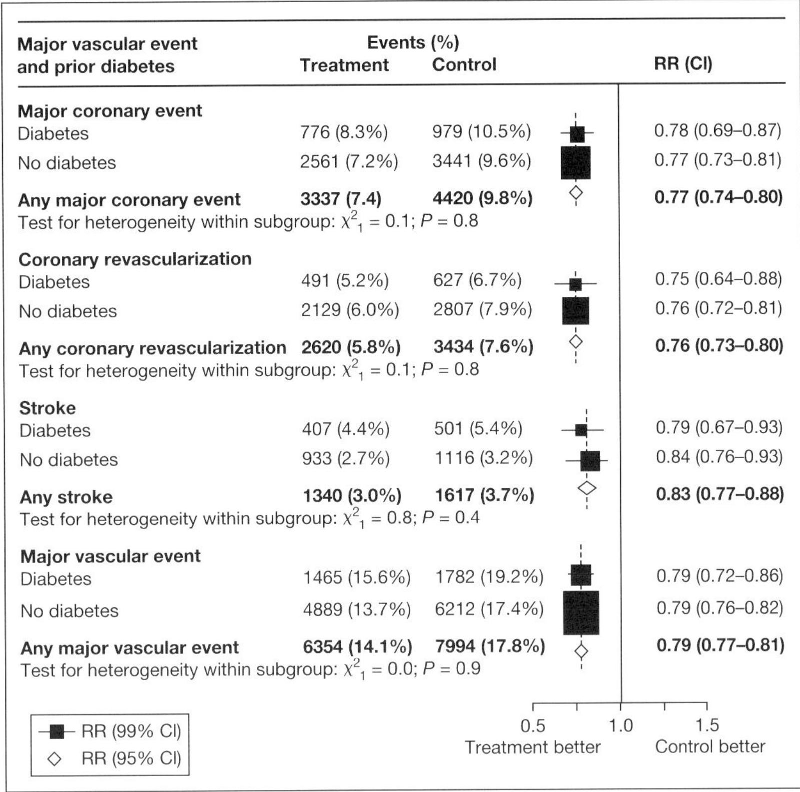

Figure 7.3 Meta-analysis of statin trials: major vascular event reduction per 1mM/l reduction in LDL-cholesterol. With permission from [9]. CI = confidence interval; DM = diabetes mellitus; RCT = randomized controlled trial; RR = relative risk

apoB are not well standardized or widely available. An alternative proposed by the National Cholesterol Education Program's Adult Treatment Panel III (NCEP ATP III) is the calculation of non-HDL-cholesterol, which estimates the cholesterol content in all atherogenic particles: VLDL, IDL, remnant particles, LDL and lipoprotein (a) (Lp(a)).

IMPLICATIONS FOR CARDIOVASCULAR OUTCOMES FROM LIPID-LOWERING TRIALS

LOW-DENSITY LIPOPROTEIN-LOWERING TRIALS

Given the heterogeneity of lipoproteins and the complexity of lipoprotein metabolism in patients with metabolic syndrome, the optimal approach for lipid management in patients with the metabolic syndrome remains to be determined. Since the mid-1990s a variety of randomized, controlled trials with HMG-CoA reductase inhibitors (statins) have established the efficacy of these LDL-lowering agents in reducing cardiovascular outcomes.

In a recent meta-analysis of 16 randomized trials of statin therapy, encompassing 90 056 individuals from various parts of the world, a mean LDL-cholesterol reduction of 1 mmol (~40 mg/dl) over 5 years resulted in a 23% reduction in MI or coronary death ($P < 0.0001$), a 17% reduction in stroke, ($P < 0.001$) and a 12% reduction in all-cause mortality ($P < 0.0001$) [8]. Similar benefits were seen in detailed analyses of patients with diabetes (n = 18 686) (Figure 7.3), or components of metabolic syndrome (HDL-cholesterol, triglycerides,

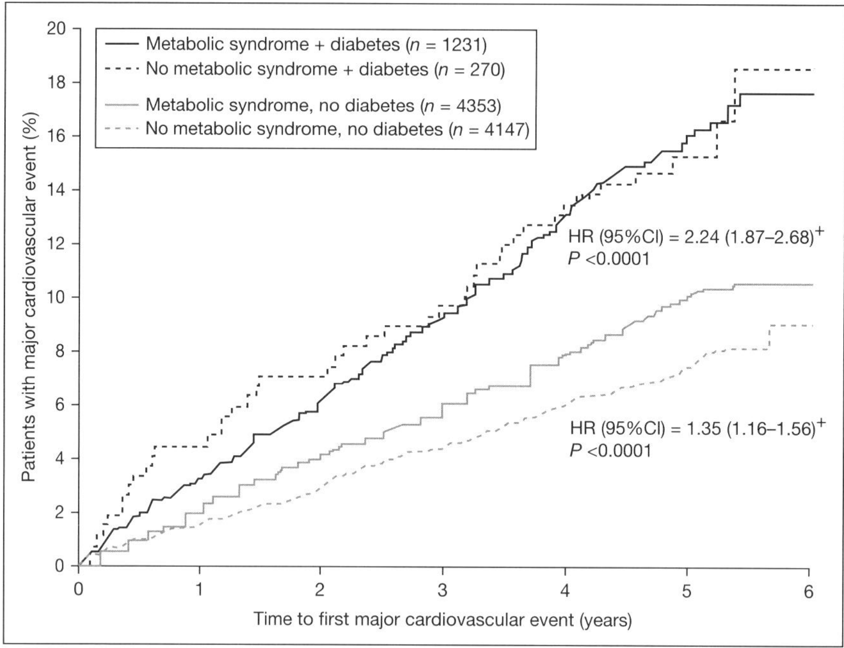

Figure 7.4 TNT: major cardiovascular events by metabolic syndrome and diabetes status. With permission from [12]. CI = confidence interval; HR = hazard ratio.

hypertension), although the absolute risk of events was greater in those with hypertriglyceridemia, low HDL-cholesterol or hypertension [9].

In another meta-analysis of twelve large, randomized trials, comparing patients with or without diabetes, similar risk reductions of 21–23% in CHD events were found in both populations in primary or secondary prevention [10]. Since the absolute baseline risk in patients with diabetes is greater, the benefit in such patients, with similar decrease in lipid levels, was correspondingly greater, especially in secondary prevention.

Although these differences in benefits with statin therapy have not been shown conclusively in patients with metabolic syndrome in the absence of diabetes, there are two studies which suggest that patients with metabolic syndrome may, in fact, have greater benefit compared to those without metabolic syndrome. The first is the sub-analysis of data from the Scandinavian Simvastatin Survival Study (4S) trial [11]. In that analysis, those with the lipid triad (high LDL, high triglyceride, low HDL) had a coronary event rate of 0.48 (confidence interval [CI] 0.33–0.69) compared to those with isolated high LDL alone, (event rate 0.86; CI 0.59–1.26). More recently, a re-analysis of the Treat to New Target (TNT) statin trial was carried out according to the presence or absence of metabolic syndrome, as defined by the revised ATP III criteria [12]. Of the 10 001 patients in this trial, comparing efficacy of atorvastatin 80 mg vs 10 mg in patients with clinically stable CHD, 5584 had metabolic syndrome. Irrespective of treatment assignment, the hazard ratio (HR) of CHD events over 5 years of follow-up in those with metabolic syndrome was 1.35 ($P < 0.001$), compared to those without (Figure 7.4).

Furthermore, there was a 30% risk reduction in CHD events with atorvastatin 80 mg vs 10 mg in patients with metabolic syndrome, in the presence or absence of diabetes (Figure 7.5),

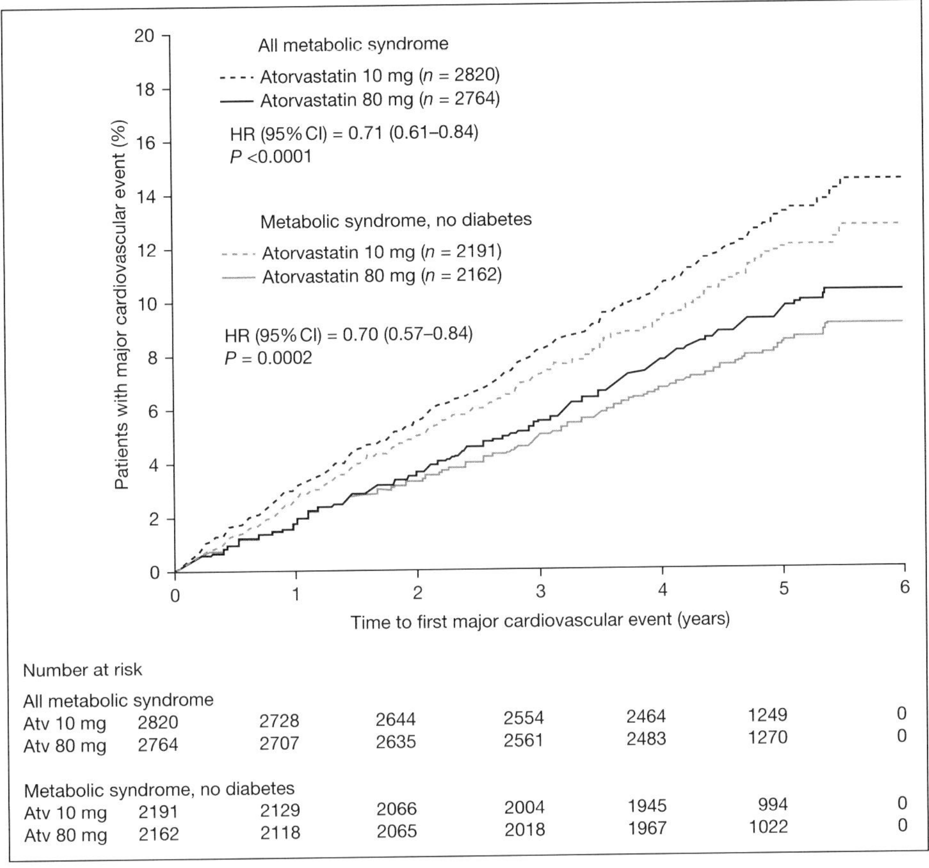

Figure 7.5 TNT: major cardiovascular events by treatment and metabolic status. With permission from [12]. Atv = atorvastatin; CI = confidence interval; HR = hazard ratio.

although patients with diabetes and metabolic syndrome were at the highest risk (Figure 7.4). It is currently debated whether the putative anti-inflammatory effects of statins may account for part of the benefits in patients with metabolic syndrome [13].

EFFICACY AND SAFETY OF INTENSIVE LIPID-LOWERING WITH STATINS

In view of the markedly increased risk of subsequent cardiovascular events (CHD and stroke) in patients with pre-existing CHD, the current update of the ATP III guidelines and American Heart Association (AHA) guidelines recommend an LDL-cholesterol goal of <70 mg/dl in all patients in this category [14]. A recent meta-analysis included four trials of intensive LDL-lowering therapy in patients with acute coronary syndromes (PROVE-IT and A-to-Z) or stable coronary artery disease (CAD) (TNT and IDEAL), involving 27 548 patients [15]. Of these, 4379 patients had diabetes. The mean LDL-cholesterol achieved by intensive therapy was 75 mg/dl, compared to 101 mg/dl by standard treatment. This analysis revealed a 16% risk reduction in coronary death or MI ($P < 0.0003$) and an 18% risk reduction in stroke ($P = 0.012$) (Figure 7.6). Similar outcomes were observed in patients with diabetes. However, these analyses were underpowered for effects on cardiovascular or total mortality. Of some concern is the small, but significant, increase in hepatic toxicity with more intensive therapy, using 80 mg

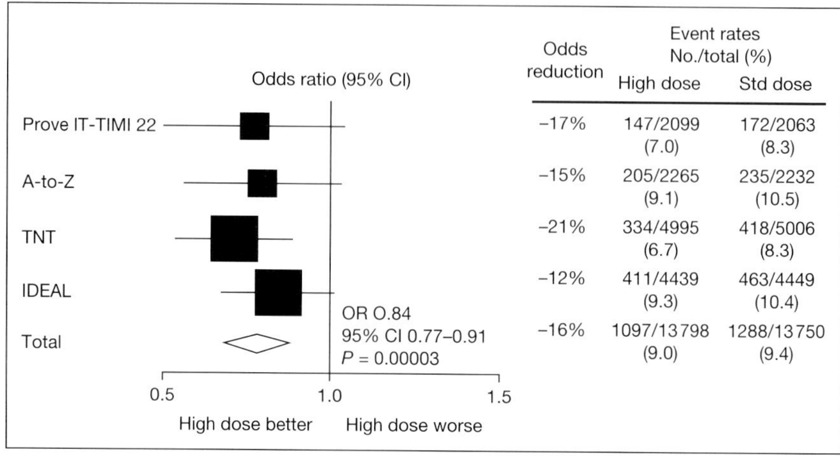

Figure 7.6 Meta-analysis of intensive statin trials: coronary death or myocardial infarction (with permission from [15]).

Table 7.1 Intensive statin trials: severe adverse events (with permission from [15])

	Rhabdomyolysis (n)*		***CK >10 × ULN (n)†***		***AST and /or ALT >33 ULN (n)‡***	
Trial	***Standard dose (%)***	***High dose (%)***	***Standard dose (%)***	***High dose (%)***	***Standard dose (%)***	***High dose (%)***
PROVE IT-TIMI-22 (2,6)(n = 4162)	0	0	0.10	0.15	1.1	3.3
A-to-Z (4)(n = 4497)	0	0.13	0.04	0.4	0.36	0.84
TNT (3)(n = 10 001)	0.06	0.04	0	0	0.18	1.2
IDEAL (5)(n = 8888)	0.07	0.05	0	0	0.16	1.37

Follow-up periods are 2 years for the PROVE IT-TIMI-22 trials and 5 years for the TNT and IDEAL trials. Percentages for all events except those in the PROVE IT-TIMI-22 trial were back-calculated from numbers presented in published manuscripts.*Cases were based on the treating physician's diagnosis for the TNT and IDEAL trials, and a definition of CK level higher than 10 000 U/I for A-to-Z . †A-to-Z reported with an additional patient with an alcohol-related rise in CK without muscle symptoms. ‡The PROVE IT-TIMI-22 trial reported elevations in ALT; IDEAL reported a number of abnormalities.
ALT = alanine aminotransferase; AST = aspartate aminotransferase; CK = creatine kinase; ULN = upper limit of normal.

dosing of both atorvastatin and simvastatin in these trials; however, there was no significant increase in the incidence of myositis or rhabdomyolysis (Table 7.1). In many patients with intolerance to higher dose statins, and consequent difficulty in achieving the LDL goal, combinations of lower dose statins with cholesterol absorption inhibitors (ezetimibe, bile acid sequestrants e.g. cholestyramine, colesevelam), or niacin are very useful strategies [16, 17]. However, in a recent trial in patients with familial hypercholesterolemia, the addition of ezetimibe to simvastatin 80mg resulted in a non-significant increase in the carotid artery intima-media thickness, compared to simvastatin alone despite a 16% greater reduction in LDL-c, after 2 years [18]. The clinical significance of this finding remains uncertain, pending ongoing studies.

	Relative risk (95% CI)
Unadjusted (21 studies)	
Men (n = 65863)	1.30 (1.25–1.35)
Women (n = 11089)	1.69 (1.45–1.97)
Adjusted for HDL-Cholesterol	
Men (n = 29105)	1.12 (1.06–1.19)
Women (n = 6345)	1.37 (1.13–1.66)

Figure 7.7 Hypertrigylceridemia and CHD: a meta-analysis of 21 studies. With permission from [19].

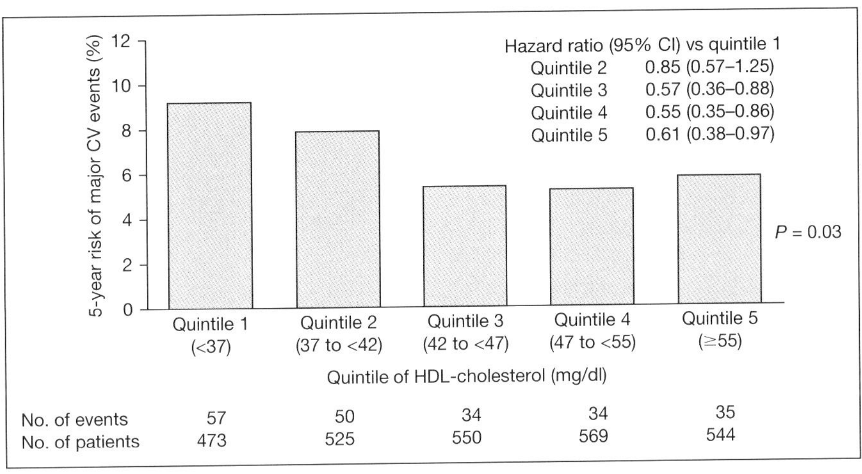

Figure 7.8 Treat to New Targets (TNT) trial subanalyses: hazard ratios for the quintiles of HDL levels on 5-year major cardiovascular events in patients achieving LDL-c level <70 mg/dl. With permission from [20].

EVIDENCE FOR THE BENEFITS OF TRIGLYCERIDE- AND HDL-INTERVENTION

The triglyceride-rich lipoproteins and low HDL-cholesterol are intimate components of the metabolic syndrome. Unlike the evidence from a plethora of trials of CHD risk reduction with statins, the direct evidence from drugs to lower triglycerides or to raise HDL-cholesterol is relatively limited. A meta-analysis of 21 observational studies suggested a significant relationship of triglycerides with CHD, even after adjustment for HDL-cholesterol, especially in women [19] (Figure 7.7). In the 4S trial, in *post-hoc* analyses, patients with the lipid triad (elevated LDL, elevated triglyceride and low HDL cholesterol) had the highest event rates in the placebo arm and the greatest risk reduction with simvastatin [11]. Similarly, the TNT trial sub-analyses strongly suggest increasing CHD risk with number of metabolic syndrome characteristics (see above). Furthermore, a recent further analysis of the TNT trial [20] revealed that in patients achieving an on-treatment LDL-cholesterol of <70 mg/dl, the risk of CHD events differed significantly by HDL-cholesterol quintiles (P = 0.003), with a 39% lower hazard ratio in patients in quintile 5 vs quintile 1 (HDL-cholesterol >55

Table 7.2 INTER-HEART: risk of acute myocardial infarction associated with risk factors in the overall population

Risk factor	*% Controls*	*% Cases*	*PAR 1 (99% CI)*	*PAR 2 (99% CI)*
apoB/apoA-1(5 v 1)	20.0	33.5	54.1 (49–58.6)	49.2 (43.8–54.5)
Current smoking	26.8	45.2	36.4 (33.9–39.0)	35.7 (32.5–39.1)
Diabetes	7.5	18.5	12.3 (11.2–13.5)	9.9 (8.5–11.5)
Hypertension	21.9	39.0	23.4 (21.7–25.1)	17.9 (15.7–20.4)
Abdominal obesity (3 v 1)	33.3	46.3	33.7 (30.2 37.4)	20.1 (15.3–26.0)
Psychosocial	–	–	28.8 (22.6–35.8)	32.5 (25.1–40.8)
Veg & fruits daily	42.4	35.8	12.9 (10.0–16.6)	13.7 (9.9–18.6)
Exercise	19.3	14.3	25.5 (20.1–31.8)	12.2 (5.5–25.1)
Alcohol	24.5	24.0	13.9 (9.3–20.2)	6.7 (2.0–20.2)
Combined	–	–	90.4 (88.1–92.4)	90.4 (80.1–92.4)

CI = confidence interval; PAR = population attributable risk.

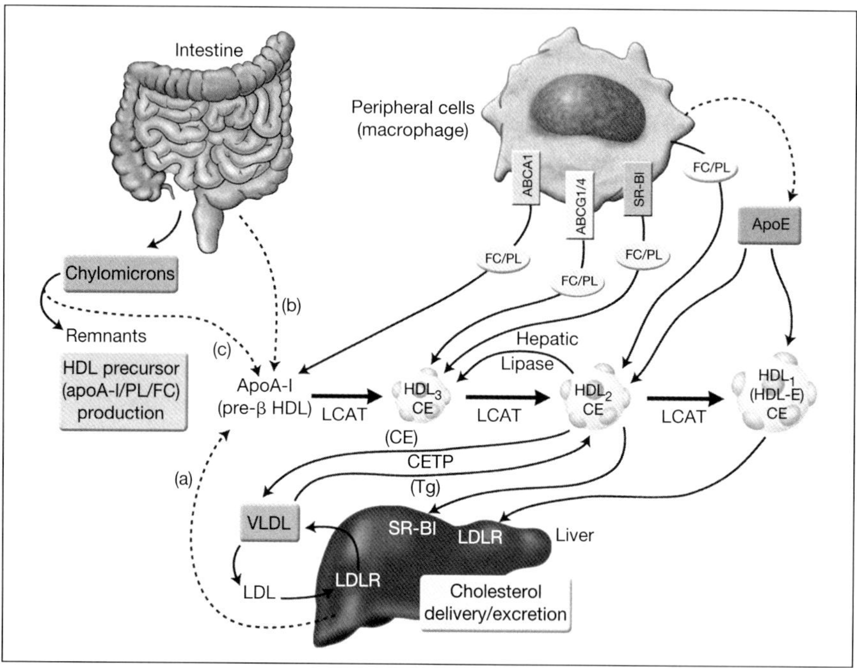

Figure 7.9 Role of HDL in the redistribution of lipids. With permission from [23].

vs <38 mg/dl) (Figure 7.8). Of note also are similar observations with triglyceride as a risk factor for CHD events in the subanalysis of the PROVE-IT trial, with a significant 37% lower hazard ratio (P <0.01) in those with triglycerides <150 vs >150 mg/dl despite achieving identical LDL-cholesterol <70mg/dl [21]. Finally, in the Interheart study, a large, case–control study of determinants of acute MI in 52 countries around the world, apoB/apoA-1 ratio, rather than either alone, was the strongest risk-determinant, along with abdominal obesity and hypertension (Table 7.2) [22].

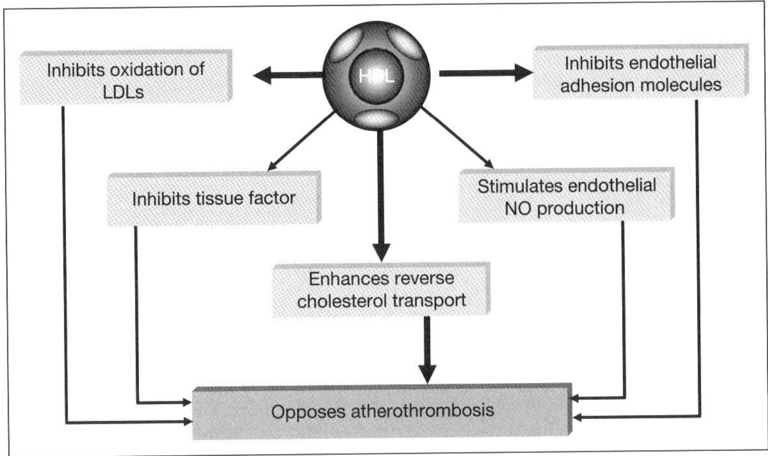

Figure 7.10 HDL effects on atherogenesis. With permission from [24]. LDL = low-density lipoprotein; NO = nitric oxide.

Table 7.3 Summary of lipid trials with fibrates in patients with diabetes or metabolic syndrome

Trial	*Drug*	*Endpoints*	*n*	*CHD*	*Outcome*	*P*
HHS	Gemfibrozil	Cardiac events/ deaths	292	No	68% reduction	<0.005
BIP	Bezafibrate	Fatal or non-fatal MI	1470	Yes	29% reduction	0.002
SENDCAP	Bezafibrate	Carotid ultrasound	328	No	No difference*	-
DAIS	Fenofibrate	Coronary stenosis on angiography	418	48% of patients	Reduced lesion progression	0.02
VA-HIT	Gemfibrozil	Fatal/non-fatal MI	769	Yes	32% reduction	<0.004
FIELD	Fenofibrate	CHD death or non-fatal MI	9975	No:7664 Yes:2131	11% reduction**	NS**

*60% fewer coronary events (P = 0.004); ** Non-fatal MI reduced by 24% (P = 0.01) and total CV events reduced by 19% in the primary cohort group (P = 0.004)
BIP = Bezafibrate Infarction Prevention; DAIS = Diabetes Atherosclerosis Intervention Study; FIELD = Fenofibrate Intervention and Event Lowering in Diabetes; HHS = Helsinki Heart Study; SENDCAP = St Mary's Ealing Northwick Park Diabetes Cardiovascular Prevention Study; VA-HIT = Veterans Administration – HDL Intervention Trial.

HDL is intimately involved in reverse cholesterol transport (Figure 7.9), and has other crucial effects in the pathogenesis of atherosclerosis (Figure 7.10) [23, 24]. The antioxidant effects of HDL may be impaired in patients with type 2 diabetes [25] in addition to enhanced activity of CETP caused by hypertriglyceridemia and insulin resistance.

Table 7.3 summarizes the lipid trials with fibrates in patients with diabetes or metabolic syndrome. In the Helsinki Heart Study, a primary prevention trial, a subgroup of 292 patients achieved a 71% decrease in CHD events with gemfibrozil over 5 years [26]. In the Bezafibrate Infarction Prevention (BIP) study, the subgroup of 1470 patients with metabolic syndrome or diabetes had a 29% risk reduction of re-infarction (P <0.02) [27]. In the St. Mary's,

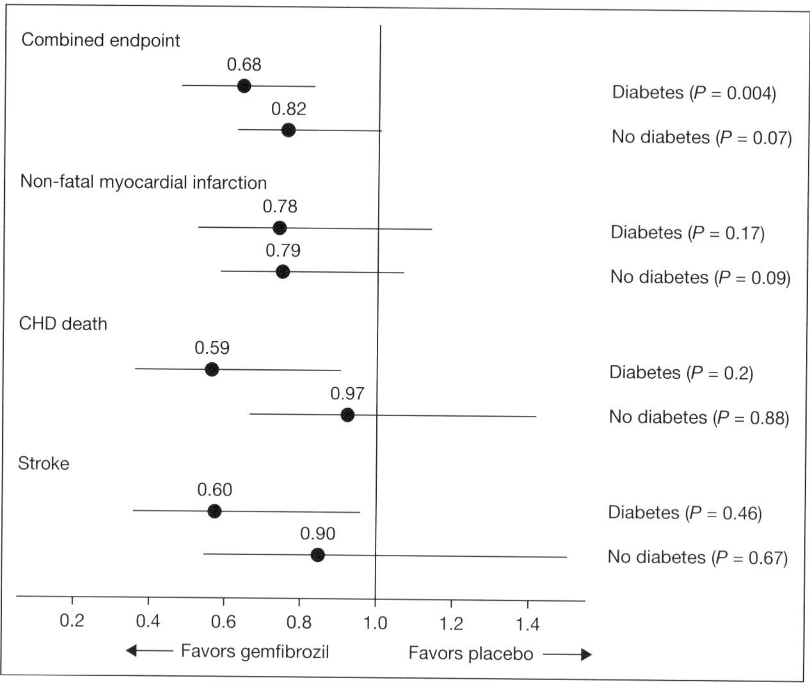

Figure 7.11 VA-HDL Intervention Trial (VA-HT): hazard ratios for major cardiovascular events with Gemfibrozil compared with placebo in non-diabetic (n = 1748) and diabetic (n = 769) subjects.

Ealing, Northwick Park Diabetes Cardiovascular Disease Prevention (SENDCAP) trial, involving 328 patients with type 2 diabetes, intervention with bezafibrate resulted in no significant difference in the primary endpoint of carotid lesions detected by ultrasound, but there were 60% fewer total coronary events over a period of 3 years ($P < 0.01$) [28]. In the Diabetes Atherosclerosis Intervention Study (DAIS), an angiographic regression trial, 418 patients with type 2 diabetes and evidence of CHD on angiography were treated with fenofibrate or placebo over at least 3 years [29]. The fenofibrate group showed significantly slower progression of disease and a trend toward fewer clinical endpoints (38 vs 50) in this relatively small trial.

Two large fibrate trials have shown somewhat discrepant results. The Veterans Affairs High-Density Lipoprotein Cholesterol Intervention Trial (VA-HIT) studied 2531 men with CHD who had LDL-cholesterol <140 mg/dl, HDL-cholesterol lower than 40 mg/dl, and triglyceride <300 mg/dl at baseline. Of these, 769 had evidence of diabetes or metabolic syndrome [30]. Treatment with gemfibrozil for a median duration of 5.1 years resulted in 24% risk reduction in the combined outcome of CHD death, MI and stroke, despite no change in LDL-cholesterol but HDL-cholesterol rose by 6% and triglyceride levels decreased by 30%. The diabetes subgroup had a greater reduction in the combined endpoints (32%), compared to the non-diabetic subjects (18%) (Figure 7.11). Subsequent analyses from the VA-HIT revealed that the outcomes in this trial were not explained by the change in triglycerides and were only partially explained by the rise in HDL-cholesterol [31]. The 5-year event rates were highly correlated with insulin resistance with or without diabetes, and the event reduction was significantly greater in those with insulin resistance and was independent of the HDL-cholesterol or triglyceride levels before or after treatment [32]. These

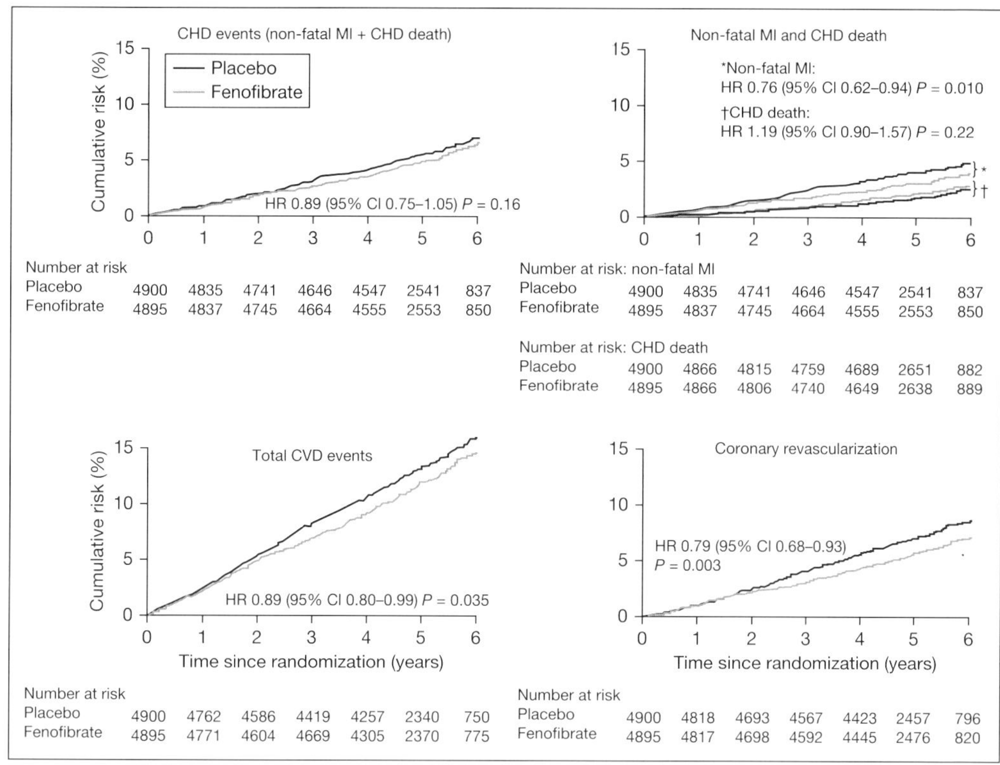

Figure 7.12 FIELD: cumulative CVD events. With permission from [34].

analyses suggest the possibility that other anti-atherogenic effects of fibrates, mediated by a variety of mechanisms, including peroxisome proliferator-activated receptor-α (PPAR-α) agonism, anti-inflammatory effects on vessel walls, and fibrinolysis, can contribute to the event reductions seen in the VA-HIT. Interestingly, evidence from the BIP study suggests an insulin sensitizing effect of fibrates [33].

The largest trial of fibrates, to date, is the FIELD trial which was conducted with fenofibrate vs placebo in 9795 patients with type 2 diabetes, of which the majority (7664) were in the primary prevention group. Overall, there was a non-significant 11% reduction in primary endpoint of CHD death or non-fatal MI ($P = 0.16$) but a significant 24% reduction in non-fatal MI ($P = 0.010$) and a significant 11% reduction in total cardiovascular events ($P = 0.035$) (Figure 7.12) [34]. Of note, 17% of placebo- and 8% of fenofibrate-treated patients were started on statins during the trial. Furthermore, only 38% of the patients had dyslipidemia and the subgroup tended to have a lower rate of CVD events. Also, the primary prevention majority had a significant 19% reduction in total CVD events ($P = 0.004$). Patients with metabolic syndrome had a higher risk of events but a similar event reduction. Of the adverse effects, there was a slight increase in creatinine that resolved after discontinuation after the end of the trial. Similarly, homocysteine concentration was higher in the fenofibrate-treated patients by 3.7 mmol/l but declined to the same level as in the placebo group after the discontinuation of the drug. Interestingly, there was significantly less progression of retinopathy requiring laser treatment and less progression of albuminuria ($P < 0.003$), despite no differences in mean fasting glucose, HbA1c or blood pressure.

Table 7.4 American Diabetes Association lipid treatment recommendations (with permission from [35])

- Lifestyle modifications
- Primary LDL-cholesterol goal <100 mg/dl; if CVD: LDL-cholesterol <70 mg/dl is an option
- Statin therapy added to lifestyle changes, regardless of baseline LDL, if:
  - overt CVD
  - without CVD but age >40 years + one or more other CVD risk factors
- Without overt CVD and age <40 years
  - consider statin if LDL-cholesterol >100 mg/dl or multiple risk factors, despite lifestyle therapy
- In drug-treated patients, a reduction in LDL-cholesterol of ~40% from baseline if LDL targets not achieved with maximum tolerated statin therapy
- Triglycerides <150 mg/dl; HDL-cholesterol >40 mg/dl(men), >50 mg/dl (women): desirable
  - Combination therapy to achieve lipid goals may be needed but outcome studies pending

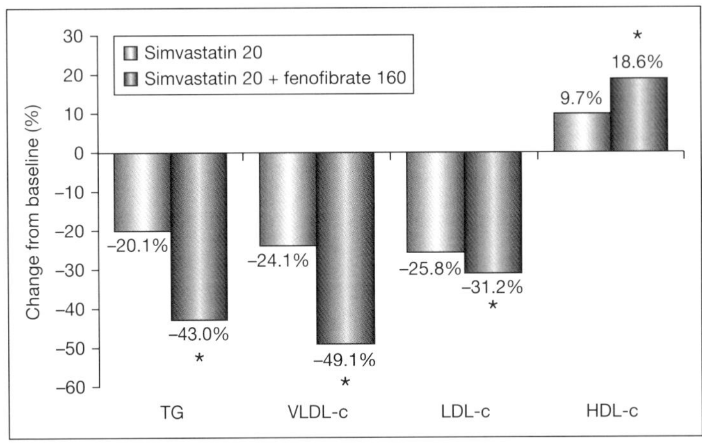

Figure 7.13 SAFARI: combination therapy in patients with combined hyperlipidemia. With permission from [36].

ROLE OF COMBINATION THERAPY IN METABOLIC SYNDROME

According to the ATP III update [14] and the American Diabetes Association (ADA) guidelines [35], combination therapy with an LDL-lowering drug, preferably a statin, plus fibrates or niacin, may be considered in high-risk patients with elevated triglycerides or low HDL-cholesterol (Table 7.4). However, despite the known pharmacologic effects of fibrates and nicotinic acid in ameliorating the underlying defects of diabetic dyslipidemia (increased triglyceride-rich lipoproteins, low HDL-cholesterol, small, dense LDL particles), the role of combining these agents with statins in preventing cardiovascular events remains inconclusive, and further clinical trials are needed.

Trials such as VA-HIT, FIELD and DAIS support the potential of adding fibrates to statins, because combined lipid disorders are very common in patients with insulin resistance and type 2 diabetes. In short-term studies, statins in combination with fibrates [36, 37] or a statin along with niacin [38] have been shown to be more effective in normalizing all lipid abnormalities, including lipid particle distribution, than either agent alone, without significant risk for adverse events, including myositis (Figures 7.13 and 7.14). However,

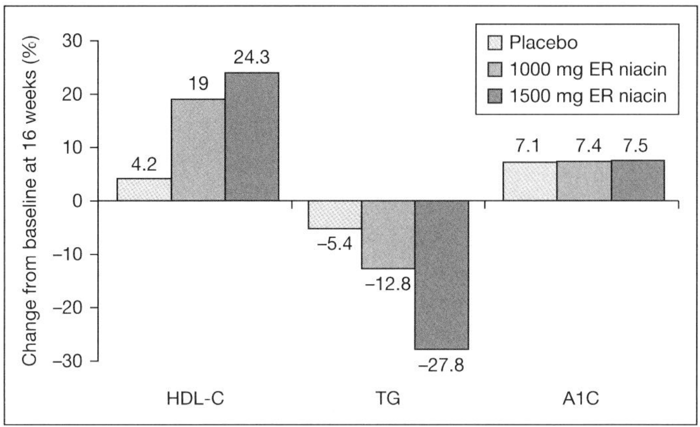

Figure 7.14 ER niacin vs placebo in people with type 2 diabetes: the ADVENT study. With permission from [38].

Table 7.5 Myopathy with statins and fibrates (adapted with permission from [39,40])

Myopathy with statins and fibrates

- Creatine kinase (CK)
    - Elevation >10 × ULN observed in 0.1% of patients at starting dose of statins.
    - Measure at baseline and monitor symptoms
- Rhabdomyolysis (incidence = 1 in 10,000 person-years).
  Renal failure may occur if drug continued
- Risk increases with dose escalation, renal disease, hypothyroidism, or in combination with gemfibrozil, cyclosporine, verapamil, amiodarone, HIV-protease inhibitors etc.
- Reversed after discontinuation

caution should be exercised in patients with potential drug interactions (e.g., cyclosporine, antifungal agents, protease inhibitors, erythromycin) and in those with renal disease (Table 7.5) [39, 40].

In a study of 160 patients with CHD and low HDL-cholesterol, the HDL Atherosclerosis Treatment Study (HATS), combining niacin with simvastatin over 3 years, resulted in an impressive reduction in angiographic progression of lesions and clinical endpoints [41]. A subgroup (16%) of these patients had diabetes. Similarly, in a recent 12-month study, with another 12 months of open-label follow-up, niacin–simvastatin combination therapy, in 167 patients with stable coronary artery disease, resulted in significantly reduced progression of carotid intima-media thickness, compared to simvastatin alone [42]. However, this study did not have the power to detect differences in clinical outcomes. Niacin was shown to significantly reduce the risk of non-fatal MI and stroke in the Coronary Drug Project (CDP), in which 40% of the patients had evidence of abnormal glucose tolerance [43]. Lovastatin in combination with extended-release niacin, in fixed-combination doses of up to 40 mg lovastatin plus 2000 mg niaspan daily, was reported to lower LDL-cholesterol and triglyceride by 47% and 41%, respectively, and to increase HDL-cholesterol by 30% [44]. Similar results were reported with the lovastatin–niaspan combination in a 20-week study of patients with type 2 diabetes [45]. The combination of statins with niacin has also been shown to

Table 7.6 Potential HDL therapies

Potential HDL therapies
Synthetic HDLs
apoA-1 mimetic peptides
Cholesteryl ester transfer protein (CETP) inhibitors
PRAR-α, PRAR-δ agonists
MK-0524A- ER niacin + statin
Cannabanoid-1 receptor antagonists

lead to a significant reduction in small, dense LDL particles, as well as a reduction in Lp(a) levels, compared to statins alone or statins in combination with ezetimibe [46]. Contrary to past studies with a larger dosage of niacin, recent evidence suggests no significant worsening of glycemic control with 1–1.5 g of niacin [38]. The non-flush over-the-counter (OTC) formulations of niacin are ineffective and their use should be discouraged. A combination pill of niacin and DP-1 receptor antagonist (MK-0524) to prevent flushing is currently in clinical trials.

In patients with diabetic lipemia or severe hypertriglyceridemia in metabolic syndrome, fibrates are the drug of choice, in addition to several concurrent measures including glycemic control, a very low-fat diet, alcohol restriction, physical activity, and weight management. Many such patients are unable to lower triglyceride levels to a safe range (<500 mg/dl) with fibrates in combination with diet and lifestyle changes, and they require the addition of niacin or fish oils, or both. Fish oils are usually required in relatively large doses to provide 3 to 6 g or more of omega-3 fatty acids – EPA and DHA [47, 48]. A high potency, ~900 mg, omega-3 ethyl ester preparation (Lovaza, formerly known as Omacor) is currently approved for use in patients with triglycerides >500 mg/dl [48].

A valid approach to raising HDL-cholesterol in patients with diabetes is the addition of a thiazolidinedione (TZD). Both of the available TZDs, rosiglitazone and pioglitazone, raise HDL-cholesterol by as much as 10–15% depending upon the baseline HDL levels [49]. Pioglitazone has been shown to have more favorable lipid effects but both agents are effective in correcting the LDL compositional abnormalities associated with insulin resistance [50]. However, the relative value of these agents in overall cardiovascular outcomes needs additional studies.

NOVEL LIPID INTERVENTION APPROACHES

Of the novel approaches to augmenting HDL effects on anti-atherogenesis (Table 7.6), CETP inhibitors, for a number of years, have been thought to be worth pursuing. CETP inhibition with recently available agents has been shown to increase HDL-cholesteol by 50–100% in dose-ranging studies [51]. However, whether the compositional changes in HDL particles brought about by this mechanism will be pro- or anti-atherogenic remains controversial [23, 24, 52]. In a population-based prospective study, a common CETP polymorphism was associated with higher HDL-cholesterol but paradoxically increased incidence of CHD [53]. A large clinical trial (ILLUMINATE) with torcetrapib, a CETP inhibitor, was halted in December 2006 due to an unexpected increase in adverse CVD outcomes in patients with CHD despite standard statin treatment [54]. A drug-specific, rather than CETP inhibition-specific effect to explain the adverse effects could not be ruled out since torcetrapib resulted in a modest but significant increase in blood pressure and mineralocorticoid activity [54]. In light of this, other CETP antagonists are currently being studied [23, 55].

Table 7.7 summarizes some of the ongoing major lipid trials in patients with or without diabetes and metabolic syndrome. In particular, the ACCORD trial is comparing long-term

Table 7.7 Major ongoing lipid trials

	n	*Drugs*	*Endpoints*
SEARCH	~ 10 000	Simvastatin 20 mg or 80 mg ± B12+ folate	MI and CAD death by aggressive LDL- and homocysteine-lowering
AURORA	~ 2700	Rosuvastation 10 mg or placebo	Major CVD endpoints in ESRD
AIM-HIGH	~ 3000	Simvastatin or simvastatin +ER niacin	Secondary prevention of CHD in metabolic syndrome
ACCORD	~ 5800	Simvastain 20 mg ± fenofibrate	CAD death or non-fatal MI by LDL- and triglyceride-lowering in DM
THRIVE	~20 000	Simvastatin ± ezetimibe ± 529A	Major CVD endpoints by HDL-raising in CHD or high risk

ACCORD = Action to Control Cardiovascular Risk in Diabetes; AIM-HIGH = Atherothrombosis Intervention in Metabolic Syndrome with low HDL/High triglycerides and Impact on Global Health Outcomes; AURORA = A Study Evaluating the Use of Rosuvastatin in Patients Requiring Ongoing Renal Dialysis; CAD = coronary artery disease; CVD = cardiovascular disease; DM = diabetes mellitus; ESRD = end-stage renal disease; LDL = low-density lipoprotein; MI = myocardial infarction; SEARCH = Study of Effectiveness of Additional Reductions in Cholesterol and Homocysteine; THRIVE = Treatment of HDL to Reduce the Incidence of Vascular Events.

benefits of simvastatin and fenofibrate, whereas AIM-HIGH is comparing simvastatin and niacin, compared to statin alone, in patients with known cardiovascular disease and dyslipidemia associated with metabolic syndrome.

SUMMARY

The metabolic syndrome, with or without diabetes, is associated with an increased incidence of cardiovascular disease. The atherogenic dyslipidemia of metabolic syndrome is characterized by insulin resistance and an increase in triglyceride-rich lipoproteins, as well as a decrease in HDL-cholesterol and compositionally abnormal lipoproteins, including smaller, denser LDL particles. The increase in pro-inflammatory and prothrombotic milieu, along with visceral obesity and endothelial dysfunction inherent in metabolic syndrome, likely contribute to the enhanced atherogenecity in the presence of dyslipidemia.

A number of clinical trials have established the benefits of LDL-lowering in individuals with increased baseline cardiovascular risk, including those with metabolic syndrome in the absence of diabetes. This has been best shown in secondary prevention trials thus far. Several epidemiologic studies as well as angiographic regression trials and clinical trials have also documented the benefits of strategies to raise HDL and lower triglyceride-rich particles. The impact of the HDL particle, as a disease modifier, is currently the subject of particularly intense scrutiny. A number of potential newer avenues to increase HDL synthesis and/or inhibit its catabolism are being pursued.

Currently, major clinical trials are in progress, exploring the benefits of combination therapy to achieve improved overall lipid profile – beyond optimal LDL – in patients with metabolic syndrome with or without diabetes in both primary as well as secondary prevention.

REFERENCES

1. Hu FB, Stampfer MJ, Haffner SM, Solomon CG, Willett WC, Manson JE. Elevated risk of cardiovascular disease prior to clinical diagnosis of type 2 diabetes. *Diabetes Care* 2002; 25:1129–1134.

2. Howard BV, Best LG, Galloway JM *et al.* Coronary heart disease risk equivalence in diabetes depends on concomitant risk factors. *Diabetes Care* 2006; 29:391–397.
3. Krauss RM. Lipids and lipoproteins in patients with type 2 diabetes. *Diabetes Care* 2004; 27:1496–1504.
4. Taskinen MR. Diabetic dyslipidaemia: from basic research to clinical practice. *Diabetologia* 2003; 46:733–749.
5. Garvey WT, Kwon S, Zheng D *et al.* Effects of insulin resistance and type 2 diabetes on lipoprotein subclass particle size and concentration determined by nuclear magnetic resonance. *Diabetes* 2003; 52:453–462.
6. Sniderman AD. Non-HDL cholesterol versus apolipoprotein B in diabetic dyslipoproteinemia: alternatives and surrogates versus the real thing. *Diabetes Care* 2003; 26:2207–2208
7. Brunzell JD, Davidson M, Furberg CD *et al.* Lipoprotein managment in patients with cardiometabolic risk. Consensus statement from the American Diabetes Association and the American College of Cardiology Foundation. *Diabetes Care* 2008; 31:811–822.
8. Baigent C, Keech A, Kearney PM *et al.* Efficacy and safety of cholesterol-lowering treatment: prospective meta-analysis of data from 90,056 participants in 14 randomised trials of statins. *Lancet* 2005; 366:1267–1278.
9. Kearney PM, Blackwell L, Collins R *et al.* Efficacy of cholesterol-lowering therapy in 18,686 people with diabetes in 14 randomised trials of statins: a meta-analysis. *Lance*t 2008; 371:117–125.
10. Costa J, Borges M, David C, Vaz CA. Efficacy of lipid lowering drug treatment for diabetic and non-diabetic patients: meta-analysis of randomised controlled trials. *Br Med J* 2006; 332:1115–1124.
11. Ballantyne CM, Olsson AG, Cook TJ, Mercuri MF, Pedersen TR, Kjekshus J. Influence of low high-density lipoprotein cholesterol and elevated triglyceride on coronary heart disease events and response to simvastatin therapy in 4S. *Circulation* 2001; 104:3046–3051.
12. Deedwania P, Barter P, Carmena R *et al.* Reduction of low-density lipoprotein cholesterol in patients with coronary heart disease and metabolic syndrome: analysis of the Treating to New Targets study. *Lancet* 2006; 368:919–928.
13. Devaraj S, Chan E, Jialal I. Direct demonstration of an antiinflammatory effect of simvastatin in subjects with the metabolic syndrome. *J Clin Endocrinol Metab* 2006; 91:4489–4496.
14. Grundy SM, Cleeman JI, Merz CN *et al.* Implications of recent clinical trials for the National Cholesterol Education Program Adult Treatment Panel III guidelines. *Circulation* 2004; 110:227–239.
15. Cannon CP, Steinberg BA, Murphy SA, Mega JL, Braunwald E. Meta-analysis of cardiovascular outcomes trials comparing intensive versus moderate statin therapy. *J Am Coll Cardiol* 2006; 48:438–445.
16. Goldberg AC, Sapre A, Liu J, Capece R, Mitchel YB. Efficacy and safety of ezetimibe coadministered with simvastatin in patients with primary hypercholesterolemia: a randomized, double-blind, placebo-controlled trial. *Mayo Clin Proc* 2004; 79:620–629.
17. Hunninghake D, Insull W, Jr, Toth P, Davidson D, Donovan JM, Burke SK. Co-administration of colesevelam hydrochloride with atorvastatin lowers LDL cholesterol additively. *Atherosclerosis* 2001; 158:407–416.
18. Kastelein JJP, Akdim F, Stores ESG *et al.* Simvastatin with or without Ezetimibe in familial hypercholesterolaemia. *N Engl J Med* 2008; 358:1431–1443.
19. Abdel-Maksoud MF, Hokanson JE. The complex role of triglycerides in cardiovascular disease. *Semin Vasc Med* 2002; 2:325–333.
20. Barter P, Gotto AM, LaRosa JC *et al.* HDL cholesterol, very low levels of LDL cholesterol, and cardiovascular events. *N Engl J Med* 2007; 357:1301–1310.
21. Miller M, Cannon CP, Murphy SA, Qin J, Ray KK, Braunwald E. Impact of triglyceride levels beyond low-density lipoprotein cholesterol after acute coronary syndrome in the PROVE IT-TIMI 22 trial. *J Am Coll Cardiol* 2008; 51:724–730.
22. Yusuf S, Hawken S, Ounpuu S *et al.* Effect of potentially modifiable risk factors associated with myocardial infarction in 52 countries (the INTERHEART study): case–control study. *Lancet* 2004; 364:937–952.
23. Mahley RW, Huang Y, Weisgraber KH. Putting cholesterol in its place: apoE and reverse cholesterol transport. *J Clin Invest* 2006; 116:1226–1229.
24. Barter P. Metabolic abnormalities: high-density lipoproteins. *Endocrinol Metab Clin North Am* 2004; 33:393–403.
25. Mastorikou M, Mackness M, Mackness B. Defective metabolism of oxidized phospholipid by HDL from people with type 2 diabetes. *Diabetes* 2006; 55:3099–3103.

26. Koskinen P, Manttari M, Manninen V, Huttunen JK, Heinonen OP, Frick MH. Coronary heart disease incidence in NIDDM patients in the Helsinki Heart Study. *Diabetes Care* 1992; 15:820–825.
27. Tenenbaum A, Motro M, Fisman EZ, Tanne D, Boyko V, Behar S. Bezafibrate for the secondary prevention of myocardial infarction in patients with metabolic syndrome. *Arch Intern Med* 2005; 165:1154–1160.
28. Elkeles RS, Diamond JR, Poulter C *et al*. Cardiovascular outcomes in type 2 diabetes. A double-blind placebo-controlled study of bezafibrate: the St. Mary's, Ealing, Northwick Park Diabetes Cardiovascular Disease Prevention (SENDCAP) Study. *Diabetes Care* 1998; 21:641–648.
29. Effect of fenofibrate on progression of coronary-artery disease in type 2 diabetes: the Diabetes Atherosclerosis Intervention Study, a randomised study. *Lancet* 2001; 357:905–910.
30. Rubins HB, Robins SJ, Collins D *et al*. Diabetes, plasma insulin, and cardiovascular disease: subgroup analysis from the Department of Veterans Affairs high-density lipoprotein intervention trial (VA-HIT). *Arch Intern Med* 2002; 162:2597–2604.
31. Robins SJ, Collins D, Wittes JT *et al*. Relation of gemfibrozil treatment and lipid levels with major coronary events: VA-HIT: a randomized controlled trial. *JAMA* 2001; 285:1585–1591.
32. Robins SJ, Rubins HB, Faas FH *et al*. Insulin resistance and cardiovascular events with low HDL cholesterol: the Veterans Affairs HDL Intervention Trial (VA-HIT). *Diabetes Care* 2003; 26:1513–1551.
33. Tenenbaum A, Fisman EZ, Boyko V *et al*. Attenuation of progression of insulin resistance in patients with coronary artery disease by bezafibrate. *Arch Intern Med* 2006; 166:737–741.
34. Keech A, Simes RJ, Barter P *et al*. Effects of long-term fenofibrate therapy on cardiovascular events in 9795 people with type 2 diabetes mellitus (the FIELD study): randomised controlled trial. *Lancet* 2005; 366:1849–1861.
35. Standards of medical care in diabetes – 2008. *Diabetes Care* 2008; 31(suppl 1):S12–S54.
36. Grundy SM, Vega GL, Yuan Z, Battisti WP, Brady WE, Palmisano J. Effectiveness and tolerability of simvastatin plus fenofibrate for combined hyperlipidemia (the SAFARI trial). *Am J Cardiol* 2005; 95:462–468.
37. Athyros VG, Papageorgiou AA, Athyrou VV, Demitriadis DS, Kontopoulos AG. Atorvastatin and micronized fenofibrate alone and in combination in type 2 diabetes with combined hyperlipidemia. *Diabetes Care* 2002; 25:1198–1202.
38. Grundy SM, Vega GL, McGovern ME *et al*. Efficacy, safety, and tolerability of once-daily niacin for the treatment of dyslipidemia associated with type 2 diabetes: results of the assessment of diabetes control and evaluation of the efficacy of niaspan trial. *Arch Intern Med* 2002; 162:1568–1576.
39. Graham DJ, Staffa JA, Shatin D *et al*. Incidence of hospitalized rhabdomyolysis in patients treated with lipid-lowering drugs. *JAMA* 2004; 292:2585–2590.
40. Antons KA, Williams CD, Baker SK, Phillips PS. Clinical perspectives of statin-induced rhabdomyolysis. *Am J Med* 2006; 119:400–409.
41. Brown BG, Zhao XQ, Chait A *et al*. Simvastatin and niacin, antioxidant vitamins, or the combination for the prevention of coronary disease. *N Engl J Med* 2001; 345:1583–1592.
42. Taylor AJ, Lee HJ, Sullenberger LE. The effect of 24 months of combination statin and extended-release niacin on carotid intima-media thickness: ARBITER 3. *Curr Med Res Opin* 2006; 22:2243–2250.
43. Canner PL, Furberg CD, Terrin ML, McGovern ME. Benefits of niacin by glycemic status in patients with healed myocardial infarction (from the Coronary Drug Project). *Am J Cardiol* 2005; 95:254–257.
44. Bays HE, Dujovne CA, McGovern ME *et al*. Comparison of once-daily, niacin extended-release/lovastatin with standard doses of atorvastatin and simvastatin (the ADvicor Versus Other Cholesterol-Modulating Agents Trial Evaluation [ADVOCATE]). *Am J Cardiol* 2003; 91:667–672.
45. Grundy SM, Vega GL, McGovern ME *et al*. Comparative effects on lipids and glycemic control of niacin extended-release/lovastatin or fenofibrate in patients with diabetic dyslipidemia. 64th Annual Scientific Sessions, Orlando, FL, June 4–8, 2004, # 29-LB.
46. Bays HE, McGovern ME. Once-daily niacin extended release/lovastatin combination tablet has more favourable effects on lipoprotein particle size and subclass distribution than atorvastatin and simvastatin. *Prev Cardiol* 2003; 6:179–188.
47. Kris-Etherton PM, Harris WS, Appel LJ. Fish consumption, fish oil, omega-3 fatty acids, and cardiovascular disease. *Arterioscler Thromb Vasc Biol* 2003; 23:e20–e30.
48. Durrington PN, Bhatnagar D, Mackness MI *et al*. An omega-3 polyunsaturated fatty acid concentrate administered for one year decreased triglycerides in simvastatin treated patients with coronary heart disease and persisting hypertriglyceridaemia. *Heart* 2001; 85:544–548.
49. Yki-Jarvinen H. Thiazolidinediones. *N Engl J Med* 2004; 351:1106–1118.

50. Goldberg RB, Kendall DM, Deeg MA *et al.* A comparison of lipid and glycemic effects of pioglitazone and rosiglitazone in patients with type 2 diabetes and dyslipidemia. *Diabetes Care* 2005; 28:1547–1554.
51. Clark RW, Sutfin TA, Ruggeri RB *et al.* Raising high-density lipoprotein in humans through inhibition of cholesteryl ester transfer protein: an initial multidose study of torcetrapib. *Arterioscler Thromb Vasc Biol* 2004; 24:490–497.
52. Fazio S, Linton MF. Sorting out the complexities of reverse cholesterol transport: CETP polymorphisms, HDL, and coronary disease. *J Clin Endocrinol Metab* 2006; 91:3273–3275.
53. Borggreve SE, Hillege HL, Wolffenbuttel BH *et al* An increased coronary risk is paradoxically associated with common cholesteryl ester transfer protein gene variations that relate to higher high-density lipoprotein cholesterol: a population-based study. *J Clin Endocrinol Metab* 2006; 91:3382–3388.
54. Barter PJ, Caulfield M, Eriksson M *et al.* Effects of torcetrapib in patients at high risk for coronary events. *N Engl J Med* 2007; 357:2109–2122.
55. Krishna R, Anderson MS, Bergman AJ *et al.* Effect of the cholesteryl ester transfer protein inhibitor, anacetrapib, on lipoproteins in patients with dyslipidaemia and on 24-h ambulatory blood pressure in healthy individuals: two double-blind, randomised placebo-controlled phase I studies. *Lancet* 2007; 370:1907–1914.

8

A potential role for insulin in management of the metabolic syndrome

P. Dandona, A. Chaudhuri, P. Mohanty, H. Ghanim

INTRODUCTION

The classical definition of the metabolic syndrome as defined by Reaven comprised obesity, insulin resistance, hypertension, hypertriglyceridemia, low high-density lipoprotein (HDL) and hyperuricemia [1]. Although this cluster of clinical features coexist frequently, and lead to a markedly enhanced risk of cardiovascular disease (CVD) and type 2 diabetes mellitus [2, 3], there is no single approach to the reversal or treatment of this complex other than an aggressive change of lifestyle accompanied by appropriate pharmacological treatment of a specific clinical feature. Only a change in lifestyle can ensure the reversal of obesity and since obesity is the major contributor to insulin resistance, hyperinsulinemia and dysglycemia as well as hypertension, efforts directed towards the reversal of obesity constitute the most important and rational measures in the reversal of this syndrome [2, 4]. Indeed, the unitary nature of this symptom complex or syndrome has been challenged on the basis that there is no single treatment that reverses this syndrome and thus it does not constitute a single disease or a syndrome [5]. However, if a disease or a syndrome is the consequence of an unhealthy lifestyle, clearly the answer must reside in the reversal of an unhealthy lifestyle.

Since obesity and overweight are the foundations of insulin resistance and the metabolic syndrome, and since insulin has recently been shown to exert powerful anti-inflammatory effects, it is important to elaborate on these effects [4, 6–10] (Table 8.1 and Figure 8.1). Each of the features of these novel effects may well be altered in this syndrome and thus may help in the understanding of the pathogenic mechanism(s) underlying this condition [4]. Similarly, macronutrient intake has recently been shown to induce a pro-inflammatory state and thus may account in part for the inflammation that characterizes the state of obesity [4]. Recent data also show that certain proteins capable of interfering with insulin signal transduction mechanisms are increased in obesity and are also acutely induced by macronutrient intake [11, 12].

The evolution of the features of the metabolic syndrome over the years has included the elevation of plasma concentrations of plasminogen activator inhibitor-1 (PAI-1) and C-reactive

Paresh Dandona, MD, PhD, FRCP, FACP, FACC, FACE, Director, Diabetes-Endocrinology Center of WNY; Chief, Division of Endocrinology SUNY at Buffalo; Distinguished Professor of Medicine, Division of Endocrinology, State University of New York at Buffalo, Millard Fillmore Hospital, Buffalo, New York, USA

Ajay Chaudhuri, MD, Division of Endocrinology, State University of New York at Buffalo, Millard Fillmore Hospital, Buffalo, New York, USA

Priya Mohanty, MD, Division of Endocrinology, State University of New York at Buffalo, Millard Fillmore Hospital, Buffalo, New York, USA

Husam Ghanim, PhD, Division of Endocrinology, State University of New York at Buffalo, Millard Fillmore Hospital, Buffalo, New York, USA

Table 8.1 Classical biological effects of insulin and classical metabolic syndrome based on resistance to the metabolic effects of insulin (with permission from [4])

	Normal insulin action	*Insulin-resistant state*
Carbohydrates	↓Hepatic glucose production ↑Glucose utilization ↑Glycogenesis	Hyperglycemia Hyperinsulinemia
Lipids	↓Lipolysis ↓FFA and glycerol ↑Lipogenesis ↑HDL ↓Triglycerides	↑Lipolysis ↑FFA and glycerol ↑Hepatic triglyceride and apoB synthesis Hypertriglyceridemia ↓HDL ↑Small dense LDL
Proteins	↓Gluconeogenesis ↓Amino acids ↑Protein synthesis	↑Gluconeogenesis ↑Protein catabolism ↓Protein synthesis
Purines	↑Uric acid clearance ↓Uric acid formation	Hyperuricemia

FFA = free fatty acids; HDL = high-density lipoprotein; LDL = low-density lipoprotein

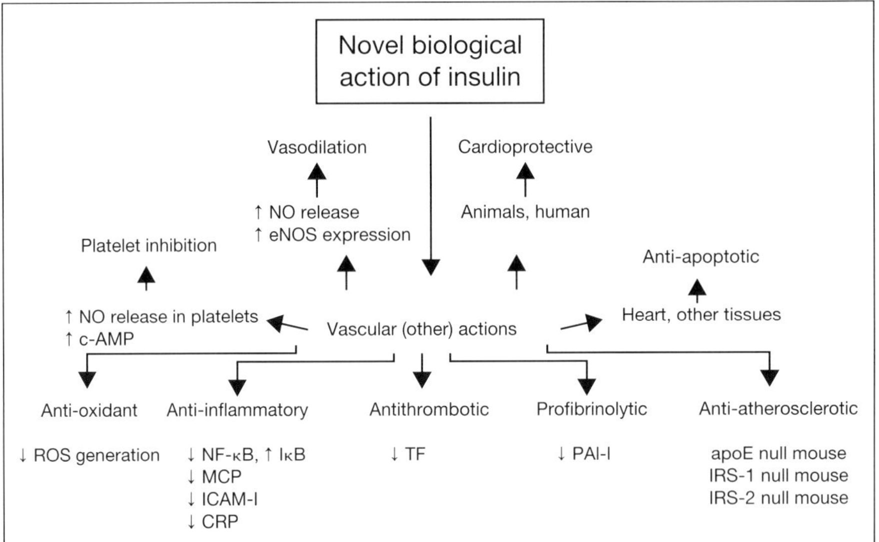

Figure 8.1 Novel biological effects of insulin targeted at endothelial cells, platelets and leucocytes resulting in vasodilation, anti-aggregatory effects on platelets, anti-inflammatory effects and other related effects. With permission from [4]. apoE = apolipoprotein E; c-AMP = cyclic AMP; CRP = C-reactive protein; eNOS = endothelial nitric oxide synthase; ICAM-1 = intracellular adhesion molecule-1; IκB = I kappa B; IRS = insulin resistance syndrome; MCP = monocyte chemotactic protein; NF-κB = nuclear factor kappa B; NO = nitric oxide; PAI = plasminogen activator inhibitor; TF = tissue factor.

protein (CRP) [2]. Although initially unexplained, the discovery that insulin exerts a potent anti-inflammatory effect and the fact that it suppresses both PAI-1 and CRP explains this phenomenon in the insulin resistance states like obesity, the metabolic syndrome, type 2 diabetes and polycystic ovary syndrome (PCOS) [4, 10, 13]. The adipose tissue secretes pro-inflammatory cytokines in obesity [14, 22]. This may lead to chronic inflammation and may also contribute to the pro-inflammatory state observed with obesity [15–21]. Both CRP and PAI-1 increases are known to be associated with an increase in cardiovascular risk [23].

ANTI-INFLAMMATORY EFFECT OF INSULIN

The discovery of the anti-inflammatory effect of insulin can be traced back to the observation that insulin exerts a vasodilatory effect in arteries, veins and capillaries (micro-circulation) [24, 25]. Since these reports also showed that this effect was due to nitric oxide (NO) generation from the endothelium, *in vivo*, a direct effect of insulin on NO release by the endothelium was investigated. The endothelium was shown to release NO in a dose-dependent fashion in response to insulin stimulation in human umbilical vein endothelial cells [26, 27]. Furthermore, the expression of endothelial NO synthase (eNOS) in response to insulin also increased in a dose-dependent fashion in human aortic endothelial cells [28].

Definitive experiments demonstrating the anti-inflammatory effects of insulin were first performed, *in vitro*, in human aortic endothelial cells. They showed that insulin suppressed the expression of the pro-inflammatory intracellular adhesion molecule-1, (ICAM-1), the chemokine, monocyte chemoattractant protein-1 (MCP-1), and the key pro-inflammatory transcription factor, nuclear factor kappa B (NF-κB) in human aortic endothelial cells at physiologically relevant concentrations [26, 28, 29]. This was followed by the demonstration that insulin infusions given at a low dose (2 units per hour) to obese subjects suppressed reactive oxygen species (ROS generation), $p47^{phox}$ expression (an indicator of NADPH oxidase, the enzyme which generates the superoxide radical action), NF-κB binding and increased inhibitor kappa B α (Iκ-Bα) expression by mononuclear cells [10]. In addition, insulin causes an acute reduction in plasma concentrations of ICAM-1, MCP-1 and another pro-inflammatory transcription factor, early growth response-1 (Egr-1), tissue factor and PAI-1 [30]. Insulin has also been shown to suppress matrix metalloproteinase-9 (MMP-9) and vascular endothelial growth factor (VEGF), two key mediators involved in the spread of inflammation and in the increase of vascular permeability [31, 32].

In a study involving patients with acute myocardial infarction (AMI), insulin was also shown to suppress CRP and serum amyloid A (SAA) by 40% within 24 h of the initiation of the insulin infusion while glucose concentrations were not allowed to change [33]. This effect of insulin was confirmed in patients with myocardial infarction and has now also been confirmed in patients undergoing coronary artery bypass grafts (CABG) in two studies [34, 35]. While this effect of insulin in post-CABG patients was apparent even earlier at 12 h after the initiation of the infusion, the magnitude of the effect on CRP and SAA concentrations was similar to that (40%) observed in AMI studies in spite of an overall increase in CRP and SAA concentrations which was 30 times greater than that observed in AMI [33–35]. One of the studies on CABG patients also demonstrated that the use of subcutaneously injected insulin to maintain normoglycemia was not able to cause a reduction in CRP concentrations [34]. Thus, it is likely that the anti-inflammatory effect of insulin is only exerted when insulin concentration is maintained at a high level using intravenous infusions supported by small amounts of glucose to prevent hypoglycemia. Treatment of AMI patients with insulin also suppresses PAI-1 and pro-MMP-1 [33, 36]. In patients treated in an intensive care unit (ICU), insulin infusions have also been shown to suppress (inducible nitric oxide synthase (iNOS) expression in the liver and to reduce plasma concentrations of nitrite and nitrate, the two metabolites of NO [37]. The anti-inflammatory effect of insulin has also been shown in patients with burns [38]. Similar anti-inflammatory effects have been observed in animals with experimental burns [39]. More recently, data demonstrating interference by insulin on signal transduction by interleukin-6 (IL-6) on adipocytes, has also been shown *in vitro*. Thus, the phosphorylation and activation of signal transducer and activator of transcription 3 (STAT-3) leads to its translocation into the nucleus and the transcriptional activation of genes regulated by STAT-3. Two major pro-inflammatory genes activated by STAT-3 are serum amyloid A and haptoglobin [40].

Another interesting aspect of the recently demonstrated effects of insulin is its ability to offer cardio-protection in patients with AMI [33, 41, 42]. Such an effect has been observed in experimental myocardial infarction in both rats and dogs in association with the suppression of pro-apoptotic factors by insulin [43–45]. In these models, insulin infused prior to reperfusion has reduced the size of the myocardial infarct by 45%. This intriguing novel effect of insulin may explain the cardioprotective effect of insulin demonstrated in clinical trials of AMI. In this context, it is of interest that the administration of CRP to rats undergoing an experimental myocardial infarct increases the size of the infarct and the prior administration of synthetic molecules, which bind CRP (and thus prevent its action), reduce the size of this infarct [46, 47]. Thus, the CRP suppressive action of insulin may also contribute to significant reduction in the size of the infarct.

In addition to these effects, insulin has also been shown to induce vasodilation in arteries and veins, and to induce increased micro-circulatory (capillary) flow [24, 25]. This effect is mediated by the stimulation of eNOS and the generation of endothelial nitric oxide leading to an increase in cyclic guanosine monophosphate (cGMP) in the vascular smooth muscle [24, 25]. The increase in micro-circulatory flow in the myocardium is reflected in an increase in myocardial blush following angioplasty [48]. Insulin has also been shown to exert an antiplatelet effect, *in vitro* and *in vivo* [49]. This effect is mediated by platelet NOS activation and the release of NO and the subsequent generation of cGMP from guanylate cyclase [50]. This effect has recently been shown to occur in patients with acute coronary syndrome following an intravenous infusion of insulin [51]. Such an antiplatelet effect of insulin would contribute further to its anti-inflammatory effect since the platelet is loaded with CD40 ligand which when bound to its receptor, CD40, activates pro-inflammatory pathways [52]. The inhibition of platelet aggregation would thus prevent the activation of a major pro-inflammatory pathway in addition to suppressing thrombotic tendencies.

In view of the various novel effects of insulin that have recently been demonstrated, one can reasonably expect to have a diminution in these effects in insulin-resistant states. Therefore, insulin-resistant states are likely to be characterized by clinical features that may result from impairment of insulin action of various magnitudes (Figure 8.2).

PRO-INFLAMMATORY EFFECTS OF GLUCOSE AND OTHER MACRONUTRIENTS

The first demonstration that glucose induces the generation of ROS and superoxide radical and the induction of $p47^{phox}$ by leucocytes upon the administration of 75 g of glucose to normal subjects was intriguing in that the concentrations of glucose in plasma were by definition normal [53]. Clearly, even a normally handled load of glucose could lead to oxidative stress. Glucose intake was also shown to cause the translocation of $p47^{phox}$ to the cell membrane in addition to causing comprehensive inflammation at the cellular and molecular level as reflected in the increase in NF-κB binding and the activation of IκB kinases α and β with a decrease in IκBα [54]. In addition, glucose intake resulted in an increase in tumor necrosis factor alpha (TNF-α) mRNA. The infusion of glucose into normal subjects results in an increase in TNF-α and IL-6 if the subject's endogenous insulin secretion is inhibited by the concomitant infusion of somatostatin [55]. Glucose intake has also been shown to increase activator protein-1 (AP-1) and Egr-1, two major pro-inflammatory transcription factors and the key genes activated by them: *MMP-2, MMP-9* and tissue factor (TF) [56]. Since TF is an activator of the extrinsic pathway of coagulation, it follows that glucose intake will promote a thrombotic tendency [57]. Glucose has also been shown to increase the expression of the adhesion molecule ICAM-3 and CD69 (Jay Friedman, PhD thesis). The latter is a receptor activator of T cells and is thus pro-inflammatory. It is of interest that its expression is increased in acute myocardial infarction and that its increase is associated with

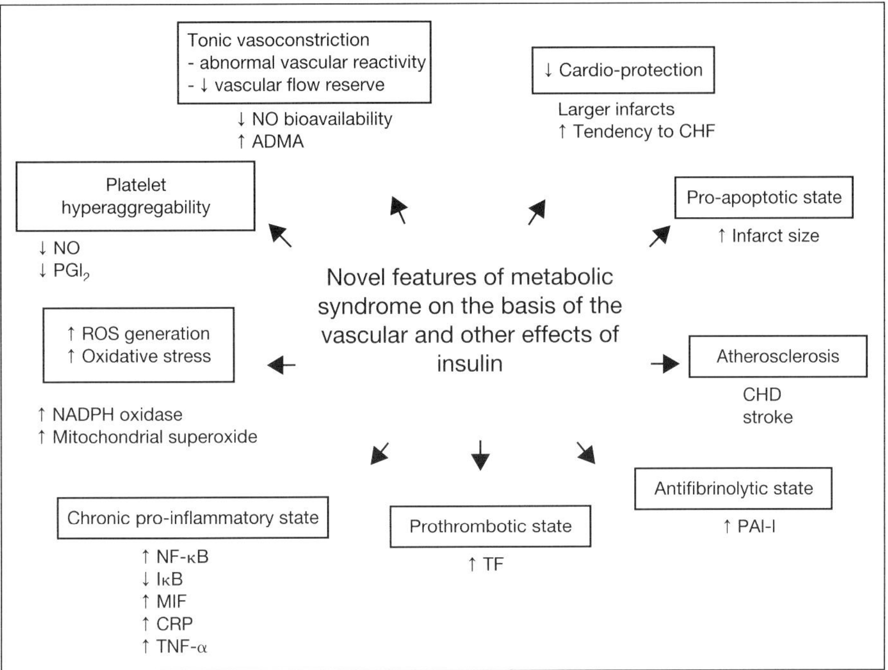

Figure 8.2 Extension of metabolic syndrome based on novel actions of insulin. With permission from [4]. ADMA = asymmetric dimethylarginine; CHD = coronary heart disease; CHF = congestive heart failure; CRP = C-reactive protein; IκB = I kappa B protein; MIF = migration inhibitory factor; NADPH = nicotinamide adenine dinucleotide phosphate; NF-κB = nuclear factor kappa B; NO = nitric oxide; PAI = plasminogen activator inhibitor; PG = prostaglandin; ROS = reactive oxygen species; TNF-α = tumor necrosis factor alpha.

an increase in cardiovascular events [58]. Glucose has been shown to increase thrombin activation in subjects with type 2 diabetes and this effect has been reduced with the administration of antioxidants [59].

The intake of saturated fat taken as cream (33 g fat = 300 calories) also results in an increase in ROS generation by leucocytes and the occurrence of inflammation at the cellular and molecular levels, similar to that described for glucose [60]. The infusion of triglyceride and heparin to raise the plasma concentration of free fatty acids (FFAs) from 200–300 μmol/l in normal subjects to 800–900 μmol/l, similar to that found in obese subjects, also leads to an increase in ROS generation, NF-κB binding and plasma concentration of migration inhibitory factor (MIF) [61]. In addition, such an infusion is also known to cause acute insulin resistance. A 900-calorie fast food meal also results in an increase in ROS generation, $p47^{phox}$, Iκ-kinases α and β, an increase in NF-κB binding and a decrease in Iκ-Bα [12]. This inflammatory response lasts for more than 3 hours. In the obese, the state of inflammation induced by a fast food meal is of a greater magnitude and lasts longer than that in normal subjects. This is probably due to the fact that the obese are in a pro-inflammatory, oxidative stress state even after fasting overnight and thus the effect of the fast food meal is additional. While discussing the pro-inflammatory effects of macronutrients, it is also important to investigate whether there are ways to avoid pro-inflammatory foods and to discover foods that are unlikely to cause oxidative or inflammatory stress. Recent work has shown that orange juice, alcohol and a meal rich in fruit and fiber do not cause inflammatory or oxidative stress [54, 62, 63]. Thus, appropriate food choices can be made to avoid oxidative and inflammatory insults.

Just as macronutrient intake results in inflammation, its withdrawal or reduction results in a decrease in oxidative stress and inflammation. Thus, a reduction in caloric intake to 1000 calories per day in a group of obese patients resulted in a marked reduction in ROS generation, lipid peroxidation, protein carbonylation and oxidative damage of the amino acid phenylalanine over the course of four weeks while subjects lost approximately 13 lbs in weight [64]. In a study involving normal subjects, a 48 h fast resulted in the reduction of ROS generation by leucocytes by 35% at 24 h and >50% at 48 h [65]. There was a concomitant decrease in the expression of $p47^{phox}$ [65]. On the basis of these observations, one can conclude that macronutrient intake is probably the single most important contributor of oxidative stress, *in vivo*. These observations have been confirmed in the obese on the basis that dietary restriction led to a significant reduction in isoprostane excretion in the urine [64]. Long-term caloric restriction with weight loss also results in the fall of the pro-inflammatory cytokine, TNF-α [14]. Weight loss and caloric restriction have also been shown to reduce other cytokines and CRP [4].

INFLAMMATION AND PATHOGENESIS OF INSULIN RESISTANCE

On the basis of the above actions of insulin, glucose and macronutrients, one can predict that insulin resistance in obesity and the metabolic syndrome are likely to be associated with an increase in oxidative stress and inflammation (Figure 8.2). Indeed, we now recognize that the indices of oxidative stress and inflammation are increased in these states [13, 16, 66–72]. These features impart to these states an increased propensity towards atherosclerosis [73–77]. The features of increased oxidative stress and inflammation are probably also the result of excessive macronutrient intake in the obese and the overweight [14, 70, 78–82]. While we consider the pathogenesis of chronic inflammatory and oxidative stress in obese and overweight subjects, it is important to ask if there is a mechanistic link between these processes and insulin resistance. Indeed, it has recently been shown that certain molecules, which may interfere with insulin signal transduction, may be generated by pro-inflammatory stimuli. Among them are the suppressor of cytokine signaling (SOCS-3) and protein kinase Cβ (PKCβ) [83–87]. SOCS-3 is induced by TNF-α and IL-6, two major NF-κB regulated pro-inflammatory cytokines. SOCS-3 interferes with insulin signal transduction by reducing the tyrosine phosphorylation of the insulin receptor, the expression of insulin receptor substrate 1 (IRS-1) and increasing the ubiquitination and the proteosomal degradation of IRS-1. It has recently been shown that SOCS-3 expression in the obese is increased markedly and that there is an inverse relationship between SOCS-3 expression on the one hand and insulin receptor phosphorylation and homeostasis model assessment-insulin resistance (HOMA-IR) on the other [11]. Furthermore, recent work shows that SOCS-3 expression is induced by macronutrient intake. Thus, the pro-inflammatory stimulus of macronutrient intake may also be responsible for SOCS-3, the factor interfering with the insulin signaling mechanism and thus contributing to insulin resistance. These data allow us to unify the mechanisms underlying post- prandial oxidative stress, inflammation, obesity and insulin resistance.

The next issue to consider is the loss of β cell function and the insulin reserve. Two factors have hitherto been recognized to affect β cell reserve in the insulin-resistant states of obesity, the metabolic syndrome and type 2 diabetes. They are lipotoxicity due to an increase in FFA concentration in obesity and in other insulin-resistant states, and glucotoxicity after hyperglycemia has set in [88–94]. The mechanisms underlying the pathogenesis of β cell loss thus become clearer with the understanding that both FFAs and glucose cause oxidative stress and inflammation [53, 61]. Oxidative stress and inflammation can lead to the activation of pro-apoptotic signals which may contribute to a loss of β cell population [95–97]. Furthermore, it has recently been shown that insulin signaling may be important in β cell function and insulin secretion since the selective deletion of the insulin receptor in the β cell leads to defects in insulin secretion [98]. As discussed above, inflammation interferes with insulin signal transduction. Thus, the pathogenesis of insulin resistance and β cell loss may in part be dependent

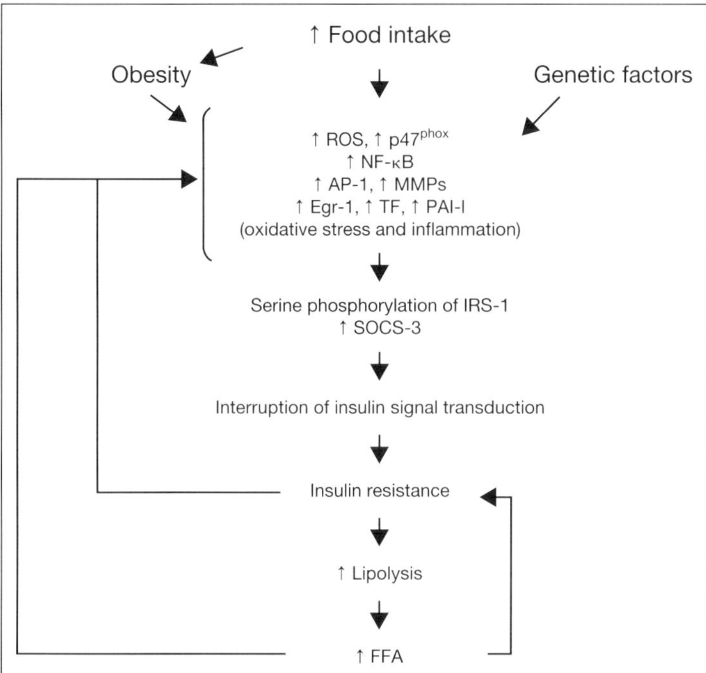

Figure 8.3 Pathogenesis of metabolic syndrome. With permission from [4].
AP-1 = activator protein-1; Egr-1 = early growth response factor-1; FFA = free fatty acids; IRS = insulin resistance syndrome; MMP = matrix metalloproteinase; NF-κB = nuclear factor kappa B; PAI = plasminogen activator inhibitor; ROS = reactive oxygen species; TF = tissue factor.

upon similar mechanisms. The former is due to the action of pro-inflammatory mediators on insulin signal transduction in insulin-responsive tissues and the latter due to the action of these mediators on the pancreatic β cell. The temporal difference in the manifestation of these two features of type 2 diabetes may be a function of the time it takes for inflammation and oxidative stress to impair insulin secretion and to induce critical apoptosis and the lack of β cell regeneration. Relative insulinopenia in type 2 diabetes is probably a function of a combination of impaired insulin secretion from the existent β cells and the declining population of β cells.

On the basis that oxidative stress may contribute significantly to insulin resistance and to β cell loss, can we produce a unified view of the pathogenesis of the metabolic syndrome? This is important since it has been argued that the metabolic syndrome is not a single disease entity in the absence of a single pathogenic mechanism. This argument is further extended by the statement that there is no single treatment strategy for this condition, reflecting the absence of a single pathogenic mechanism. In addition, resistance to the known metabolic actions of insulin, result in hyperlipidemia, hypertension, a tendency towards hyperglycemia and diabetes (Table 8.1). The metabolic syndrome is also likely to have other features related to impaired insulin action. It would thus appear that starting with an increase in macronutrient intake and the induction of acute oxidative and inflammatory stress, followed by the induction of pro-inflammatory molecules which interfere with insulin signal transduction, it is possible to build a hypothesis explaining the pathogenesis of the metabolic syndrome based on lifestyle. The addition of factors originating from genetic influences would complete this picture (Figure 8.3).

MANAGEMENT OF VARIOUS FEATURES OF THE METABOLIC SYNDROME

The major goals for the management of the metabolic syndrome are to reduce the risk for atherosclerotic cardiovascular disease and the development of type 2 diabetes mellitus. These goals are met by assessing both the short-term risk of atherosclerotic disease and by trying to modify the various components of the metabolic syndrome in an effort to reduce the long-term risk of cardiovascular events. Lifestyle modification is therefore an essential component of management irrespective of the short-term risk of cardiovascular disease, while pharmacological therapy and goals for treatment of dyslipidemia and hypertension are primarily driven by the risk for CVD. Subjects with established CVD and diabetes mellitus are at high risk for developing a cardiac event and should receive intensive intervention. In the absence of these clinical conditions, choice and intensity of risk factor modification should be guided by the Framingham risk scoring assessment for developing CVD.

MANAGEMENT OF THE METABOLIC SYNDROME: A ROLE FOR INSULIN

If indeed insulin resistance is the essential component of the metabolic syndrome and inflammation is a major mechanism underlying insulin resistance, insulin can be a potential therapeutic agent in the treatment of this syndrome in view of its anti-inflammatory properties. The classical experiments showing an improvement in insulin sensitivity following the treatment of badly controlled insulin-taking diabetics with intensive insulin therapy have hitherto been explained on the basis of a reduction in glucotoxicity [99–101]. However, it is possible that it is partly due to the anti-inflammatory and potentially insulin sensitizing effect of insulin. In this light, it would in future be important to investigate the effects of insulin on the expression of the putative molecules which interfere with insulin signal transduction: SOCS-3, PKCβ2 and TRB3. Although it sounds strange, insulin may well have a role as a potential insulin sensitizer. It may also play a role in β cell preservation through its ROS suppressive and anti-inflammatory effects and its suppressive effects on glucose and FFA concentrations. The latter two effects would remove the potential toxic effects of glucose and FFA at the β cell level. Finally, the provision of exogenous insulin may also rest the β cell.

The discussion above would justify a trial of insulin in patients with prediabetes or the metabolic syndrome. Such patients may potentially be prevented from becoming diabetic through a reduction in insulin resistance and the preservation of the β cell.

Indeed, a trial is currently being conducted in patients with either impaired glucose tolerance (IGT) or impaired fasting glucose (IFG), with graded doses of a basal insulin, glargine, to investigate whether:

- their progression to type 2 diabetes can be prevented; and
- the incidence of cardiovascular events can be reduced.

This study, called ORIGIN, aims to reduce fasting plasma concentrations of glucose to less than 85 mg/dl over a period of 5 years. The results of this study will emerge in 2010 and will obviously be of great interest for both clinical and scientific reasons.

While the use of insulin is an interesting investigative approach, the mainstays of the treatment of the metabolic syndrome must remain:

- lifestyle change with caloric restriction, exercise and weight loss; and
- specific drug therapy for the various components of the syndrome like hypertension and hyperlipidemia.

In addition, as far as the treatment of hyperglycemia in diabetic patients with the metabolic syndrome is concerned, insulin remains the most potent agent with an unlimited ability to reduce glucose concentrations. In this respect, insulin can either be used as monotherapy or in combination with other oral anti-diabetic drugs like metformin and thiazolidinediones.

REFERENCES

1. Reaven GM. Banting lecture 1988. Role of insulin resistance in human disease. *Diabetes* 1988; 37:1595–1607.
2. Grundy SM, Cleeman JI, Daniels SR *et al*. Diagnosis and management of the metabolic syndrome: an American Heart Association/National Heart, Lung, and Blood Institute Scientific Statement. *Circulation* 2005; 112:2735–2752.
3. Klein BE, Klein R, Lee KE. Components of the metabolic syndrome and risk of cardiovascular disease and diabetes in Beaver Dam. *Diabetes Care* 2002; 25:1790–1794.
4. Dandona P, Aljada A, Chaudhuri A, Mohanty P, Garg R. Metabolic syndrome: A comprehensive perspective based on interactions between obesity, diabetes, and inflammation. *Circulation* 2005; 111:1448–1454.
5. Kahn R, Buse J, Ferrannini E, Stern M. The metabolic syndrome: time for a critical appraisal: joint statement from the American Diabetes Association and the European Association for the Study of Diabetes. *Diabetes Care* 2005; 28:2289–2304.
6. Carr DB, Utzschneider KM, Hull RL *et al*. Intra-abdominal fat is a major determinant of the National Cholesterol Education Program Adult Treatment Panel III criteria for the metabolic syndrome. *Diabetes* 2004; 53:2087–2094.
7. Ferrannini E, Haffner SM, Mitchell BD, Stern MP. Hyperinsulinaemia: the key feature of a cardiovascular and metabolic syndrome. *Diabetologia* 1991; 34:416–422.
8. Lemieux I, Pascot A, Couillard C *et al*. Hypertriglyceridemic waist: A marker of the atherogenic metabolic triad (hyperinsulinemia; hyperapolipoprotein B; small, dense LDL) in men? *Circulation* 2000; 102:179–184.
9. Park YW, Zhu S, Palaniappan L, Heshka S, Carnethon MR, Heymsfield SB. The metabolic syndrome: prevalence and associated risk factor findings in the US population from the Third National Health and Nutrition Examination Survey, 1988–1994. *Arch Intern Med* 2003; 163:427–436.
10. Dandona P, Aljada A, Mohanty P *et al*. Insulin inhibits intranuclear nuclear factor kappaB and stimulates kappa B in mononuclear cells in obese subjects: evidence for an anti-inflammatory effect? *J Clin Endocrinol Metab* 2001; 86:3257–3265.
11. Ghanim H, Aljada A, Daoud N, Deopurkar R, Chaudhuri A, Dandona P. Role of inflammatory mediators in the suppression of insulin receptor phosphorylation in circulating mononuclear cells of obese subjects. *Diabetologia* 2007; 50:278–285.
12. Aljada A, Mohanty P, Ghanim H *et al*. Increase in intranuclear nuclear factor kappa B and decrease in inhibitor kappa B in mononuclear cells after a mixed meal: evidence for a proinflammatory effect. *Am J Clin Nutr* 2004; 79:682–690.
13. Dandona P, Aljada A, Bandyopadhyay A. Inflammation: the link between insulin resistance, obesity and diabetes. *Trends Immunol* 2004; 25:4–7.
14. Dandona P, Weinstock R, Thusu K, Abdel-Rahman E, Aljada A, Wadden T. Tumor necrosis factor-alpha in sera of obese patients: fall with weight loss. *J Clin Endocrinol Metab* 1998; 83:2907–2910.
15. Hotamisligil GS, Shargill NS, Spiegelman BM. Adipose expression of tumor necrosis factor-alpha: direct role in obesity-linked insulin resistance. *Science* 1993; 259:87–91.
16. Ghanim H, Aljada A, Hofmeyer D, Syed T, Mohanty P, Dandona P. Circulating mononuclear cells in the obese are in a proinflammatory state. *Circulation* 2004; 110:1564–1571.
17. Kern PA, Ranganathan S, Li C, Wood L, Ranganathan G. Adipose tissue tumor necrosis factor and interleukin-6 expression in human obesity and insulin resistance. *Am J Physiol Endocrinol Metab* 2001; 280:E745–E751.
18. Pradhan AD, Manson JE, Rifai N, Buring JE, Ridker PM. C-reactive protein, interleukin 6, and risk of developing type 2 diabetes mellitus. *JAMA* 2001; 286:327–334.
19. Vozarova B, Weyer C, Hanson K, Tataranni PA, Bogardus C, Pratley RE. Circulating interleukin-6 in relation to adiposity, insulin action, and insulin secretion. *Obes Res* 2001; 9:414–417.
20. Xu H, Barnes GT, Yang Q *et al*. Chronic inflammation in fat plays a crucial role in the development of obesity-related insulin resistance. *J Clin Invest* 2003; 112:1821–1830.
21. La Cava A, Alviggi C, Matarese G. Unraveling the multiple roles of leptin in inflammation and autoimmunity. *J Mol Med* 2004; 82:4–11.
22. Ukkola O, Santaniemi M. Adiponectin: a link between excess adiposity and associated comorbidities? *J Mol Med* 2002; 80:696–702.
23. Libby P, Ridker PM, Maseri A. Inflammation and atherosclerosis. *Circulation* 2002; 105:1135–1143.

24. Grover A, Padginton C, Wilson MF, Sung BH, Izzo JL, Jr, Dandona P. Insulin attenuates norepinephrine-induced venoconstriction. An ultrasonographic study. *Hypertension* 1995; 25:779–784.
25. Steinberg HO, Brechtel G, Johnson A, Fineberg N, Baron AD. Insulin-mediated skeletal muscle vasodilation is nitric oxide dependent. A novel action of insulin to increase nitric oxide release. *J Clin Invest* 1994; 94:1172–1179.
26. Aljada A, Saadeh R, Assian E, Ghanim H, Dandona P. Insulin inhibits the expression of intercellular adhesion molecule-1 by human aortic endothelial cells through stimulation of nitric oxide. *J Clin Endocrinol Metab* 2000; 85:2572–2575.
27. Zeng G, Quon MJ. Insulin-stimulated production of nitric oxide is inhibited by wortmannin. Direct measurement in vascular endothelial cells. *J Clin Invest* 1996; 98:894–898.
28. Aljada A, Dandona P. Effect of insulin on human aortic endothelial nitric oxide synthase. *Metabolism* 2000; 49:147–150.
29. Aljada A, Ghanim H, Saadeh R, Dandona P. Insulin inhibits NFkappaB and MCP-1 expression in human aortic endothelial cells. *J Clin Endocrinol Metab* 2001; 86:450–453.
30. Aljada A, Ghanim H, Mohanty P, Kapur N, Dandona P. Insulin inhibits the pro-inflammatory transcription factor early growth response gene-1 (Egr)-1 expression in mononuclear cells (MNC) and reduces plasma tissue factor (TF) and plasminogen activator inhibitor-1 (PAI-1) concentrations. *J Clin Endocrinol Metab* 2002; 87:1419–1422.
31. Dandona P, Aljada A, Mohanty P, Ghanim H, Bandyopadhyay A, Chaudhuri A. Insulin suppresses plasma concentration of vascular endothelial growth factor and matrix metalloproteinase-9. *Diabetes Care* 2003; 26:3310–3314.
32. Weis S, Shintani S, Weber A *et al.* Src blockade stabilizes a Flk/cadherin complex, reducing edema and tissue injury following myocardial infarction. *J Clin Invest* 2004; 113:885–894.
33. Chaudhuri A, Janicke D, Wilson MF *et al.* Anti-inflammatory and profibrinolytic effect of insulin in acute ST-segment-elevation myocardial infarction. *Circulation* 2004; 109:849–854.
34. Koskenkari JK, Kaukoranta PK, Rimpilainen J *et al.* Anti-inflammatory effect of high-dose insulin treatment after urgent coronary revascularization surgery. *Acta Anaesthesiol Scand* 2006; 50:962–969.
35. Visser L, Zuurbier CJ, Hoek FJ *et al.* Glucose, insulin and potassium applied as perioperative hyperinsulinaemic normoglycaemic clamp: effects on inflammatory response during coronary artery surgery. *Br J Anaesth* 2005; 95:448–457.
36. Chaudhuri A, Janicke D, Wilson MF, Ghanim H, Aljada A, Dandona P. Free Fatty Acid Suppressive, Pro- MMP-1 lowering and cardioprotective effect of insulin in STEMI. *Diabetes* 2005; 54:A182:739-P.
37. Langouche L, Vanhorebeek I, Vlasselaers D *et al.* Intensive insulin therapy protects the endothelium of critically ill patients. *J Clin Invest* 2005; 115:2277–2286.
38. Herndon DN, Tompkins RG. Support of the metabolic response to burn injury. *Lancet* 2004; 363:1895–1902.
39. Jeschke MG, Einspanier R, Klein D, Jauch KW. Insulin attenuates the systemic inflammatory response to thermal trauma. *Mol Med* 2002; 8:443–450.
40. Andersson CX, Sopasakis VR, Wallerstedt E, Smith U. Insulin antagonizes IL-6 signaling and is anti-inflammatory in 3T3-L1 adipocytes. *JBC* 2007; 282:9430–9435.
41. Cheung NW, Wong VW, McLean M. The Hyperglycemia: Intensive Insulin Infusion in Infarction (HI-5) study: a randomized controlled trial of insulin infusion therapy for myocardial infarction. *Diabetes Care* 2006; 29:765–770.
42. Malmberg K, Ryden L, Efendic S *et al.* Randomized trial of insulin-glucose infusion followed by subcutaneous insulin treatment in diabetic patients with acute myocardial infarction (DIGAMI study): effects on mortality at 1 year. *J Am Coll Cardiol* 1995; 26:57–65.
43. Gao F, Gao E, Yue TL *et al.* Nitric oxide mediates the antiapoptotic effect of insulin in myocardial ischemia-reperfusion: the roles of PI3-kinase, Akt, and endothelial nitric oxide synthase phosphorylation. *Circulation* 2002; 105:1497–1502.
44. Jonassen AK, Brar BK, Mjos OD, Sack MN, Latchman DS, Yellon DM. Insulin administered at reoxygenation exerts a cardioprotective effect in myocytes by a possible anti-apoptotic mechanism. *J Mol Cell Cardiol* 2000; 32:757–764.
45. Zhang HX, Zang YM, Huo JH *et al.* Physiologically tolerable insulin reduces myocardial injury and improves cardiac functional recovery in myocardial ischemic/reperfused dogs. *J Cardiovasc Pharmacol* 2006; 48:306–313.
46. Griselli M, Herbert J, Hutchinson WL *et al.* C-reactive protein and complement are important mediators of tissue damage in acute myocardial infarction. *J Exp Med* 1999; 190:1733–1740.

47. Pepys MB, Hirschfield GM, Tennent GA *et al.* Targeting C-reactive protein for the treatment of cardiovascular disease. *Nature* 2006; 440:1217–1221.
48. Bucciarelli-Ducci C, Bianchi M, De Luca L *et al.* Effects of glucose-insulin-potassium infusion on myocardial perfusion and left ventricular remodeling in patients treated with primary angioplasty for ST-elevation acute myocardial infarction. *Am J Cardiol* 2006; 98:1349–1353.
49. Trovati M, Massucco P, Mattiello L, Mularoni E, Cavalot F, Anfossi G. Insulin increases guanosine-3′,5′-cyclic monophosphate in human platelets. A mechanism involved in the insulin anti-aggregating effect. *Diabetes* 1994; 43:1015–1019.
50. Trovati M, Anfossi G, Massucco P *et al.* Insulin stimulates nitric oxide synthesis in human platelets and, through nitric oxide, increases platelet concentrations of both guanosine-3′, 5′-cyclic monophosphate and adenosine-3′, 5′-cyclic monophosphate. *Diabetes* 1997; 46:742–749.
51. Worthley MI, Holmes AS, Willoughby SR *et al.* The deleterious effects of hyperglycemia on platelet function in diabetic patients with acute coronary syndromes: mediation by superoxide production, resolution with intensive insulin administration. *J Am Coll Cardiol* 2007; 49:304–310.
52. Libby P, Simon DI. Inflammation and thrombosis: the clot thickens. *Circulation* 2001; 103:1718–1720.
53. Mohanty P, Hamouda W, Garg R, Aljada A, Ghanim H, Dandona P. Glucose challenge stimulates reactive oxygen species (ROS) generation by leucocytes. *J Clin Endocrinol Metab* 2000; 85:2970–2973.
54. Dhindsa S, Tripathy D, Mohanty P *et al.* Differential effects of glucose and alcohol on reactive oxygen species generation and intranuclear nuclear factor-kappaB in mononuclear cells. *Metabolism* 2004; 53:330–334.
55. Esposito K, Nappo F, Marfella R *et al.* Inflammatory cytokine concentrations are acutely increased by hyperglycemia in humans: role of oxidative stress. *Circulation* 2002; 106:2067–2072.
56. Aljada A, Ghanim H, Mohanty P, Syed T, Bandyopadhyay A, Dandona P. Glucose intake induces an increase in activator protein 1 and early growth response 1 binding activities, in the expression of tissue factor and matrix metalloproteinase in mononuclear cells, and in plasma tissue factor and matrix metalloproteinase concentrations. *Am J Clin Nutr* 2004; 80:51–57.
57. Mackman N. Role of tissue factor in hemostasis, thrombosis, and vascular development. *Arterioscler Thromb Vasc Biol* 2004; 24:1015–1022.
58. Steppich BA, Moog P, Matissek C *et al.* Cytokine profiles and T cell function in acute coronary syndromes. *Atherosclerosis* 2007; 190:443–451.
59. Ceriello A, Giacomello R, Stel G *et al.* Hyperglycemia-induced thrombin formation in diabetes. The possible role of oxidative stress. *Diabetes* 1995; 44:924–928.
60. Mohanty P, Ghanim H, Hamouda W, Aljada A, Garg R, Dandona P. Both lipid and protein intakes stimulate increased generation of reactive oxygen species by polymorphonuclear leukocytes and mononuclear cells. *Am J Clin Nutr* 2002; 75:767–772.
61. Tripathy D, Mohanty P, Dhindsa S *et al.* Elevation of free fatty acids induces inflammation and impairs vascular reactivity in healthy subjects. *Diabetes* 2003; 52:2882–2887.
62. Mohanty P, Daoud N, Ghanim H *et al.* Absence of oxidative stress and inflammation following the intake of a 900 kcalorie meal rich in fruit and fiber. *Diabetes* 2004; 53:A405.
63. Ghanim H, Mohanty P, Pathak R, Chaudhuri A, Sia CL, Dandona P. Orange juice or fructose intake does not induce oxidative and inflammatory response. *Diabetes Care* 2007; 30:1406–1411.
64. Dandona P, Mohanty P, Ghanim H *et al.* The suppressive effect of dietary restriction and weight loss in the obese on the generation of reactive oxygen species by leukocytes, lipid peroxidation, and protein carbonylation. *J Clin Endocrinol Metab* 2001; 86:355–362.
65. Dandona P, Mohanty P, Hamouda W *et al.* Inhibitory effect of a two day fast on reactive oxygen species (ROS) generation by leucocytes and plasma ortho-tyrosine and meta-tyrosine concentrations. *J Clin Endocrinol Metab* 2001; 86:2899–2902.
66. Hotamisligil GS, Arner P, Caro JF, Atkinson RL, Spiegelman BM. Increased adipose tissue expression of tumor necrosis factor-alpha in human obesity and insulin resistance. *J Clin Invest* 1995; 95:2409–2415.
67. Mohanty P, Khurana U, Chaudhuri A, Thusu K, Aljada A. Non-suppressibility of reactive oxygen species (ROS) generation by mononuclear cells (MNC) in obesity. *Diabetes* 1996; 45(suppl 1):171A (abstract).
68. Baynes JW. Role of oxidative stress in development of complications in diabetes. *Diabetes* 1991; 40:405–12.
69. Vincent HK, Powers SK, Stewart DJ, Shanely RA, Demirel H, Naito H. Obesity is associated with increased myocardial oxidative stress. *Int J Obes Relat Metab Disord* 1999; 23:67–74.

70. Dandona P, Mohanty P, Ghanim H *et al.* The suppressive effect of dietary restriction and weight loss in the obese on the generation of reactive oxygen species by leukocytes, lipid peroxidation, and protein carbonylation. *J Clin Endocrinol Metab* 2001; 86:355–362.
71. Engstrom G, Hedblad B, Stavenow L, Lind P, Janzon L, Lindgarde F. Inflammation-sensitive plasma proteins are associated with future weight gain. *Diabetes* 2003; 52:2097–2101.
72. Bistrian BR, Khaodhiar L. Chronic systemic inflammation in overweight and obese adults. *JAMA* 2000; 283:2235; author reply 2236.
73. Festa A, D'Agostino R, Jr, Howard G, Mykkanen L, Tracy RP, Haffner SM. Chronic subclinical inflammation as part of the insulin resistance syndrome: the Insulin Resistance Atherosclerosis Study (IRAS). *Circulation* 2000; 102:42–47.
74. DeGraba TJ. Expression of inflammatory mediators and adhesion molecules in human atherosclerotic plaque. *Neurology* 1997; 49:S15–S19.
75. Teramoto S, Yamamoto H, Ouchi Y. Increased C-reactive protein and increased plasma interleukin-6 may synergistically affect the progression of coronary atherosclerosis in obstructive sleep apnea syndrome. *Circulation* 2003; 107:E40.
76. Brand K, Page S, Rogler G *et al.* Activated transcription factor nuclear factor-kappa B is present in the atherosclerotic lesion. *J Clin Invest* 1996; 97:1715–1722.
77. Ross R. Atherosclerosis – an inflammatory disease. *N Engl J Med* 1999; 340:115–126.
78. Ceriello A, Bortolotti N, Motz E *et al.* Meal-generated oxidative stress in type 2 diabetic patients. *Diabetes Care* 1998; 21:1529–1533.
79. Talior I, Yarkoni M, Bashan N, Eldar-Finkelman H. Increased glucose uptake promotes oxidative stress and PKC-delta activation in adipocytes of obese, insulin-resistant mice. *Am J Physiol Endocrinol Metab* 2003; 285:E295–E302.
80. Aljada A, Mohanty P, Ghanim H *et al.* Increase in intranuclear nuclear factor kappaB and decrease in inhibitor kappaB in mononuclear cells after a mixed meal: evidence for a proinflammatory effect. *Am J Clin Nutr* 2004; 79:682–690.
81. Ziccardi P, Nappo F, Giugliano G *et al.* Reduction of inflammatory cytokine concentrations and improvement of endothelial functions in obese women after weight loss over one year. *Circulation* 2002; 105:804–809.
82. Tuomilehto J, Lindstrom J, Eriksson JG *et al.* Prevention of type 2 diabetes mellitus by changes in lifestyle among subjects with impaired glucose tolerance. *N Engl J Med* 2001; 344:1343–1350.
83. Rui L, Yuan M, Frantz D, Shoelson S, White MF. SOCS-1 and SOCS-3 block insulin signaling by ubiquitin-mediated degradation of IRS1 and IRS2. *J Biol Chem* 2002; 277:42394–42408.
84. Senn JJ, Klover PJ, Nowak IA *et al.* Suppressor of cytokine signaling-3 (SOCS-3), a potential mediator of interleukin-6-dependent insulin resistance in hepatocytes. *J Biol Chem* 2003; 278:13740–13746.
85. Emanuelli B, Peraldi P, Filloux C *et al.* SOCS-3 inhibits insulin signaling and is up-regulated in response to tumor necrosis factor-alpha in the adipose tissue of obese mice. *J Biol Chem* 2001; 276:47944–47949.
86. Standaert ML, Bandyopadhyay G, Galloway L *et al.* Effects of knockout of the protein kinase C beta gene on glucose transport and glucose homeostasis. *Endocrinology* 1999; 140:4470–4477.
87. Bossenmaier B, Mosthaf L, Mischak H, Ullrich A, Haring HU. Protein kinase C isoforms beta 1 and beta 2 inhibit the tyrosine kinase activity of the insulin receptor. *Diabetologia* 1997; 40:863–866.
88. Maedler K, Spinas GA, Dyntar D, Moritz W, Kaiser N, Donath MY. Distinct effects of saturated and monounsaturated fatty acids on beta-cell turnover and function. *Diabetes* 2001; 50:69–76.
89. Maedler K, Oberholzer J, Bucher P, Spinas GA, Donath MY. Monounsaturated fatty acids prevent the deleterious effects of palmitate and high glucose on human pancreatic beta-cell turnover and function. *Diabetes* 2003; 52:726–733.
90. Grill V, Bjorklund A. Dysfunctional insulin secretion in type 2 diabetes: role of metabolic abnormalities. *Cell Mol Life Sci* 2000; 57:429–440.
91. Harmon JS, Gleason CE, Tanaka Y, Poitout V, Robertson RP. Antecedent hyperglycemia, not hyperlipidemia, is associated with increased islet triacylglycerol content and decreased insulin gene mRNA level in Zucker diabetic fatty rats. *Diabetes* 2001; 50:2481–2486.
92. Poitout V, Robertson RP. Minireview: Secondary beta-cell failure in type 2 diabetes – a convergence of glucotoxicity and lipotoxicity. *Endocrinology* 2002; 143:339–342.
93. Dubois M, Kerr-Conte J, Gmyr V *et al.* Non-esterified fatty acids are deleterious for human pancreatic islet function at physiological glucose concentration. *Diabetologia* 2004; 47:463–469.

94. Marchetti P, Del Prato S, Lupi R, Del Guerra S. The pancreatic beta-cell in human Type 2 diabetes. *Nutr Metab Cardiovasc Dis* 2006; 16 (suppl 1):S3–S6.
95. Nakamura U, Iwase M, Uchizono Y *et al.* Rapid intracellular acidification and cell death by H_2O_2 and alloxan in pancreatic beta cells. *Free Radic Biol Med* 2006; 40:2047–2055.
96. Wu L, Nicholson W, Knobel SM *et al.* Oxidative stress is a mediator of glucose toxicity in insulin-secreting pancreatic islet cell lines. *J Biol Chem* 2004; 279:12126–12134.
97. Piro S, Anello M, Di Pietro C *et al.* Chronic exposure to free fatty acids or high glucose induces apoptosis in rat pancreatic islets: possible role of oxidative stress. *Metabolism* 2002; 51:1340–1347.
98. Otani K, Kulkarni RN, Baldwin AC *et al.* Reduced beta-cell mass and altered glucose sensing impair insulin-secretory function in betaIRKO mice. *Am J Physiol Endocrinol Metab* 2004; 286:E41–E49.
99. Garvey WT, Olefsky JM, Griffin J, Hamman RF, Kolterman OG. The effect of insulin treatment on insulin secretion and insulin action in type II diabetes mellitus. *Diabetes* 1985; 34:222–234.
100. Ryan EA, Imes S, Wallace C. Short-term intensive insulin therapy in newly diagnosed type 2 diabetes. *Diabetes Care* 2004; 27:1028–1032.
101. Li Y, Xu W, Liao Z *et al.* Induction of long-term glycemic control in newly diagnosed type 2 diabetic patients is associated with improvement of beta-cell function. *Diabetes Care* 2004; 27:2597–2602.

9

Suppressing inflammation: a novel approach to treating the metabolic syndrome

A. D. Rao, V. Fonseca

INTRODUCTION

It is becoming clear that inflammatory processes may underlie the interrelated conditions of diabetes, the metabolic syndrome, and cardiovascular disease (CVD). CVD continues to be the leading cause of mortality in patients with diabetes, despite considerable advances in its prevention and treatment [1–3]. Both diabetes and the metabolic syndrome are risk factors for CVD.

Recent studies suggest that a state of chronic, subacute inflammation, specifically mediated by the IKKβ/NF-κB pathway, might be both involved in the pathogenesis of insulin resistance and provide new targets for its reversal [4–6]. These concepts are supported by epidemiological results looking at correlates and potential causes of type 2 diabetes [7–9]. Furthermore, relationships between insulin resistance and mediators of inflammation, including the pro-inflammatory cytokines, interleukin (IL)-6 and IL-1β and possibly tumor necrosis factor (TNF)-α have been described [8, 9].

Subacute inflammation may also play a role in the development of the associated dyslipidemia and hypertension and thus play a central role in this syndrome. Together, insulin resistance (with or without hyperglycemia), dyslipidemia, and hypertension all increase risk for atherosclerosis, which is itself increasingly thought to be a disease of chronic subacute inflammation [10]. Furthermore, targeting inflammation may have an impact on both hyperglycemia as well as other cardiovascular risk factors that constitute the metabolic syndrome. The various biomarkers of inflammation such as inflammatory cytokines (TNF-α, IL-6, and IL-1β), chemokines (monocyte chemoattractant protein-1 [MCP-1] and IL-8) and C-reactive protein (CRP) are increased in obesity and correlate with insulin resistance and CVD.

In this chapter, we discuss clinical data on the efficacy of various drugs such as metformin, peroxisome proliferator-activated receptor (PPAR) agonists and anti-inflammatory agents in amelioration of inflammation in subjects with metabolic syndrome, and finally examine the possibility of suppressing inflammation with anti-inflammatory drugs to treat diabetes mellitus and metabolic syndrome.

CHEMICAL MARKERS OF INFLAMMATION

The acute phase protein, C-reactive protein (CRP), is produced by the liver (Figure 9.1) in response to injury and inflammation, and this is predictive of (sometimes major) coronary

Ajay D. Rao, MD, Fellow, Endocrinology, Section of Endocrinology, Tulane University Health Sciences Center, New Orleans, Louisiana, USA

Vivian Fonseca, MD, FRCP, Professor of Medicine and Pharmacology, Tullis Tulane Alumni Chair in Diabetes; Chief, Section of Endocrinology, Department of Medicine, Tulane University Health Sciences Center, New Orleans, Louisiana, USA

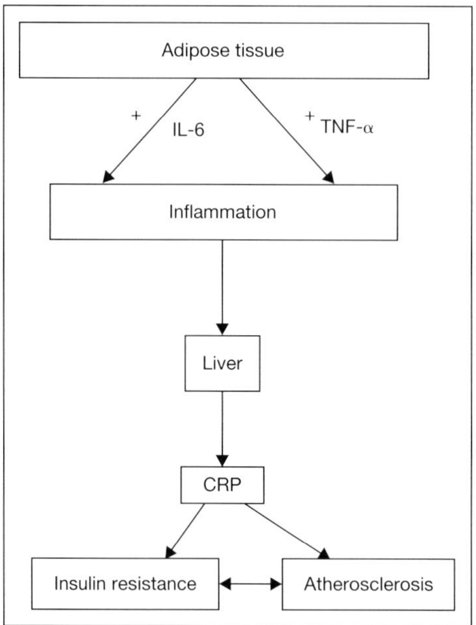

Figure 9.1 Schematic representation of the interactions between inflammation, insulin resistance and atherosclerosis. CRP = reactive protein; IL-6 = interleukin 6; TNF-α = tumor necrosis factor alpha.

events in apparently healthy people [11, 12]. It is also of prognostic value in patients with acute coronary syndromes [13]. Data are also emerging that CRP may be an independent risk factor for hypertension [14], and also a marker of carotid atherosclerotic activity in early carotid atherosclerosis [15].

In 2003, the American Heart Association and the Centers for Disease Control and Prevention issued a statement on inflammatory markers and CVD [16]. The statement concluded that if inflammatory markers were to be measured as markers of risk, highly sensitive-CRP (hs-CRP) would be the first choice. The statement also stratified patients into three relative risk categories based on average hs-CRP levels: low risk – hs-CRP <1 mg/l; average risk – hs-CRP 1–3 mg/l and high risk – >3 mg/l.

High plasma CRP levels have been seen in overweight and obese adults [17]. A study of 16 616 men and women from the third National Health and Nutrition Examination Survey (NHANES) in 1988–1994 looked at elevated CRP levels (<0.22 mg/dl) according to body mass index (BMI) [17]. Elevated CRP levels were more common in overweight (BMI 25–29 kg/m^2) and obese (BMI <30 kg/m^2) subjects, particularly women, compared with those of normal weight (BMI <25 kg/m^2). Elevated serum CRP was more common with increasing BMI. The same observations were made in healthy, non-smoking, non-estrogen using adults aged 17–39 years. Adiponectin is an anti-inflammatory compound produced by adipocytes, low levels of which are associated with insulin resistance [18]. Low levels of adiponectin were seen in obese healthy women and were inversely correlated with IL-6 and hs-CRP [19].

The National Health and Nutrition Survey (carried out in the former West Germany from 1987 to 1988) assessed the association between CRP and features of the metabolic syndrome in 1703 healthy subjects [20]. Features were total cholesterol, high-density lipoprotein (HDL)-cholesterol, triglycerides, uric acid, BMI and prevalence of diabetes and hypertension. There was a statistically significant positive correlation between CRP and the features of the metabolic syndrome. As many subjects had more than one feature of metabolic syndrome, the CRP levels were measured according to the number of defining features. There was a statistically

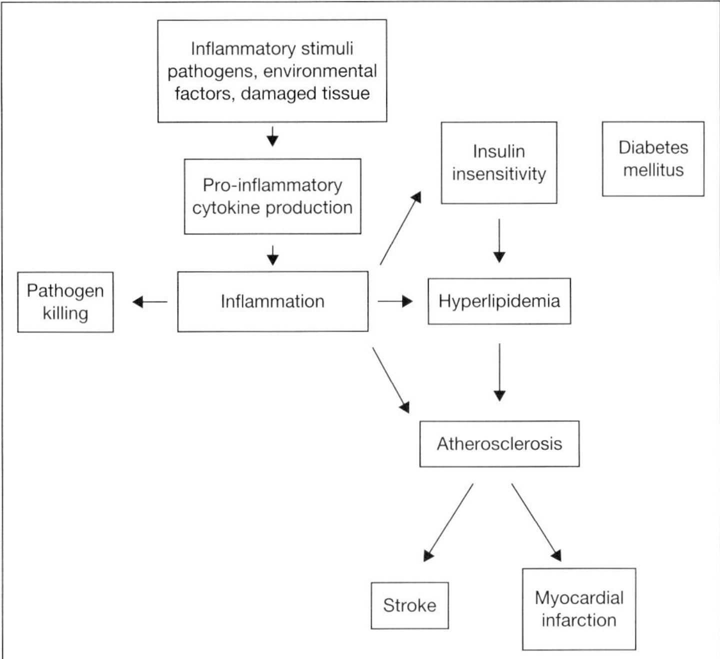

Figure 9.2 Linkages between the response to pathogens and disorders and diseases where chronic inflammation participates in the pathogenesis.

significant increase in CRP levels with increasing number of features of the metabolic syndrome. Data from an eight-year follow up of 14 719 initially healthy women in the US further confirmed that measuring CRP gives clinically relevant prognostic information on the future risk of CVD in patients with and without metabolic syndrome [12].

Obesity is an established risk factor for diabetes, and it is interesting to note that adipose tissue is thought to be the source of pro-inflammatory agents such as IL-6 and TNF-α. The Women's Health Study in the US investigated the relationship between IL-6, CRP and type 2 diabetes [8]. Baseline levels of IL-6 and CRP were significantly higher ($P < 0.001$) in women who developed type 2 diabetes over 4 years than in diabetes-free controls. Chronic inflammation and increased levels of inflammatory mediators have been shown to precede type 2 diabetes. The Insulin Resistance Atherosclerosis Study investigated the relationship between the concentrations of the acute phase proteins (CRP and fibrinogen) and plasminogen activator inhibitor type 1 (PIA-1), and the incidence of type 2 diabetes [21]. Baseline levels of CRP, fibrinogen and PIA-1 were higher in those who developed diabetes during 5 years of follow up than in those who did not. Figure 9.2 shows the effects of chronic production of pro-inflammatory cytokines [22]. To summarize, inflammatory markers are linked to increases in BMI, the features of metabolic syndrome and the incidence of diabetes, which probably lead to a higher risk of CVD and, ultimately, decreased survival.

PRO-INFLAMMATORY CYTOKINES, ENDOTHELIAL ACTIVATION, MONOCYTES/MACROPHAGES AND THE METABOLIC SYNDROME

Pro-inflammatory cytokines, including IL-1β, IL-6 and TNF-α, are produced in cells involved in immunity and inflammation, such as macrophages and monocytes, and in adipose tissue and liver, particularly in response to over-nutrition. The cytokines (IL-1β, IL-6 and TNF-α) also act on liver to produce a characteristic dyslipidemia associated with type 2 diabetes, increased very low-density lipoprotein (VLDL) and decreased HDL, and to promote the release of acute-phase proteins which are atherosclerotic risk factors, such as fibrinogen. Circulating cytokines may act on the endothelium to promote atherogenesis and they may impair β cell insulin secretion.

Elevations in components of the acute-phase response and of inflammation more generally occur in type 2 diabetes and predict risk for its occurrence [8, 23–25]. Elevated markers include PAI1, CRP, fibrinogen, leukocyte count, sialic acid, IL-6 and IL-1β. However, the big question in the field has been whether these are simply correlative markers for the process or causatively involved in its pathogenesis. It is clear that pro-inflammatory cytokines such as IL-6 and TNF-α can cause insulin resistance in animal models [26–28]. However, in order to prove a true cause and effect relationship in human disease it may be necessary to demonstrate amelioration of the disease process by specific inhibitors of these cytokines. Such data are beginning to emerge with anti-inflammatory agents, as discussed below. On the other hand, a specific monoclonal antibody against TNF-α, which suppresses inflammation and is used to treat other inflammatory diseases, has had very little, if any, effect on diabetes or the metabolic syndrome [29, 30]. Nevertheless, elucidating this pro-inflammatory role of TNF-α led to the discovery of other bioactive substances that further confirmed that fat was a site for the production of cytokines. Implicated cytokines have included leptin, IL-6, resistin, MCP-1, PAI-1, angiotensinogen, visfatin, retinol-binding-4, serum amyloid A (SAA), and others [31, 35].

Cytokines, in particular IL-1, TNF and IL-6, are the main inducers of the acute-phase response [36]. Several lines of evidence indicate that IL-6 is the central mediator of the inflammatory response and promotes insulin resistance [37]. In addition, IL-6 administered to humans subcutaneously induces an acute inflammatory response [38]. In fact, IL-6 is believed to be the main driver of CRP release from hepatocytes [39]. A very tight correlation exists between IL-6 and CRP; such a strong correlation does not exist for other cytokines. Furthermore, IL-6 and hs-CRP are associated with visceral adiposity and 30% of circulating IL-6 is derived from human adipose tissue [40]. Moreover, baseline IL-6 levels independently predict future cerebrovascular events (CVE) [11]. Pickup *et al.* [41] have shown increased levels of IL-6 in subjects with more than two features of the metabolic syndrome. Furthermore, in type 2 diabetes, monocyte release of IL-6 is significantly increased when compared to non-diabetic controls [42].

Data suggest that the transcription factor NF-κB is a central integrator of pro-inflammatory signals and a key regulator of genes involved in inflammation, innate immunity, and apoptosis, as highlighted by Shoelson and Goldfine [4]. Numerous signals that activate NF-κB in addition to pro-inflammatory cytokines include bacterial cell wall and viral products, double-standed DNA (dsDNA), mitogens and oxidative stress (Figure 9.3) [43]. Toll-like receptors, the gatekeepers of innate immunity, activate NF-κB. IκB proteins sequester NF-κB in the cytoplasm of resting cells. Activation of the kinase IKKβ promotes IκBα phosphorylation, ubiquitination, and proteasomal degradation. Table 9.1 lists some of the genes regulated by NF-κB that have been implicated in the pathogenesis of insulin resistance, type 2 diabetes and CVD.

Many of the gene products regulated by NF-κB have been implicated as markers or mediators of insulin resistance and type 2 diabetes (Table 9.1). It has been suggested that NF-κB orchestrates the transcription of a constellation of genes, some known and others yet to be discovered, that coordinately mediate obesity-induced insulin resistance.

DIABETES TREATMENTS AND INFLAMMATION

THERAPEUTIC LIFESTYLE INTERVENTION AND MODULATION OF INFLAMMATION

Therapeutic lifestyle change (TLC), including diet and exercise, is the cornerstone of therapy for the metabolic syndrome. Thus, the first step in reducing the excess cardiovascular risk

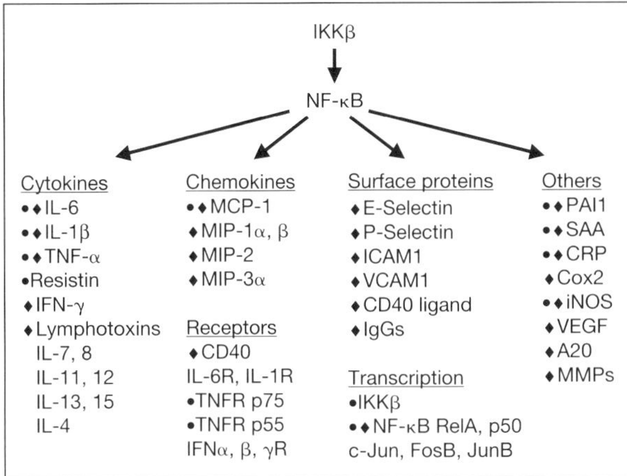

Figure 9.3 Selected NF-κB responsive genes with potential roles in insulin resistance and type 2 diabetes (●) or CHD (◆). Collectively, these could be considered mediators of the metabolic syndrome.

Table 9.1 The metabolic syndrome: evidence for a pro-inflammatory state

↑Acute phase proteins (hs-CRP and SAA)
↓Adiponectin
↑Pro-inflammatory status (IL-6, IL-18 and TNF-α)
↑Leptin
↑Chemokines (MCP-1 and IL-8)
↓Anti-inflammatory cytokines (IL-10)
hs-CRP = highly sensitive C-reactive protein; IL = interleukin; MCP-1 = monocyte chemottractant protein-1; SAA = serum amyloid A; TNF-α = tumor nerosis factor alpha.

associated with the presence of the metabolic syndrome is the adoption of a healthier lifestyle (particularly reducing body weight and increasing physical activity). The beneficial effects of TLC with regards to modulation of metabolic syndrome features have been convincingly shown in various diabetes prevention studies [44, 45]. Although, TLC, including diet and exercise is the cornerstone and foremost therapy for the treatment of metabolic syndrome, at times TLC is not effective because of patient compliance. Moreover, obesity is a chronic and relapsing disease and, therefore, many patients find it difficult to lose weight and maintain weight loss with lifestyle therapy alone. Furthermore, many people are not able to fully reverse existing metabolic risk factors with TLC, and as risk factors worsen with advancing age, there is an increased need for drugs to manage particular risk factors. In view of this, we will discuss here the pharmacologic therapy of obesity-related inflammation and the associated implications of the metabolic syndrome.

PHARMACOLOGIC MODULATION OF METABOLIC SYNDROME AND ITS IMPACT ON INFLAMMATION

As stated previously, obesity-related inflammation and the associated metabolic syndrome features can be reduced by a variety of drugs such as metformin, statins, PPAR-α agonists (fibrate class of anti-dyslipidemic drugs), PPAR-γ agonists (insulin-sensitizing thiazolidinediones), angiotensin receptor blockers (ARBs) and the endocannabinoid receptor-1 blocker (rimonabant).

Metformin

Metformin, an antihyperglycemic agent, appears to decrease adiposity and improve hepatic insulin resistance. Kay and co-workers [46] reported a greater reduction in weight and body mass following 8 weeks of metformin therapy (850 mg bid) along with low-caloric, low-glycemic diet in obese (BMI >30 kg/m^2) adolescents with hyperinsulinemia as compared to placebo ($n = 12$/group). Notably, metformin combined with standard lifestyle advice was one of the treatments evaluated in the Diabetes Prevention Program (DPP) clinical trial, a population with a high prevalence of the metabolic syndrome [45]. In the DPP, metformin reduced CRP compared with the placebo group, but was still less effective than lifestyle change. In men, the median changes in CRP from baseline to 1 year were –33% in the lifestyle group, –7% in the metformin group, and +5% in the placebo group. In women, the changes in CRP from baseline to follow-up were –29% in the lifestyle group, –14% in the metformin group, and 0% in the placebo group. Dandona and colleagues [47] have reported the suppressive action of metformin 1g (Glucophage XR; 1000 mg twice daily for 6 weeks) in reducing plasma macrophage migration inhibitory factor (MIF) concentrations in obese subjects as compared to non-obese healthy subjects. More studies are required with metformin in the context of various other cardiovascular risk factors in metabolic syndrome subjects.

PPAR-α agonists and lipid-lowering drugs

Currently there are three fibrates available – gemfibrozil, fenofibrate and bezafibrate treat atherogenic dyslipidemia and can also be used in dyslipidemia of the metabolic syndrome. These drugs are useful in that they impact two of the components of the definition of the syndrome. However, their impact on inflammation appears to be minor – although this has not been well studied. Fenofibrate-induced increase of HDL-cholesterol is reported to be associated with a significant reduction of plasma intracellular adhesion molecule-1 (sICAM-1) and sE-selectin concentrations in the low-HDL subjects [48]. Furthermore, Després and co-workers [49] confirmed the efficacy of gemfibrozil (600 mg bd for 6 months) on reduction of CRP levels (~32%) with no effect on IL-6 and TNF levels in abdominally obese patients with metabolic syndrome.

In patients with hypercholesterolemia, fibrates decrease IL-6 and CD40 ligand as well as MCP-1 [50]. Furthermore, in a study in dyslipidemic obese (with features of metabolic syndrome), fibrates resulted in a significant reduction in CRP [51]. Thus, in addition to their favorable effects on lipid profiles, evidence is mounting that benefits may also stem from the anti-inflammatory and anti-atherosclerotic properties of the PPAR-α activators. In patients with angiographically established atherosclerosis, fenofibrate treatment decreased the circulating levels of IL-6 and lowered the plasma levels of CRP and fibrinogen [52, 53]. In addition, fenofibrate treatment significantly reduced plasma interferon (IFN) and TNF levels in patients with type IIb hyperlipoproteinemia [54]. Similar effects were observed in hypertriglyceridemic patients after bezafibrate administration [55]. Fenofibrate treatment also led to a reduction in ICAM-1, MCP-1 and α-macroglobulin and plasminogen plasma levels in patients with hyperlipoproteinemia [56, 57].

In this context it is important to note that some of the clinically available statins have been shown to downregulate the transcriptional activities of NF-κB, activator protein-1 (AP-1), and hypoxia-inducible factor-1α (HIF-1α). These studies have also shown a resultant reduction in the prothrombotic and pro-inflammatory cytokines [58]. However, none of the statins appear to significantly influence either insulin resistance or glycemia.

PPAR-γ agonists

PPAR-γ agonists, which are insulin sensitizers, have been the focus of much research in the last decade and are discussed in detail elsewhere in this book.

PPAR-γ is expressed by macrophages and recent studies suggest that thiazolidinediones (TZDs) may have broad effects on suppressing macrophage-mediated inflammation [58]. All these findings put together suggest that PPAR-γ agonists have inhibitory effects on inflammatory processes. Several studies have demonstrated a significant reduction in a variety of inflammatory markers in patients with the metabolic syndrome with or without diabetes mellitus [59–66].

Overall, it appears that PPAR-γ agonists have a wide range of anti-inflammatory effects in non-diabetic patients. Potential mechanisms underlying this anti-inflammatory effect include insulin sensitization and direct modulation of transcriptional activity in the vessel wall.

Specific anti-inflammatory agents

Numerous molecular pathways have been implicated in the link between inflammation and insulin resistance. As early as a century ago, high doses of sodium salicylate were first demonstrated to diminish glycosuria in diabetic patients [67, 68]. This connection between the antihyperglycemic and anti-inflammatory effects of salicylates and the pathogenesis of insulin resistance was not realized until recently.

Salicylates

Treating diabetes using high-dose salicylates is an old method and one that is accompanied by insulin sensitization. Furthermore, it has been shown during short-term trials that salicylate therapy markedly lowers circulating glucose, triglycerides, free fatty acids and cholesterol, and that all of these effects are mediated by the IKKβ/NF-κB pathway [4].

Early studies suggested effects of aspirin were centered around glucose metabolism, while more recent trials have shown a detrimental effect of aspirin therapy on insulin sensitivity [68]. Some recent studies have shown that high-dose aspirin improved multiple metabolic measures in patients with type 2 diabetes, including substantial reductions in fasting and post-prandial glucose, triglycerides, and FFAs. Non-acetylated salicylates, also inhibit NF-κB, due to inhibition of IKKβ. In a study by Hundal *et al.*, nine type 2 diabetics were exposed to high-dose treatment of aspirin (7 g/day) and underwent mixed-meal tolerance tests and hyperinsulinemic-euglycemic clamps. The results showed that there was a reduction in inflammatory markers (CRP), lipid profiles and, most importantly, fasting plasma glucose. Clinical trials to test efficacy, tolerability and durability of salsalate are currently being undertaken in the National Institutes of Health (NIH)-funded TINSAL-T2D and CVD trials. In addition, other anti-inflammatory strategies are also being considered, including the potential use of specific Jun N-terminal Kinase (JNK) or IKKβ inhibitors and compounds that block TNF-α, IL-6, toll-like receptor (TLR), or chemokine signaling.

Anti-inflammatory drugs are conveniently separated into the glucocorticoids and non-steroidal anti-inflammatory drugs (NSAIDs). The actions of the glucocorticoids are mediated by the glucocorticoid receptor, a member of the nuclear receptor family. Since glucocorticoids promote insulin resistance, these do not provide much promise as potential treatments for type 2 diabetes or CHD. NSAIDs are chemically distinct and among the most commonly used drugs. Nearly all of the NSAIDs inhibit one or both of the cyclooxygenase enzymes, Cox1 and Cox2.

Aspirin (ASA, acetylsalicylic acid), the acetylated form of salicylate, is the prototypical NSAID. Aspirin very efficiently inhibits the Cox enzymes through irreversible, covalent transacetylation of an active site residue, i.e. aspirin's acetyl group covalently modifies Cox. Aspirin is antithrombotic even at low doses of 80–100 mg/day, because it irreversibly modifies Cox1 in platelets. Since platelets are non-nucleated and cannot resynthesize Cox1, this inactivates platelets for their lifetimes. Aspirin at the typical analgesic/antipyretic/anti-inflammatory dose of 650 mg inhibits both Cox1 and Cox2 in most cells and tissues. In this case, aspirin is dosed more frequently, every 4–6 h up to 4 doses per day. Other non-selective NSAIDs, including ibuprofen, naprosyn, ketoprofen and indomethacin, also inhibit Cox1 and Cox2 in most cells and tissues.

Salicylate has a distinct mechanism of action. At the high doses necessary for therapeutic efficacy (3–7 g/day), salicylates inhibit NF-κB [69], apparently by binding IKKβ and inhibiting IκB phosphorylation [70]. Salicylate is a very weak inhibitor of Cox1 or Cox2, because it lacks the acetyl group necessary for transacetylation and covalent modification. Aspirin, on the other hand, appears to be equivalent to salicylate in inhibiting NF-κB. However, gastrointestinal toxicity and risk of life-threatening bleeds limit aspirin's use at high doses.

IL-1 antagonists

Recently, IL-1β, a pro-inflammatory cytokine has been implicated in β-cell destruction leading to type 1 diabetes. Interestingly, findings have also shown its role in type 2 diabetes, including intra-islet production of inflammatory mediators. Larsen, and co-workers looked at IL-1β as a potential therapeutic target for preserving β-cell mass and function in patients with this condition [71]. Interleukin-1 receptor antagonist, a naturally occurring competitive inhibitor of interleukin-1 binding to the type I receptor [72], protects human β cells from glucose-induced functional impairment and apoptosis [73]. Interleukin-1 receptor antagonist is reported to have no agonistic activity [74, 75]. The expression of interleukin-1 receptor antagonist is decreased in β cells obtained from patients with type 2 diabetes [76]. Given these observations, it has been hypothesized that intervening in the islet balance between interleukin-1 receptor antagonist and interleukin-1 β might improve β-cell function and glycemic control in patients with type 2 diabetes.

Hydroxychloroquine

Antimalarials have been used for autoimmune diseases such as rheumatoid arthritis (RA) and systemic lupus erythematosus (SLE) and have anti-inflammatory effects. In the past, hypoglycemia was identified as an adverse effect during treatment with these agents. A recent study investigated the association between one of these agents (hydroxychloroquine) and the incidence of diabetes [77]. There was a reduction in diabetes risk up to 77% for patients taking hydroxychloroquine for more than 4 years. The pathophysiological basis for its antihyperglycemic effect may be related to the increase of insulin secretion and/or inhibition of its clearance [78]. It is important to note that more prospective studies are needed in this area.

SUMMARY

Recent research has highlighted the importance of inflammation-induced insulin resistance and CVD. Several mediators of inflammation have been identified and mechanistic pathways elucidated. Some of these may serve as surrogate biomarkers for diabetes and CVD risk. Several interventions in diabetes and CVD suppress inflammation and, in specific anti-inflammatory drugs, have antidiabetic effects. Thus, approaches that target inflammation may provide benefit for the large number of persons that will be affected by the obesity epidemic.

REFERENCES

1. Wilson PW. Diabetes mellitus and coronary heart disease. *AJKD* 1998; 32:S89–S100.
2. Wilson PW, D'Agostino R, Levy D, Belanger AM, Silbershatz H, Kannel WB. Prediction of coronary heart disease using risk factor categories. *Circulation* 1998; 97:1837–1847.

3. Geiss LS, Herman WH, Smith PJ, National Diabetes Data Group. *Diabetes in America*. National Institute of Diabetes and Digestive and Kidney Diseases, 1995; 233–257.
4. Shoelson SE, Lee J, Goldfine AB. Inflammation and insulin resistance. *Journal of Clinical Investigation* 2006; 116:1793–1801.
5. Cai D, Frantz DF, Melendez PA, Hansen L, Lee J, Shoelson SE. Local and systemic insulin resistance resulting from hepatic activation of IKKβ and NF-κB. *Nat Med* 2005; 11:183–190.
6. Kim JK, Kim YJ, Fillmore JJ *et al*. Prevention of fat-induced insulin resistance by salicylate. *JCI* 2001; 108:437–446.
7. Pickup JC, Crook MA. Is type II diabetes mellitus a disease of the innate immune system? *Diabetologia* 1998; 41:1241–1248.
8. Pradhan AD, Manson JE, Rifai N, Buring JE, Ridker PM. C-reactive protein, interleukin 6, and risk of developing type 2 diabetes mellitus. *JAMA* 2001; 286:327–334.
9. Spranger J, Kroke A, Mohlig M *et al*. Inflammatory cytokines and the risk to develop type 2 diabetes: Results of the prospective population-based European Prospective Investigation into Cancer and Nutrition (EPIC) – Potsdam Study. *Diabetes* 2003; 52:812–817.
10. Libby P. Inflammation in atherosclerosis. *Nature* 2002; 420:868–874.
11. Ridker PM, Hennekens CH, Buring JE, Rifai N. C-reactive protein and other markers of inflammation in the prediction of cardiovascular disease in women. *NEJM* 2000; 342:836–843.
12. Ridker PM, Buring JE, Cook NR, Rifai N. C-reactive protein, the metabolic syndrome, and risk of incident cardiovascular events: an 8-year follow-up of 14719 initially healthy American women. *Circulation* 2003; 107:391–397.
13. Abbate A, Biondi-Zoccal GC, Brugaletta S, Liuzzo G, Biasucci LM. C-reactive protein and other inflammatory biomarkers as predictors of outcome following acute coronary syndromes. *Seminars in Vascular Medicine* 2003; 3:375–384.
14. Bautista LE, Lopez-Jaramillo P, Vera LM, Casas JP, Otero AP, Guaracao AI. Is C-reactive protein an independent risk factor for essential hypertension? *Journal of Hypertension* 2001; 19:857–861.
15. Hashimoto H, Kitagawa K, Hougaku H *et al*. C-reactive protein is an independent predictor of the rate of increase in early carotid atherosclerosis. *Circulation* 2001; 104:63–67.
16. Pearson TA, Mensah GA, Alexander RW *et al*. Markers of inflammation and cardiovascular disease: Application to clinical and public health practice: A statement for healthcare professionals from the Centers for Disease Control and Prevention and the American Heart Association. *Circulation* 2003; 107:499–511.
17. Visser M, Bouter LM, McQuillan GM, Wener MH, Harris TB. Elevated C-reactive protein levels in overweight and obese adults. *JAMA* 1999; 282:2131–2135.
18. Weyer C, Funahashi T, Tanaka S *et al*. Hypoadiponectinemia in obesity and type 2 diabetes: Close association with insulin resistance and hyperinsulinemia. *JCEM* 2001; 86:1930–1935.
19. Engeli S, Feldpausch M, Gorzelniak K *et al*. Association between adiponectin and mediators of inflammation in obese women. *Diabetes* 2003; 52:942–947.
20. Frohlich M, Imhof A, Berg G *et al*. Association between C-reactive protein and features of the metabolic syndrome. *Diabetes Care* 2000; 23:1835–1839.
21. Festa A, D'Agostino R, Tracy RP, Haffner SM. Elevated levels of acute-phase proteins and plasminogen activator inhibitor-1 predict the development of type 2 diabetes: the insulin resistance atherosclerosis study. *Diabetes* 2002; 51:1131–1137.
22. Grimble RF. Inflammatory status and insulin resistance. *Curr Opin Clin Nutr Metab Care* 2002; 5:551–559.
23. Barzilay JI, Freedland ES. Inflammation and its relationship to insulin resistance, type 2 diabetes mellitus, and endothelial dysfunction. *Metabolic Syndrome* 2003; 1:55–67.
24. Pickup JC. Inflammation and activated innate immunity in the pathogenesis of type 2 diabetes. *Diabetes Care* 2004; 27:813–823.
25. Barzilay JI, Abraham L, Heckbert SR *et al*. The relation of markers of inflammation to the development of glucose disorders in the elderly: the Cardiovascular Health Study. *Diabetes* 2001; 50:2384–2389.
26. Hotamisligil GS, Murray DL, Choy LN, Spiegelman BM. Tumor necrosis factor alpha inhibits signaling from the insulin receptor. *Proc Natl Acad Sci* 1994; 91:4854–4858.
27. Hotamisligil GS, Shargill NS, Spiegelman BM. Adipose expression of tumor necrosis factor-alpha: Direct role in obesity-linked insulin resistance. *Science* 1993; 259:87–91.
28. Klover PJ, Zimmers TA, Koniaris LG, Mooney RA. Chronic exposure to interleukin-6 causes hepatic insulin resistance in mice. *Diabetes* 2003; 52:2784–2789.

29. Dominguez H, Storgaard H, Rask-Madsen C *et al*. Metabolic and vascular effects of tumor necrosis factor-alpha blockade with etanercept in obese patients with type 2 diabetes. *J Vasc Res* 2005; 42:517–525.
30. Gonzalez-Gay MA, De Matias JM, Gonzalez-Juanatey C *et al*. Anti-tumor necrosis factor-alpha blockade improves insulin resistance in patients with rheumatoid arthritis. *Clin Exp Rheumatol* 2006; 24:83–86.
31. Zhang Y, Proenca R, Maffei M, Barone M, Leopold L, Friedman JM. Positional cloning of the mouse obese gene and its human homologue. *Nature* 1994; 372:425–432.
32. Fried SK, Bunkin DA, Greenberg AS. Omental and subcutaneous adipose tissues of obese subjects release interleukin-6: Depot difference and regulation by glucocorticoid. *JCEM* 1998; 83:847–850.
33. Steppan CM, Bailey ST, Bhat S *et al*. The hormone resistin links obesity to diabetes. *Nature* 2001; 409:307–312.
34. Shimomura I *et al*. Enhanced expression of PAI-1 in visceral fat: Possible contributor to vascular disease in obesity. *Nat Med* 1996; 2:800–803.
35. Fukuhara A, Matsuda M, Nishizawa M *et al*. Visfatin: A protein secreted by visceral fat that mimics the effects of insulin. *Science* 2005; 307:426–430.
36. Baumann H, Goldie J. The acute phase response. *Immunol Today* 1994; 15:74–80.
37. Heinrich PC, Castell JV, Andus T. Interleukin-6 and the acute phase response. *Biochem J* 1990; 265:621–636.
38. Banks RE, Forbes MA, Storr M *et al*. The acute phase protein response in patients receiving subcutaneous IL-6. *Clin Exp Immunol* 1995; 102:217–223.
39. Li SP, Goldman ND. Regulation of human C-reactive protein gene expression by two synergistic IL-6 responsive elements. *Biochemistry* 1996; 35:9060–9068.
40. Aldhahi W, Hamdy O. Adipokines, inflammation, and the endothelium in diabetes. *Curr Diab Rep* 2003; 3:293–298.
41. Pickup JC, Mattock MB, Chusney GD, Burt D. NIDDM as a disease of the innate immune system: Association of acute-phase reactants and interleukin-6 with metabolic syndrome X. *Diabetologia* 1997; 40:1286–1292.
42. Devaraj S, Jialal I. Alpha tocopherol supplementation decreases serum C-reactive protein and monocyte interleukin-6 levels in normal volunteers and type 2 diabetic patients. *Free Radic Biol Med* 2000; 29:790–792.
43. Baeuerle PA, Baltimore D. NF-kappa B: Ten years after. *Cell* 1996; 87:13–20.
44. Diabetes Prevention Program (DPP) Research Group. The Diabetes Prevention Program (DPP): Description of lifestyle intervention. *Diabetes Care* 2002; 25:2165–2171.
45. Orchard TJ, Temprosa M, Goldberg R *et al*. The effect of metformin and intensive lifestyle intervention on the metabolic syndrome: the Diabetes Prevention Program randomized trial. *Ann Intern Med* 2005; 142:611–619.
46. Kay JP, Alemzadeh R, Langley G, D'Angelo L, Smith P, Holshouser S. Beneficial effects of metformin in normoglycemic morbidly obese adolescents. *Metabolism* 2001; 50:1457–1461.
47. Dandona P, Aljada A, Ghanim H *et al*. Increased plasma concentration of macrophage migration inhibitory factor (MIF) and MIF mRNA in mononuclear cells in the obese and the suppressive action of metformin. *JCEM* 2004; 89:5043–5047.
48. Calabresi L, Gomaraschi M, Villa B, Omoboni L, Dmitrieff C, Franceschini G. Elevated soluble cellular adhesion molecules in subjects with low HDL-cholesterol. *Arterioscler Thromb Vasc Biol* 2002; 22:656–661.
49. Després JP, Lemieux I, Pascot A *et al*. Gemfibrozil reduces plasma C-reactive protein levels in abdominally obese men with the atherogenic dyslipidemia of the metabolic syndrome. *Arterioscler Thromb Vasc Biol* 2003; 23:702–703.
50. Undas A, Celinska-Lowenhoff M, Domagala TB *et al*. Early antithrombotic and anti-inflammatory effects of simvastatin versus fenofibrate in patients with hypercholesterolemia. *Thromb Haemost* 2005; 94:193–199.
51. Coban E, Sari R. The effect of fenofibrate on the levels of high sensitivity C-reactive protein in dyslipidemic obese patients. *Endocr Res* 2004; 30:343–349.
52. Zambon A, Gervois P, Pauletto P, Fruchart JC, Staels B. Modulation of hepatic inflammatory risk markers of cardiovascular diseases by PPAR-alpha activators: Clinical and experimental evidence. *Arterioscler Thromb Vasc Biol* 2006; 26:977–986.
53. Gervois P, Kleemann R, Pilon A *et al*. Global suppression of IL-6-induced acute phase response gene expression after chronic in vivo treatment with the peroxisome proliferator-activated receptor-alpha activator fenofibrate. *J Biol Chem* 2004; 279:16154–16160.

54. Madej A, Okopien B, Kowalski J *et al*. Effects of fenofibrate on plasma cytokine concentrations in patients with atherosclerosis and hyperlipoproteinemia IIb. *Int J Clin Pharmacol Ther* 1998; 36:345–349.
55. Jonkers IJ, Mohrschladt MF, Westendorp RG, van der Laarse A, Smelt AH. Severe hypertriglyceridemia with insulin resistance is associated with systemic inflammation: Reversal with bezafibrate therapy in a randomized controlled trial. *Am J Med* 2002; 112:275–280.
56. Kowalski J, Okopien B, Madej A *et al*. Effects of atorvastatin, simvastatin, and fenofibrate therapy on monocyte chemoattractant protein-1 secretion in patients with hyperlipidemia. *Eur J Clin Pharmacol* 2003; 59:189–193.
57. Kowalski J, Okopien B, Madej A *et al*. Effects of fenofibrate and simvastatin on plasma sICAM-1 and MCP-1 concentrations in patients with hyperlipoproteinemia. *Int J Clin Pharmacol Ther* 2003; 41:241–247.
58. Castrillo A, Tontonoz P. Nuclear receptors in macrophage biology: At the crossroads of lipid metabolism and inflammation. *Annu Rev Cell Dev Biol* 2004; 20:455–480.
59. Ghanim H, Garg R, Aljada A *et al*. Suppression of nuclear factor-kappaB and stimulation of inhibitor kappaB by troglitazone: Evidence for an anti-inflammatory effect and a potential antiatherosclerotic effect in the obese. *JCEM* 2001; 86:1306–1312.
60. Sidhu JS, Cowan D, Kaski JC. The effects of rosiglitazone, a peroxisome proliferator-activated receptor-gamma agonist, on markers of endothelial cell activation, C-reactive protein, and fibrinogen levels in non-diabetic coronary artery disease patients. *JACC* 2003; 42:1757–1763.
61. Garg R, Kumbkarni Y, Aljada A *et al*. Troglitazone reduces reactive oxygen species generation by leukocytes and lipid peroxidation and improves flow-mediated vasodilation in obese subjects. *Hypertension* 2000; 36:430–435.
62. Sidhu JS, Cowan D, Kaski JC. Effects of rosiglitazone on endothelial function in men with coronary artery disease without diabetes mellitus. *AJC* 2004; 94:151–156.
63. Mohanty P, Aljada A, Ghanim H *et al*. Evidence for a potent antiinflammatory effect of rosiglitazone. *JCEM* 2004; 89:2728–2735.
64. Yu JG, Javorschi S, Hevener AL *et al*. The effect of thiazolidinediones on plasma adiponectin levels in normal, obese, and type 2 diabetic subjects. *Diabetes* 2002; 51:2968–2974.
65. Szapary PO, Bloedon LT, Samaha FF *et al*. Effects of pioglitazone on lipoproteins, inflammatory markers, and adipokines in nondiabetic patients with metabolic syndrome. *Arterioscler Thromb Vasc Biol* 2006; 26:182–188.
66. Samaha FF, Szapary PO, Iqbal N *et al*. Effects of rosiglitazone on lipids, adipokines, and inflammatory markers in nondiabetic patients with low high-density lipoprotein cholesterol and metabolic syndrome. *Arterioscler Thromb Vasc Biol* 2006; 26:624–630.
67. Yuan M, Konstantopoulos N, Lee J *et al*. Reversal of obesity- and diet-induced insulin resistance with salicylates or targeted disruption of IKKβ. *Science* 2001; 293:1673–1677.
68. Hundal RS, Petersen KF, Mayerson AB *et al*. Mechanism by which high-dose aspirin improves glucose metabolism in type 2 diabetes. *JCI* 2002; 109:1321–1326.
69. Kopp E, Ghosh S. Inhibition of NF-kappa B by sodium salicylate and aspirin. *Science* 1994; 265:956–959.
70. Yin MJ, Yamamoto Y, Gaynor RB. The anti-inflammatory agents aspirin and salicylate inhibit the activity of IκB kinase-β. *Nature* 1998; 396:77–80.
71. Larsen CM, Faulenbach M, Vaag A *et al*. Interleukin-1-receptor antagonist in type 2 diabetes mellitus. *NEJM* 2007; 356:1517–1526.
72. Dinarello CA. The role of the interleukin-1-receptor antagonist in blocking inflammation mediated by interleukin-1. *NEJM* 2000; 343:732–734.
73. Maedler K, Sergeev P, Ehses JA *et al*. Leptin modulates beta cell expression of IL-1 receptor antagonist and release of IL-1beta in human islets. *Proc Natl Acad Sci USA* 2004; 101:8138–8143.
74. Dinarello CA. Biologic basis for interleukin-1 in disease. *Blood* 1996; 87:2095–2147.
75. Zumsteg U, Reimers JI, Pociot F *et al*. Differential interleukin-1 receptor antagonism on pancreatic beta and alpha cells: Studies in rodent and human islets and in normal rats. *Diabetologia* 1993; 36:759–766.
76. Maedler K, Sergeev P, Ris F *et al*. Glucose-induced beta-cell production of IL-1beta contributes to glucotoxicity in human pancreatic islets. *JCI* 2002; 110:851–860.
77. Wasko MC, Hubert HB, Lingala VB *et al*. Hydroxychloroquine and risk of diabetes in patients with rheumatoid arthritis. *JAMA* 2007; 298:187–193.
78. Powrie JK, Smith GD, Shojaee-Moradie F, Sonksen PH, Jones RH. Mode of action of chloroquine in patients with non-insulin-dependent diabetes mellitus. *Am J Physiol* 1991; 260:E897–E904.

10

GLP-1 analogues, DPP-IV inhibitors and the metabolic syndrome

A. H. Stonehouse, J. H. Holcombe, D. M. Kendall

INTRODUCTION

Type 2 diabetes and obesity are increasingly common metabolic diseases. Both represent significant public health concerns and are reported at epidemic proportions in both the industrialized and developing worlds. Both disorders are characterized by an attendant increase in the risk for cardiovascular (CV) disease. Type 2 diabetes also carries the additional risk of microvascular complications associated with hyperglycemia. These complications have potentially profound effects on both life expectancy and quality of life. Both type 2 diabetes and obesity are associated with other common CV risk factors – the same risk factors that characterize the metabolic syndrome.

The 'metabolic syndrome' was originally defined in 1923, when the Swedish physician Eskil Kylin identified a characteristic cluster of metabolic disorders including the co-existence of hypertension, hyperglycemia, and hyperuricemia in obese individuals [1]. Over the past several decades, the definition of the metabolic syndrome has been further refined – and now includes hyperglycemia, measures of central obesity and a series of significant CV risk factors – all of which are common in patients with type 2 diabetes and CV disease. These risk factors include hypertension and dyslipidemia, including hypertriglyceridemia and high concentrations of low-density lipoprotein (LDL)-cholesterol. Furthermore, many of the risk factors portend a significantly higher risk for the future development of type 2 diabetes even in individuals with normal or only modestly impaired baseline glucose concentrations. As noted throughout this book, CV risk factors occur more frequently than would be expected by chance alone [1].

The impact of the metabolic syndrome on public health is considerable. As such, there has been substantial interest in early identification of patients at risk of developing the metabolic syndrome and on the use of both established and novel therapies alongside established lifestyle interventions to limit the future risk of both CV disease and type 2 diabetes.

Over the past decade, the definitions of the metabolic syndrome have been broadly debated. The most widely accepted criteria are those proposed by the National Cholesterol Education Program Adult Treatment Panel III (NCEP ATP III) and the World Health Organization (WHO) [2, 3]. Both criteria provide similar estimates of prevalence as they share some common features (approximately 25% of adults in the United States and a

Anthony H. Stonehouse, PhD, Medical Affairs Scientist, Amylin Pharmaceuticals, Inc., San Diego, California, USA
John H. Holcombe, MD, Medical Fellow, Lilly Research Laboratories, Eli Lilly and Company, Indianapolis, Indiana, USA
David M. Kendall, MD, Executive Director, Medical Affairs, Amylin Pharmaceuticals, Inc., San Diego, California, USA

Table 10.1 International Diabetes Federation definition of the metabolic syndrome

	Criteria
Central obesity	Waist circumference ≥94 cm (37 in) in Europid men and ≥80 cm (31.5 in) in Europid women
Requirements for diagnosis	Metabolic syndrome is defined as central obesity plus any two of the following four factors
Serum triglyceride	Triglyceride ≥1.7 mmol/l (150 mg/dl) or specific treatment for this lipid abnormality
Serum HDL-cholesterol	HDL-cholesterol <1.0 mmol/l (40 mg/dl) in men, <1.3 mmol/l (50 mg/dl) in women or specific treatment for this lipid abnormality
Hypertension	Blood pressure ≥130/85 mmHg or treatment of previously diagnosed hypertension
Fasting plasma glucose glucose (FPG)	FPG ≥5.6 mmol/l (100 mg/dl) or previously diagnosed type 2 diabetes

slightly lower percentage affected in Europe) [4, 5]. More recently, the International Diabetes Federation (IDF) and WHO have proposed a definition of the metabolic syndrome that provides criteria more commonly identified in clinical practice. This definition is also applicable to a variety of population groups, including individuals of European, Asian, African, and Hispanic origin (Table 10.1) [6].

PATHOPHYSIOLOGY OF THE METABOLIC SYNDROME: A FOCUS ON OBESITY AND GLUCOSE INTOLERANCE

Obesity – specifically central or visceral adiposity – is broadly recognized as a major contributor to the development of the metabolic syndrome. Obesity also increases the risk of developing both type 2 diabetes and CV disease. Adipose tissue itself is thought to be a metabolically active and dynamic endocrine organ. Adipocytes secrete a number of regulatory cytokines, known as adipokines, which include leptin, adiponectin, and tumor necrosis factor (TNF)-α. Adipokines are believed to play a role in the development of several features of the metabolic syndrome including dyslipidemia, insulin resistance, and abnormal vascular behavior. These compounds exert myriad effects on energy expenditure, food intake and body weight, in addition to effects on muscle, liver, pancreatic islets, vascular endothelium and heart [7]. Inflammatory cytokines, such as TNF-α, are not only secreted from adipose tissues, but also may directly alter vascular behavior, increasing the risk for vascular disease. In addition, these compounds may impair both insulin action and pancreatic β-cell function, thereby increasing the risk of glucose intolerance. Leptin, an adipose tissue-derived peptide, may protect the body during periods of mild calorie surplus by regulating fat deposition in both adipose and extra-adipose tissues. It has been speculated that certain pre-disposed individuals develop leptin resistance as part of a maladaptive response to sustained calorie excess (often seen in individuals who develop the metabolic syndrome). The consequences of leptin resistance, in the presence of ongoing calorie excess, is uncontrolled fat accumulation in adipose stores and extra-adipose tissues, which can further worsen insulin resistance and other features of the metabolic syndrome [8].

Whether adipose tissue plays a critical central role in the metabolic syndrome remains to be fully elucidated. However, there is little doubt that obesity and central fat deposition play at least a permissive role in the development of the metabolic syndrome. In addition, obesity and glucose intolerance are closely linked. The remainder of this chapter will focus on the possible link between obesity and glucose intolerance – and review the potential role of newer therapies for diabetes in individuals with glucose intolerance and co-existent features of the metabolic syndrome.

MEDICAL MANAGEMENT OF INDIVIDUALS WITH THE METABOLIC SYNDROME

There is significant controversy over whether the metabolic syndrome can be considered to be more than the sum of its collective parts. This controversy is, in part, the lack of a unified and broadly accepted definition of the metabolic syndrome. However, there is strong evidence that the metabolic syndrome should be considered as a discrete clinical entity. It is well established that there is incremental risk and geometric amplification of CV risk when multiple risk factors are present. This is exemplified by the treatment of hypertension on a background of the metabolic syndrome. Typically, treatment is less effective than would be anticipated from historic blood pressure-lowering clinical studies and is possibly explained by the interplay of risk factors associated with the metabolic syndrome. This observation suggests that other interrelated risk factors may offset the beneficial effects of a specific pharmacological intervention, and strengthens the argument for the management of the metabolic syndrome as a cluster of risk factors, rather than focusing solely on individual components. With this understanding, there is little doubt that therapies that improve glycemic control, reduce body weight, and improve both dyslipidemia and hypertension may be useful in treating the metabolic syndrome [9].

Even with these controversies, there can be little doubt as to the benefit of several therapies for patients with the metabolic syndrome. Weight loss and increased physical activity in individuals with the metabolic syndrome have been shown to substantially reduce the risk of progression to type 2 diabetes [10–12]. Furthermore, specific therapies (such as lipid-lowering and weight reduction) have significantly greater impact in those with the metabolic syndrome than in those without – supporting the use of interventions that provide additional improvement in each component of the syndrome. Management of patients with the metabolic syndrome currently focuses on four major categories of therapy and includes:

- dietary and lifestyle modification;
- specific treatment of obesity and overweight;
- treatment of individual CV risk factors;
- treatment of hyperglycemia in type 2 diabetes [9].

DIETARY AND LIFESTYLE MODIFICATION

A number of clinical studies have demonstrated the benefits of achieving moderate weight loss, through calorie restriction and increasing physical activity, in reducing the likelihood of developing the metabolic syndrome and reducing both CV disease risk and the risk of developing type 2 diabetes [10–12]. Epidemiological data from the National Health and Nutrition Examination Survey III (NHANES III) reported a substantially lower risk of developing the metabolic syndrome in subjects who maintain a non-obese body mass index (BMI) and remain physically active [11]. The landmark Diabetes Prevention Program (DPP) demonstrated that even modest weight loss and increased physical activity markedly reduced the risk of developing type 2 diabetes and the metabolic syndrome in high-risk patients [10]. Intensive lifestyle changes also reduced the persistence of the metabolic syndrome in patients with the syndrome at study baseline [10]. The specific effect of intensive weight loss on the future risk of diabetes-related macrovascular and microvascular complications in patients with type 2 diabetes and the metabolic syndrome is currently being investigated in the Action for Health in Diabetes (Look AHEAD) clinical trial [13].

Beyond specific outcomes trials, there are numerous studies that support the role of weight loss and increased physical activity in the management of the metabolic syndrome. These studies suggest that moderate weight loss and increased exercise can improve dyslipidemia, reduce blood pressure, and improve insulin sensitivity and glucose tolerance [11]. However, independent of specific clinical endpoints, patients who modify their lifestyle tend to experience improvements in virtually all components of the metabolic syndrome [11]. Additionally, diagnoses of the metabolic syndrome are less common in individuals with a BMI of $<30\,kg/m^2$ [11].

MEDICAL TREATMENT OF OBESITY: POTENTIAL IMPACT ON THE METABOLIC SYNDROME

With the increasingly well-recognized role for adiposity and obesity in the development of the metabolic syndrome, it is logical to assume that weight loss alone may decrease the risk for CV risk and progression to type 2 diabetes in patients with the metabolic syndrome. Given the difficulties with which lifestyle changes are both implemented and maintained, medical management of obesity has attracted substantial attention in recent years. Achieving and maintaining significant weight loss through lifestyle changes is difficult. Therefore, drug therapies to assist with weight management have been considered as one component for the management of patients with obesity and the metabolic syndrome. Unfortunately, few data exist on the impact of currently available therapies (such as phentermine, sibutramine and orlistat) on features of the metabolic syndrome. These agents are approved for both short- and long-term use for the management of obesity. Any single therapy can generally achieve weight loss of approximately 5% of the initial body weight. Beyond the common desire for weight loss in many patients with the metabolic syndrome, weight loss of this magnitude is associated with modest improvements in some, but not all, features of the metabolic syndrome. Phentermine, an adrenergic agent known to limit appetite and increase satiety, has been available for over 50 years and is approved for the treatment of obesity [14]. Phentermine has been reported to reduce mean body weight by an average of more than 3 kg in short-term clinical trials [14]. Sibutramine, a serotonin and noradrenergic reuptake inhibitor that acts on the central nervous system to suppress appetite, is reported to reduce body weight by approximately 4.5 kg after 1 year of treatment [15]. Orlistat inhibits gut lipase action, thereby reducing absorption of dietary fat. After one year of treatment with orlistat, obese patients experienced a weight loss of nearly 3 kg [15]. Additional studies indicate that orlistat improves cardiometabolic risk, potentially reducing the incidence of the metabolic syndrome and the progression to type 2 diabetes, but with significant gastrointestinal side-effects [16–18]. In addition to the currently available anti-obesity agents, the endocannabinoid system has been recognized as contributing to the regulation of food intake and lipid and glucose metabolism, these effects being mediated by the central and peripheral nervous systems [19]. Rimonabant, an antagonist of the cannabinoid-1 receptor, is in late-phase clinical development. In a 1-year placebo-controlled study, rimonabant reduced body weight and mean waist circumference (an indirect measure of intra-abdominal adiposity) by –6.9 kg and –7.1 cm, respectively. In addition, HDL-cholesterol, triglycerides, and fasting insulin improved from baseline by +19%, –13%, and –1.7 μU/ml, respectively, with no improvement in low-density lipoprotein (LDL)-cholesterol [20]. Moreover, a significant increase of +2.2 μg/ml in adiponectin concentrations (a predictive risk measure for CV disease and type 2 diabetes) was reported [20]. Data from a 2-year trial with rimonabant reported sustained reductions of body weight and waist circumference of –7.6 kg and –7.8 cm, respectively [21]. These changes were associated with significant improvements in HDL-cholesterol (+6.3%) and triglycerides (–8.5%) from baseline [21]. However, there was no significant change in fasting plasma glucose [21]. In 2006, rimonabant was approved in the European Union for the treatment of obesity with associated risk factors such as type 2 diabetes and dyslipidemia. The use of rimonabant with the future development of other cannabinoid-1 receptor antagonists may result in useful agents for the treatment of the metabolic syndrome.

In obese patients with type 2 diabetes, sibutramine treatment in conjunction with a low-calorie diet has been reported to improve glucose control [22]. After 2 years of treatment, patients experienced reductions in both body weight and hemoglobin A1C (HbA1c). These reductions were –4.6 kg and –0.5%, respectively. Furthermore, improvements in other measures associated with obesity and the metabolic syndrome were reported, including a reduction in BMI (–1.6 kg/m^2), reduced body fat (–2.0 kg) and lower systolic blood pressure (–7 mmHg) [22]. These data suggest that weight loss can improve glycemic control and cardiometabolic risk factors associated with both type 2 diabetes and the metabolic syndrome.

TARGETED TREATMENT OF INDIVIDUAL CV RISK FACTORS

Traditionally, the approach to patients with the metabolic syndrome has focused on intensive medical management of specific CV risk factors. While few arguments exist over the potential benefit of managing obesity, the management of hypertension, dyslipidemia, and hyperglycemia have been shown to reduce the risk of complications from CV disease and type 2 diabetes. Many clinicians continue to argue that both prevention of, and treatment for, the metabolic syndrome itself is not well supported and in fact aggressive treatment of individual risk factors must be the focus of management. Studies suggest that the treatment of hypertension, the aggressive management of lipid disorders (particularly LDL-cholesterol lowering), and lowering of blood glucose significantly benefit patients with the metabolic syndrome [5, 11–23].

The dyslipidemia of the metabolic syndrome is characterized by low levels of HDL-cholesterol and elevated triglyceride concentrations. In addition, patients with the metabolic syndrome have an increase in the fraction of small, dense and atherogenic LDL-cholesterol particles. Treatment with 3-hydroxy-3-methylglutaryl coenzyme A (HMG-CoA) reductase inhibitors, the 'statins', is of unquestioned benefit – particularly in patients with existing CV disease, type 2 diabetes and/or the metabolic syndrome. A focus on decreasing LDL-cholesterol with a statin is supported by numerous clinical studies [5, 24]. Although treatment with either fibrates or niacin can improve both HDL-cholesterol and triglycerides [25], outcome trials have not provided unequivocal support for such therapy. For example, the presence or absence of insulin resistance may be more clinically important than low HDL-cholesterol and high triglycerides, and the presence of other lipid-lowering drugs may mask the effectiveness of fibrates in reducing the incidence of coronary events [26, 27]. The combination of statin therapy with a fibrate (simvastatin and fenofibrate) is very effective in treating the metabolic syndrome – specifically dyslipidemia [28]. Statin/fibrate combination therapy is under active investigation on a background of good blood glucose control in the Action to Control Cardiovascular Risk in Diabetes (ACCORD) clinical trial.

Recently, a meta-analysis of six major primary prevention trials involving over 45 000 patients – many of whom were apparently healthy, but others undoubtedly with the metabolic syndrome – demonstrated the favorable effects of aspirin with statistically significant reductions in the risk of total coronary heart disease, non-fatal myocardial infarction, and total CV events [29].

TREATMENT OF HYPERGLYCEMIA: TYPE 2 DIABETES AND THE METABOLIC SYNDROME

Hyperglycemia is the hallmark of type 2 diabetes and remains the primary focus of treatment to limit microvascular complications. Glucose intolerance is also a characteristic of the metabolic syndrome and has received increasing attention as a primary target for treatment in patients with the syndrome. Hyperglycemia in both type 2 diabetes and the metabolic syndrome has also been associated with increased CV risk and has been the focus of attention in a number of diabetes prevention trials [9, 30].

Given that management of hyperglycemia in patients with type 2 diabetes is of established benefit, there is little doubt that all therapies that can help achieve and sustain near-normal glucose levels warrant discussion. There is also little doubt that incretin-based therapies now play an increasingly important role in the clinical management of hyperglycemia. Since up to 85% of patients with the metabolic syndrome also have type 2 diabetes, the two disorders are closely linked [31]. Current therapeutic approaches for the treatment of type 2 diabetes are based on reducing insulin resistance, decreasing hepatic glucose output, limiting glucose absorption from the intestine, or replacing insulin, either through stimulating its endogenous secretion or through exogenous replacement.

Traditional therapies, such as exogenous insulin and insulin secretagogues (e.g. sulfonylureas), reduce glycemia and can reduce microvascular risk in patients with type 2 diabetes. The reduction of glycemia in patients with type 2 diabetes has also been reported to improve macrovascular disease risk [32]. However, insulin and sulfonylureas are traditionally associated with weight gain, which may worsen several CV risk factors in the metabolic syndrome (including hypertension and lipids) [30]. Weight gain is generally greater with exogenous insulin compared to sulfonylureas, particularly when insulin treatment is intensified with multiple injection regimens. At present, it is not known whether the weight gain seen with more intensive therapies can adversely affect cardiometabolic risk. Ongoing trials will address the possible benefits of weight loss in those with established diabetes – many of whom also meet criteria for the metabolic syndrome [13].

The biguanide metformin is now considered the first-line treatment of choice for most patients with type 2 diabetes. The early use of metformin is, in great part, the consequence of its beneficial effects on glycemic control, body weight, and CV risk. While metformin has been shown to be equally effective with regard to reduction in plasma glucose (and hence reduction in microvascular risk), metformin achieves this same glucose-lowering without an increase in body weight [33]. Moreover, metformin has been reported to have modest but beneficial effects on other cardiometabolic risk factors such as triglycerides, LDL-cholesterol, and total cholesterol [33–35]. Beyond these effects in patients with type 2 diabetes, the neutral weight effect of metformin has prompted study of its possible use in patients at risk for developing type 2 diabetes. The DPP reported that metformin therapy in individuals with impaired glucose tolerance (as seen in the metabolic syndrome) could reduce the risk of progression to type 2 diabetes when compared to placebo [12]. This reduction in diabetes risk was achieved with no substantial weight gain [12]. The role of such therapies in patients with prediabetes and the metabolic syndrome requires further study; however, the possible benefits on both CV risk and body weight combined with the blood glucose-lowering potential of metformin make it an attractive initial therapy in type 2 diabetes and of probable benefit for individuals with prediabetes.

Thiazolidinediones (TZDs) are agonists of peroxisome proliferator-activated receptor gamma (PPAR-γ), a nuclear receptor expressed in adipose tissue where it regulates the expression of genes involved in lipid and carbohydrate metabolism. These insulin-sensitizing agents are commonly used for the treatment of type 2 diabetes. In addition to their glucose-lowering effects, TZDs have been shown to significantly improve a number of common CV risk factors. The TZDs rosiglitazone and pioglitazone have demonstrated their efficacy by improving hyperglycemia in several long-term clinical studies [36, 37]. The TZDs have also been shown to improve dyslipidemia, modestly decrease blood pressure, and improve abnormal vascular reactivity and prothrombotic risk factors [38]. Because of these effects, TZDs have been investigated for their potential ability to decrease cardiometabolic risk. For example, treatment with pioglitazone has been reported to increase HDL-cholesterol, improve particle distribution of LDL-cholesterol lipoproteins, and decrease triglycerides [39]. Rosiglitazone is reported to improve HDL-cholesterol and LDL-cholesterol particle size, but increases LDL-cholesterol concentration [40]. Pioglitazone, when added to conventional hyperglycemia therapies, did not reduce the composite macrovascular outcome but did improve the risk of non-fatal myocardial infarction and stroke [41].

Other studies have investigated the effect of TZDs in delaying or preventing the progression to type 2 diabetes in at-risk individuals, such as women with a previous history of gestational diabetes mellitus. In the Troglitazone in the Prevention of Diabetes (TRIPOD) study, treatment with troglitazone was associated with improved insulin sensitivity in women with insulin resistance, and the incidence of type 2 diabetes over a 4-year period was significantly reduced [42, 43]. Improved insulin sensitivity was also observed with pioglitazone treatment in the Pioglitazone in the Prevention of Diabetes (PIPOD) study. Subjects in the PIPOD study with prior treatment with troglitazone were reported to have improved β-cell function [43]. Similarly, the Diabetes Reduction Assessment with Ramipril and Rosiglitazone Medication (DREAM) study demonstrated that the incidence of type 2 diabetes in subjects with impaired fasting glucose, impaired glucose tolerance, or both, was significantly reduced by treatment with rosiglitazone [44]. These studies suggest that TZDs may prevent the development of type 2 diabetes in some subjects who have impaired glucose tolerance. Although TZDs decrease insulin resistance and improve glucose metabolism, their effects on the metabolic syndrome other than the component contributed by type 2 diabetes have not been reported.

Despite their salutary effects on glucose, and the possibility of improving CV risk and reducing risk of progression to type 2 diabetes, TZDs are known to cause significant weight gain [45]. In addition, TZD treatment increases the risk of peripheral oedema and heart failure. The weight gain observed with the use of a TZD is caused by increased adiposity and a redistribution of body fat (increased subcutaneous fat and decreased visceral fat). The possible risk–benefit on both type 2 diabetes and CV risk of significant weight gain, associated with reduced visceral adiposity, remains unknown.

Additional therapies for hyperglycemia in type 2 diabetes and the metabolic syndrome are being developed. With the recent introduction of the incretin mimetic, exenatide, and the approval of other incretin-based therapies that leverage the beneficial effects of the incretin hormones, glucagon-like peptide-1 (GLP-1) has received increased attention. Each of these therapies can significantly improve blood glucose levels. GLP-1 agonists/incretin mimetics can also significantly reduce body weight, even in the setting of improved glucose control. These therapies may also have favorable effects on a number of other features of the metabolic syndrome.

THE INCRETIN EFFECT AND THE INCRETIN HORMONE: GLP-1

The incretin effect was initially described in the 1960s when investigators noted that oral administration of glucose provoked a significantly greater insulin secretory response when compared to an isoglycemic glucose load given intravenously. This significant increase in insulin secretion following gut delivery was named '**in**testinal se**cret**ion of **in**sulin' and hence, the '**incretin**' effect. The incretin effect was ultimately ascribed to the potent insulinotropic effect of gut hormones, such as GLP-1 and glucose-dependent insulinotropic peptide. These gut peptides are now referred to as 'incretin' hormones [46–49].

GLP-1 is the best characterized of the incretin hormones and appears to be the key incretin hormone involved in carbohydrate metabolism. In response to glucose challenge or the consumption of a meal, GLP-1 is secreted by the intestinal L-cells lining the colon and ileum [50–52]. Established glucoregulatory effects of GLP-1 include enhanced glucose-dependent secretion of insulin, suppression of glucagon secretion (particularly in the post-meal state) and the regulation (or delay) of gastric emptying, which can be accelerated in

Table 10.2 Glucoregulatory effects of GLP-1

	Glucoregulatory effects
GLP-1	Enhancement of glucose-dependent insulin secretion Suppression of inappropriately elevated glucagon secretion Regulation of gastric emptying Suppression of appetite leading to reduction in food intake Reduction in body weight Promotion of β-cell proliferation and neogenesis (*in vitro* and animal models)

some patients with type 2 diabetes [51, 53–56]. GLP-1 enhances the post-prandial satiety signal, suppresses food intake and reduces appetite, probably through centrally mediated mechanisms [57–59]. Moreover, in cell lines, primary islet cultures, and in animal models, GLP-1 has been shown to both maintain and to increase pancreatic β-cell mass by promoting neogenesis, proliferation, and transformation of non-insulin secreting cells into cells capable of secreting insulin (Table 10.2) [60–64].

INCRETIN MIMETICS AND DPP-IV INHIBITORS

The hyperglycemia of both type 2 diabetes and the metabolic syndrome (in the case of prediabetes) is characterized by a complex series of hormonal abnormalities including insulin resistance, impaired β-cell responses to glucose, and a decline in circulating levels of GLP-1. New therapies are being developed that leverage the known effects of GLP-1 on β-cell function, regulation of stomach empting, and carbohydrate metabolism. Whether other unique actions of incretin-based therapies will be of benefit in those with the metabolic syndrome is not clearly understood.

The half-life of GLP-1 in the plasma is exceedingly short – generally estimated at less than 2 min. As a result of rapid degradation by the ubiquitous protease, dipeptidyl peptidase-IV (DPP-IV), GLP-1 is considered to have limited therapeutic potential [53, 65–67]. Even with this short half-life, much is known of the physiological effect of GLP-1. Infusion of GLP-1 can significantly improve glycemic control, improve insulin secretion, and produce progressive reduction in body weight [53, 68].

To leverage the glucoregulatory effects of GLP-1, the issue of the short half-life of GLP-1 is being addressed in two ways. Firstly, by developing incretin mimetics that share several glucoregulatory effects with GLP-1, but inherently resist degradation by DPP-IV, and secondly, by developing oral agents known as DPP-IV inhibitors. The latter group of compounds limit the proteolytic action of DPP-IV, sufficient to increase the concentration of endogenous GLP-1 (Table 10.3). The so-called 'incretin mimetics', such as synthetic exendin-4 (exenatide), mimic many of the characteristics of native GLP-1 (Table 10.2) but have a prolonged circulating half-life, making them suitable for clinical use (Table 10.3). The incretin mimetic exenatide has been shown to restore first-phase insulin secretion in response to intravenous glucose and improve β-cell function during mixed meals [69]. Despite the intriguing preclinical data suggesting enhanced β-cell mass with incretin-based therapies, the long-term effects of the incretin mimetics on β-cell function have yet to be fully investigated.

Leveraging the effect of incretin mimetics in the metabolic syndrome

The incretin mimetic exenatide is currently the only therapy in this class available for clinical use. Exenatide was approved by the United States Food and Drug Administration (FDA) for

Table 10.3 Modes of action of incretin mimetics and DPP-IV inhibitors

Drug	*Mode of action*
Incretin mimetics	Enhancement of glucose-dependent insulin secretion Suppression of inappropriately elevated glucagon secretion Regulation of gastric emptying Reduction of food intake Reduction in body weight (exenatide only) Increases β-cell mass in animal models, improvement of β-cell function in humans
DPP-IV inhibitors	Inhibition of DPP-IV proteolysis, suppressing degradation of endogenous GLP-1, thereby facilitating glucoregulatory effects

the treatment of type 2 diabetes in 2005. Extensive clinical data are now available assessing the clinical utility of incretin mimetics – with the vast majority of these data derived from studies with exenatide. As a result of its extensive clinical use at the time of this publication, much of this discussion will focus on exenatide and its use in treating type 2 diabetes and its potential role in treating the metabolic syndrome. Where available, data from other incretin mimetics and the DPP-IV inhibitors will also be included.

Incretin mimetics can be categorized into two groups. One group includes those agents that naturally resist DPP-IV proteolysis, such as exenatide (synthetic exendin-4), and the GLP-1 analogue BIM-51077 [70, 71]. Exenatide and BIM-51077 share glucoregulatory functions with GLP-1, but have half-lives in the circulation of greater than 2 h, thereby facilitating administration by less frequent injection [70, 71]. The second group includes compounds in development, such as CJC-1131/CJC-1134 and liraglutide. These agents have undergone chemical modification that confers resistance to DPP-IV proteolysis [72–74].

Exenatide is currently indicated as an adjunct therapy for patients with type 2 diabetes who are unable to achieve adequate glycemic control with metformin, a sulfonylurea, or a combination of both agents. Exenatide is not approved for use in patients with the metabolic syndrome nor has it been tested extensively in patients with more modest degrees of glucose intolerance (impaired glucose tolerance, impaired fasting glucose or both). Exenatide is a synthetic form of the naturally occurring peptide exendin-4, a peptide constituent of Gila monster saliva [70, 75]. Exendin-4 binds to and fully activates the mammalian GLP-1 receptor and shares many of the glucoregulatory effects with native GLP-1 *in vitro* [54, 70]. Despite their comparable glucoregulatory effects and 53% amino acid similarity, GLP-1 and exendin-4 are transcribed from unique genes in the Gila monster [76]. As a consequence of its peptide structure, exenatide resists proteolysis by DPP-IV in the circulation, resulting in a half-life of 2.4 h in humans. Furthermore, exenatide is detectable in the circulation for up to 10 h after subcutaneous injection [52, 77].

In animal and human studies, exenatide enhances glucose-dependent insulin secretion [54, 78, 79], suppresses elevated levels of glucagon – both effects regulated in a glucose-dependent manner [79, 80], and exenatide also slows gastric emptying [79, 81]. Moreover, in clinical trials and *in vivo* models, exenatide administration reduces food intake and reduces body weight – observations also seen with GLP-1 infusions (Table 10.3) [81–83]. *In vivo* studies with exenatide have demonstrated acute effects on β-cell secretory function and have suggested that β-cell mass may be increased by exposure to this incretin mimetic. Exenatide promotes β-cell proliferation and neogenesis [60, 61, 63, 84]. Using either acute or chronic administration of exenatide in patients with type 2 diabetes improves glucose-induced insulin secretion. In patients with type 2 diabetes rendered hyperglycemic by an

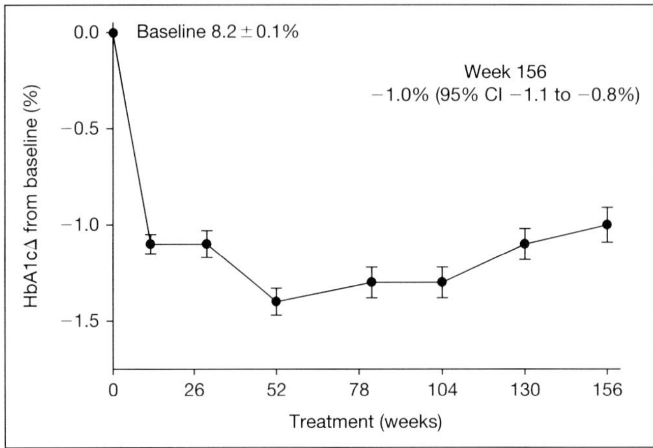

Figure 10.1 Mean (±SE) change from baseline for HbA1c after 3 years of exenatide treatment with an oral agent (metformin, a sulfonylurea, or a combination of both drugs) was -1.0% in patients with type 2 diabetes ($n = 217$). With permission from [89].

intravenous bolus of glucose, exenatide infusion restored first- and second-phase insulin secretion [69]. These data support a role for exenatide in achieving acute improvements in β-cell function in patients with type 2 diabetes [69]. Further, studies have demonstrated that although exenatide infusion suppressed inappropriate secretion of glucagon during hyperglycemia, exenatide did not adversely affect counter-regulatory glucagon responses during hypoglycemia [85].

The safety and efficacy of exenatide has been extensively investigated in three long-term, pivotal phase 3 clinical trials [86–88]. In these trials, patients with type 2 diabetes unable to achieve adequate glycemic control with traditional oral agents (metformin and/or a sulfonylurea) were randomized to receive placebo, 5 μg, or 10 μg exenatide bid in addition to their oral agent therapy. No additional changes in either diabetes medication or education/diet were made for each patient. Specifically, no drug withdrawals were necessary prior to initiation of exenatide therapy nor were specific dietary instructions provided to alter food intake over the 30 weeks of study [86–88]. After 30 weeks of treatment with exenatide and oral agent therapy, significant reductions in mean HbA1c and mean reductions in body weight were observed. Both measures improved significantly from baseline and were significantly greater than those observed with placebo treatment. At the maximal dose of exenatide (10 μg bid), HbA1c was lowered by approximately –1% from baseline, and the decline in HbA1c was coupled to body weight reductions of –2 kg to –3 kg [86–88]. In a subsequent open-label extension study, patients treated with exenatide for 3 years maintained durable mean reductions in HbA1c of –1.0% (Figure 10.1) with progressive reductions in mean body weight of –5.3 kg (Figure 10.2) [89]. Mean changes from baseline for HbA1c and body weight after 3 years of exenatide treatment in an open-label extension study are shown in Table 10.4.

Analysis of patients participating in this open-label extension study demonstrated that 3.5 years of exenatide treatment was associated with improvements in several CV risk factors, including increased HDL-cholesterol, reduced plasma triglycerides, and reduced diastolic blood pressure (Table 10.5) [89]. More recently, data from this same cohort suggested that treatment with exenatide for 82 weeks improved HbA1c and reduced body weight, and was associated with a 44% decrease in median C-reactive protein concentration relative to

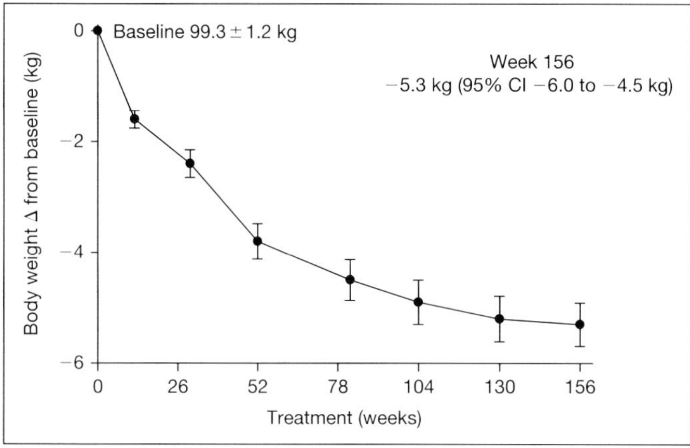

Figure 10.2 Mean (±SE) change from baseline for body weight after 3 years of exenatide treatment with an oral agent (metformin, a sulfonylurea, or a combination of both drugs) was -5.3 kg in patients with type 2 diabetes (n = 217). With permission from [89]. CI = confidence interval.

Table 10.4 Effect on HbA1c and body weight after 3 years of treatment with exenatide (n = 217, ± SE)

Time (weeks)	*Baseline*	*12*	*30*	*52*	*82*	*104*	*130*	*156*
HbA1c (%)	8.2±0.1	-1.1±0.1	-1.1±0.1	-1.4±0.1	-1.3±0.1	-1.3±0.1	-1.1±0.1	-1.0±0.1
Body weight (kg)	99.3±1.2	-1.6±0.2	-2.4±0.2	-3.8±0.3	-4.5±0.4	-4.9±0.4	-5.2±0.4	-5.3±0.4

Table 10.5 Effect on selected cardiometabolic risk factors after 3.5 years of exenatide treatment (n = 151)

Parameter	*Mean baseline*	*Mean change from baseline*
HDL-cholesterol	1 mmol/l (38.6 mg/dl)	+0.22 mmol/l (+8.5 mg/dl)
Serum triglyceride	2.5 mmol/l (225.1 mg/dl)	-0.50 mmol/l (-44.4 mg/dl)
Diastolic blood pressure	79.2 mmHg	-3.3 mmHg

baseline [90]. These data may be quite relevant to the treatment of the metabolic syndrome because the improved glycemic control and reduced body weight were associated with improvements in three of the four CV risk factors in the IDF definition of the metabolic syndrome (Table 10.1) [89].

In a placebo-controlled study, the addition of exenatide to patients with type 2 diabetes failing to achieve adequate glycemic control with a TZD and/or metformin demonstrated that exenatide improved HbA1c, increased the percentage of patients achieving the HbA1c goal of 7%, lowered fasting plasma glucose (FPG), and reduced body weight [91]. The relative effects on HbA1c have been found to be similar when exenatide or insulin glargine were compared in patients with type 2 diabetes with poor glycemic control [92]. In this direct comparator study, however, treatment with exenatide resulted in significant body weight reduction compared with insulin glargine – albeit with a higher incidence of gastrointestinal side-effects [92]. Whether the relative effect of therapies, such as exenatide on body weight, will uniformly and beneficially affect the other components of the metabolic syndrome has not been determined. However, weight loss alone is, as noted above, associated with myriad improvements in features of the metabolic syndrome. More recent data have also demonstrated that patients with type 2 diabetes and the metabolic syndrome are at risk for modest elevations of liver enzyme function and non-alcoholic steatohepatitis [93]. In patients with type 2 diabetes treated with exenatide for 3 years, elevated hepatic alanine aminotransferase (ALT, baseline 30 IU/l) significantly improved ALT concentration by −4.5 IU/L. This improvement in liver enzyme concentration was associated with a significant reduction in body weight of −5.3 kg (baseline 99 kg) [89].

While the favorable effects of exenatide on both glucose control and body weight have been consistently observed in clinical trials, it should be noted that these data were derived from studies in patients with type 2 diabetes – not from individuals with the metabolic syndrome. If these observations can be replicated in individuals with the metabolic syndrome, then incretin-based therapies like exenatide may play a role in treating that disorder – perhaps as adjunctive therapy combined with more traditional treatments (such as statins and anti-hypertensives). Exenatide once-weekly (a long-acting formulation of exenatide) is now in late-phase development and has been shown to significantly improve HbA1c and reduce body weight by −1.7% and −3.8 kg from baseline, respectively, in a 15-week study. That study provided evidence that sustained exposure to GLP-1-based therapies may also play a role in diabetes management and could theoretically be used for those with hyperglycemia and the metabolic syndrome [94].

Exenatide treatment is associated with the occurrence of transient nausea which decreases over time – reported on at least one occasion by approximately 44% of patients treated in blinded clinical trials treated for 30 weeks (versus nausea reported in 18% of subjects receiving placebo – Amylin Pharmaceuticals Inc., and Eli Lilly and Company – data on file). Severe nausea was rare and the incidence of mild-to-moderate nausea declined over time [68, 86–88]. During clinical trials, increasing the dose of exenatide after 4 weeks from 5 μg to 10 μg bid increased the incidence of nausea; however, the incidence of nausea further declined with longer exposure to exenatide [68, 86–88, 95]. During treatment with exenatide, the risk of mild-to-moderate hypoglycemia was accentuated by the use of a sulfonylurea, but that risk was reduced if the dose of sulfonylurea was decreased upon exenatide initiation [88]. In contrast, the risk of hypoglycemia was not increased when metformin was administered with exenatide [68, 87].

Other compounds in development that bind directly to the GLP-1 receptor include BIM-51077, an analog of GLP-1 with natural resistance to DPP-IV proteolysis; CJC-1134 an analog of exendin-4 covalently bound to serum albumin; and liraglutide, an acylated analog of GLP-1. The acylation facilitates binding of liraglutide to serum albumin *in vivo*, thus increasing the half-life to approximately 13 h in the circulation. Few or no data are available from the long-term use of these compounds in type 2 diabetes and very limited data on the effect of these compounds on features of the metabolic syndrome are currently available.

BIM-51077 is currently in phase 2 clinical trials. Clinical data have reported reduced blood glucose and glucagon concentrations associated with increased insulin concentration; however, no additional long-term clinical trial data are available for BIM-51077 [71]. CJC-1131 is a GLP-1-albumin complex possessing some of the glucoregulatory effects of GLP-1. CJC-1131 demonstrated resistance to proteolysis by DPP-IV with a drug half-life of approximately 10 days [72, 96–98]. However, pharmacokinetic and pharmacodynamic profiles of this compound, and limited tolerability, led to the suspension of its development in favor of CJC-1134, an exendin-4-albumin complex (ConjuChem press releases: 30/09/05 and 27/02/06). During a 6-week, phase 1/phase 2 clinical trial using CJC-1134, plasma glucose-lowering effects were reported in association with a drug half-life of approximately 8 days in patients with type 2 diabetes (ConjuChem press release: 26/04/06). Essentially no data are available on the effects of this compound on body weight and other markers of CV risk, and its place in the treatment of either type 2 diabetes or the metabolic syndrome remain to be determined. Liraglutide is currently in phase 3 clinical trials, and with its relatively long half-life, liraglutide is formulated to be suitable for single, daily injection in clinical use. Data published in an early-phase clinical trial in patients with type 2 diabetes reported that the highest dose of liraglutide (1.9 mg/day) decreased HbA1c by −1.7% from baseline over 14 weeks [99]. Liraglutide also improved, but did not normalize glucose-dependent insulin secretion, but improved fasting and post-prandial plasma glucose, reduced glucagon secretion, and slowed the rate of gastric emptying [73, 74, 100–105]. Liraglutide has also been reported to improve β-cell function, as demonstrated by improved measures of homeostasis model assessment – pancreatic B-cell function (HOMA-B) and proinsulin/insulin ratio [74, 100]. In early-phase clinical trials, liraglutide was investigated as an add-on therapy to oral agents. These studies reported that superior glycemic control was achieved by liraglutide when used as an add-on therapy to metformin compared to a sulfonylurea [104]. Although early-phase clinical trials suggest that liraglutide treatment leads to modest body weight loss, the effects of liraglutide on food consumption and body weight have not been fully investigated. In short-term trials of up to 12 weeks, reduction in body weight versus placebo averaged approximately –1.5 kg [101, 103, 104]. Liraglutide may also favorably influence cardiometabolic risk factors – with a single report demonstrating reductions in blood pressure, improved triglycerides and plasminogen activator inhibitor-1 concentrations in short-term trials [106]. At the time of publication of this chapter, there are no published data from several large liraglutide pivotal trials although initial press release information has been reported (Novo Nordisk LEAD press releases). The most commonly reported adverse events with liraglutide, in common with GLP-1 and other incretin mimetics, were gastrointestinal in nature, with minimal rates of nausea noted during drug initiation. Increased rates of diarrhoea (up to 20%) seen with liraglutide suggest that incretin hormones share a similar short-term risk for mild-to-moderate gastrointestinal intolerance [53, 68, 101, 103–105].

The incretin-based therapies described above have all been shown, albeit to varying degrees, to improve glycemic control, with some also showing modest reduction in body weight over time. Exenatide and to a lesser degree liraglutide (due to limited published data available) have demonstrated improved cardiometabolic risk factors in type 2 diabetes [89, 106]. The salutary effects of incretin mimetics on glucose, lipids, blood pressure and body weight suggest that studies of their utility should be carried out in individuals with the metabolic syndrome.

DPP-IV INHIBITORS

The use of native GLP-1 as pharmacological therapy is significantly limited by its rapid proteolysis by the enzyme DPP-IV. While the clinical effects of GLP-1 have been investigated using continuous infusion in healthy subjects and patients with type 2 diabetes, this method of drug delivery is considered to be impractical for long-term clinical use. An alternative approach is to inhibit degradation of circulating GLP-1, which can be accomplished by inhibiting endogenous DPP-IV (Table 10.3) [107]. At the time this chapter was being prepared, the DPP-IV inhibitors, vildagliptin and sitagliptin, had been approved for commercial use in the European Union (vildagliptin and sitagliptin) and the United States (sitagliptin only). In clinical studies in patients with type 2 diabetes, the DPP-IV inhibitors vildagliptin and sitagliptin improve glycemic control, but their effects on body weight are neutral, in contrast to the observations with incretin mimetics [108].

Two DPP-IV inhibitors – sitagliptin (MK-0431) and vildagliptin (LAF237) – have completed extensive late-phase clinical testing programs. Sitagliptin has been reported to increase the concentration of post-prandial GLP-1 by approximately 2-fold; this was achieved by the inhibition of up to 80% of plasma DPP-IV activity in healthy human subjects [109]. Sitagliptin was shown to increase plasma C-peptide and insulin concentrations during both mixed-meal and oral glucose tolerance testing [110]. Sitagliptin also reduced glucagon secretion, increased the concentration of the active form of GLP-1, and lowered HbA1c [110].

Large-scale clinical trials have recently reported that sitagliptin monotherapy improved HbA1c and FPG, with no significant change in body weight [111, 112]. In these studies, a fraction of patients underwent drug washout from prior diabetes therapy. In three other recent reports, patients with type 2 diabetes who failed to achieve adequate glycemic control with metformin or pioglitazone were treated with sitagliptin for 24 weeks [113–115]. These studies reported significant improvements in HbA1c and FPG, with no significant changes in body weight [113–115]. In a further 24-week study, sitagliptin improved HbA1c and FPG as an add-on therapy to glimepiride or glimepiride and metformin. However, the addition of sitagliptin resulted in a modest increase in body weight [116]. In a 52-week study, vildagliptin was reported to achieve non-inferiority versus glipizide in patients with type 2 diabetes who were unable to achieve adequate glycemic control with metformin alone. Patients treated with metformin and sitagliptin were reported to achieve similar improvements in HbA1c compared to patients treated with metformin and glipizide. Significantly, patients treated with metformin and sitagliptin did not experience significant changes in body weight [117].

Vildagliptin has also reported data from late-phase clinical studies. Patients with type 2 diabetes experienced improved post-prandial glucose and insulin concentrations, and lowered HbA1c compared to placebo when treated for 12 weeks with 50 mg/day or 100 mg/day vildagliptin. These improvements in glycemic control were associated with no change in body weight [118]. In a 52-week study in patients with type 2 diabetes, treatment with 50 mg/day vildagliptin and concomitant metformin produced similar improvements in glycemic control [119]. Vildagliptin was also reported to lower HbA1c and FPG over 24 weeks in patients with type 2 diabetes who were unable to achieve adequate glycemic control with metformin alone [120]. In a similar 24-week study, vildagliptin was reported to improve HbA1c and fasting plasma glucose in drug-naïve patients with type 2 diabetes [121]. In both these studies, vildagliptin treatment was associated with neutral effects on body weight. To date, DPP-IV inhibitors report excellent tolerability of their once-daily, orally administered compounds. In contrast to incretin mimetics, these compounds do not appear to increase the risk of gastrointestinal adverse events. The most commonly reported adverse events in DPP-IV inhibitor studies were mild hypoglycemia, nasopharyngitis, and headache [118–121]. However, post-marketing reports for sitagliptin have described serious hypersensitivity and allergic reactions including angioedema, anaphylaxis, and exfoliative skin conditions such as Stevens-Johnson syndrome.

Based on the recent approval by the United States FDA of sitagliptin and the limited clinical data currently available, there is little doubt that DPP-IV inhibitors will prove to be effective agents for the treatment of type 2 diabetes – both when used alone or in combination with other glucose-lowering therapies. The short-term side-effect profile of DPP-IV inhibitors appears to be quite favorable. HbA1c reductions with these agents are in keeping with other incretin-based therapies – with HbA1c changes of 0.6% –1.0% generally reported. In contrast to incretin mimetic therapy, however, DPP-IV inhibitor therapy is not associated with consistent reductions in body weight. There are essentially no data assessing the impact of these compounds on CV risk factors. The neutral body weight effect, coupled with the absence of data on CV risk factors at present, makes it difficult to assess the possible role of DPP-IV inhibitors for the treatment of the features of the metabolic syndrome. DPP-IV inhibitors may modestly improve β-cell function (in both human and in preclinical studies). However, few long-term data are currently available to hypothesize a role for patients early in the course of hyperglycemia. A number of ongoing clinical trials are underway that will expand our understanding of the mechanism of action of DPP-IV inhibitors, and assess what effects, if any, DPP-IV inhibitors may have on dyslipidemia and hypertension as well as body weight.

SUMMARY

The metabolic syndrome and type 2 diabetes are metabolic disorders that remain inextricably intertwined. The emergence of obesity, type 2 diabetes, and CV disease as significant clinical and public health concerns in both the developed and developing worlds has further increased the awareness of the metabolic syndrome as a potential target for treatment in hopes of reducing the future risk of both progression of hyperglycemia and CV events in this population. The improved identification and treatment of individuals with the metabolic syndrome will require therapies that possess myriad effects on all components of the syndrome. Therapies for hyperglycemia (including metformin, TZDs, and the incretin mimetics) have demonstrated a broad array of potentially favorable effects.

Currently, the cardiometabolic risk factors, including obesity, glucose intolerance, dyslipidemia and hypertension, identified by IDF as critical components of the metabolic syndrome, are only treated either individually or targeted with compounds that specifically target weight loss. Most anti-diabetes agents improve glycemic control but are hampered by their association with body weight gain. The availability of the incretin mimetic exenatide, and potentially other incretin-based therapies, along with the DPP-IV inhibitors, represent a hopeful and novel approach to the treatment of type 2 diabetes. Most notably, the incretin mimetics (currently represented by exenatide) offer the hope for sustained improvement in glycemic control with progressive reduction in body weight, both very valuable characteristics, particularly for the type 2 diabetes patient with the metabolic syndrome. Whether these effects on glucose and body weight will also be seen in those with the metabolic syndrome in the absence of type 2 diabetes is not currently known. However, the reduction in body weight with concomitant improvement in cardiometabolic risk factors in patients treated with exenatide may have a potentially beneficial role for treatment of the metabolic syndrome in the years ahead. Further study in this population will obviously be required before such an approach to therapy can be advocated for individuals without a diagnosis of type 2 diabetes.

Disclosure

Anthony H. Stonehouse and David M. Kendall are employees and stockholders of Amylin Pharmaceuticals, Inc. John H. Holcombe is an employee and stockholder of Eli Lilly and Company. Amylin Pharmaceuticals, Inc. has a global agreement with Eli Lilly and Company to collaborate on the development and commercialization of exenatide.

REFERENCES

1. Sarafidis PA, Nilsson PM. The metabolic syndrome: a glance at its history. *J Hypertens* 2006; 24:621–626.
2. Expert Panel on the Detection, Evaluation, and Treatment of High Blood Cholesterol in Adults: Executive Summary of the Third Report of the National Cholesterol Education Program (NCEP) Expert Panel on Detection, Evaluation, and Treatment of High Blood Cholesterol in Adults (Adult Treatment Panel III). *JAMA* 2001; 285:2486–2497.

3. World Health Organization: Definition, diagnosis and classification of diabetes mellitus and its complications: report of a WHO Consultation. Geneva: World Health Organization, 1999.
4. Ford ES, Giles WH, Dietz WH. Prevalence of the metabolic syndrome among US adults: findings from the third National Health and Nutrition Examination Survey. *JAMA* 2002; 287:356–359.
5. Sarti C, Gallagher J. The metabolic syndrome: prevalence, CHD risk, and treatment. *J Diabetes Complications* 2006; 20:121–132.
6. International Diabetes Federation. The IDF consensus worldwide definition of the metabolic syndrome. Available from: http://www.idf.org/webdata/docs/idf_Metasyndrome_definition.pdf
7. Hutley L, Prins JB. Fat as an endocrine organ: relationship to the metabolic syndrome. *Am J Med Sci* 2005; 330:280–289.
8. Unger RH. Hyperleptinemia: protecting the heart from lipid overload. *Hypertension* 2005; 45:1031–1034.
9. Darsow T, Kendall DM, Maggs DG. Is the metabolic syndrome a real clinical entity and should it receive drug treatment? *Curr Diab Rep* 2006; 6:357–364.
10. Orchard TJ, Temprosa M, Goldberg R *et al.*; for the Diabetes Prevention Program Research Group. The effect of metformin and intensive lifestyle intervention on the metabolic syndrome: the Diabetes Prevention Program randomized trial. *Ann Intern Med* 2005; 142:611–619.
11. Zhu S, St-Onge MP, Heshka S, Heymsfield SB. Lifestyle behaviours associated with lower risk of having the metabolic syndrome. *Metabolism* 2004; 53:1503–1511.
12. Knowler WC, Barrett-Connor E, Fowler SE *et al.* For the Diabetes Prevention Program Research Group. Reduction in the incidence of type 2 diabetes with lifestyle intervention or metformin. *N Engl J Med* 2002; 346:393–403.
13. Ryan DH, Espeland MA, Foster GD *et al.* Look AHEAD Research Group. Look AHEAD (Action for Health in Diabetes): design and methods for a clinical trial of weight loss for the prevention of cardiovascular disease in type 2 diabetes. *Control Clin Trials* 2003; 24:610–628.
14. Pi-Sunyer FX. Use of lifestyle changes treatment plans and drug therapy in controlling cardiovascular and metabolic risk factors. *Obesity (Silver Spring)* 2006; 14(suppl 3):135–142.
15. Li Z, Maglione M, Tu W *et al.* Meta-analysis: pharmacologic treatment of obesity. *Ann Intern Med* 2005; 142:532–546.
16. Reaven G, Segal K, Hauptman J, Boldrin M, Lucas C. Effect of orlistat-assisted weight loss in decreasing coronary heart disease risk in patients with syndrome X. *Am J Cardiol* 2001; 87:827–831.
17. Torgerson JS, Hauptman J, Boldrin MN, Sjostrom L. XENical in the prevention of diabetes in obese subjects (XENDOS) study: a randomized study of orlistat as an adjunct to lifestyle changes for the prevention of type 2 diabetes in obese patients. *Diabetes Care* 2004; 27:155–161.
18. Hajdukovic Z, Jovelic A, Zivotic-Vanovic M, Raden S. Influence of orlistat therapy on serum insulin level and morphological and functional parameters of peripheral arterial circulation in obese patients. *Vojnosanit Preg* 2005; 62:803–810.
19. Ravinet TC, Arnone M, Delgorge C *et al.* Anti-obesity effect of SR141716, a CB1 receptor antagonist, in diet-induced obese mice. *Am J Physiol Regul Integr Comp Physiol* 2003; 284:R345–R353.
20. Despres JP, Golay A, Sjostrom L. Rimonabant in Obesity-Lipids Study Group. Effects of rimonabant on metabolic risk factors in overweight patients with dyslipidemia. *N Engl J Med* 2005; 353:2121–2134.
21. Pi-Sunyer FX, Aronne LJ, Heshmati HM, Devin J, Rosenstock J. RIO-North America Study Group. Effect of rimonabant, a cannabinoid-1 receptor blocker, on weight and cardiometabolic risk factors in overweight or obese patients. *JAMA* 2006; 295:761–775.
22. Redmon JB, Reck KP, Raatz SK *et al.* Two-year outcome of a combination of weight loss therapies for type 2 diabetes. *Diabetes Care* 2005; 28:1311–1315.
23. Nickenig G. Should angiotensin II receptor blockers and statins be combined? *Circulation* 2004; 110:1013–1020.
24. Grundy SM, Cleeman JI, Daniels SR *et al.* American Heart Association; National Heart, Lung, and Blood Institute. Diagnosis and management of the metabolic syndrome: an American Heart Association/National Heart, Lung, and Blood Institute Scientific Statement. *Circulation* 2005; 112:2735–2752.
25. Grundy SM, Cleeman JI, Merz CN *et al.* National Heart, Lung, and Blood Institute; American College of Cardiology Foundation; American Heart Association. Implications of recent clinical trials for the National Cholesterol Education Program Adult Treatment Panel III guidelines. *Circulation* 2004; 110:227–239.
26. Robins SJ, Rubins HB, Faas FH *et al.* Veterans Affairs HDL Intervention Trial (VA-HIT). Insulin resistance and cardiovascular events with low HDL cholesterol: the Veterans Affairs HDL Intervention Trial (VA-HIT). *Diabetes Care* 2003; 26:1513–1517.

27. Keech A, Simes RJ, Barter P *et al.*; FIELD study investigators. Effects of long-term fenofibrate therapy on cardiovascular events in 9795 people with type 2 diabetes mellitus (the FIELD study): randomised controlled trial. *Lancet* 2005; 366:1849–1861.
28. Athyros VG, Mikhailidis DP, Papageorgiou AA *et al.*; GREACE Study Collaborative Group. Effect of statins and ACE inhibitors alone and in combination on clinical outcome in patients with coronary heart disease. *J Hum Hypertens* 2004; 18:781–788.
29. Bartolucci AA, Howard G. Meta-analysis of data from the six primary prevention trials of cardiovascular events using aspirin. *Am J Cardiol* 2006; 98:746–750.
30. UK Prospective Diabetes Study (UKPDS) Group. Intensive blood-glucose control with sulphonylureas or insulin compared with conventional treatment and risk of complications in patients with type 2 diabetes (UKPDS 33). *Lancet* 1998; 352:837–853.
31. Alexander CM, Landsman PB, Teutsch SM, Haffner SM. Third National Health and Nutrition Examination Survey (NHANES III); National Cholesterol Education Program (NCEP). NCEP-defined metabolic syndrome, diabetes, and prevalence of coronary heart disease among NHANES III participants age 50 years and older. *Diabetes* 2003; 52:1210–1214.
32. Stratton IM, Adler AI, Neil HA *et al.* Association of glycaemia with macrovascular and microvascular complications of type 2 diabetes (UKPDS 35): prospective observational study. *Br Med J* 2000; 321:405–412.
33. UK Prospective Diabetes Study (UKPDS) Group. Effect of intensive blood-glucose control with metformin on complications in overweight patients with type 2 diabetes (UKPDS 34). *Lancet* 1998; 352:854–865.
34. Nagi DK, Yudkin JS. Effects of metformin on insulin resistance, risk factors for cardiovascular disease, and plasminogen activator inhibitor in NIDDM subjects. A study of two ethnic groups. *Diabetes Care* 1993; 16:621–629.
35. Charles MA, Eschwege E, Grandmottet P *et al.* Treatment with metformin of non-diabetic men with hypertension, hypertriglyceridaemia and central fat distribution: the BIGPRO 1.2 trial. *Diabetes Metab Res Rev* 2000; 16:2–7.
36. Rosenblatt S, Miskin B, Glazer NB, Prince MJ, Robertson KE. The impact of pioglitazone on glycemic control and atherogenic dyslipidemia in patients with type 2 diabetes mellitus. *Coron Artery Dis* 2001; 12:413–423.
37. Mayerson AB, Hundal RS, Dufour S *et al.* The effect of rosiglitazone on insulin sensitivity, lipolysis, and hepatic and skeletal muscle triglyceride content in patients with type 2 diabetes. *Diabetes* 2002; 51:797–802.
38. Parulkar AA, Pendergrass ML, Granda-Ayala R, Lee TR, Fonseca VA. Nonhypoglycemic effects of thiazolidinediones. *Ann Intern Med* 2001; 134:61–71.
39. Rajagopalan R, Iyer S, Khan M. Effect of pioglitazone on metabolic syndrome risk factors: results of double-blind, multicenter, randomized clinical trials. *Curr Med Res Opin* 2005; 21:163–172.
40. Derosa G, Cicero AF, Gaddi A *et al.* Metabolic effects of pioglitazone and rosiglitazone in patients with diabetes and metabolic syndrome treated with glimepiride: a twelve-month, multicenter, double-blind, randomized, controlled, parallel-group trial. *Clin Ther* 2004; 26:744–754.
41. Dormandy JA, Charbonnel B, Eckland DJ *et al.*; for the PROactive investigators. Secondary prevention of macrovascular events in patients with type 2 diabetes in the PROactive Study (PROspective pioglitAzone Clinical Trial In macroVascular Events): a randomised controlled trial. *Lancet* 2005; 366:1279–1289.
42. Azen SP, Peters RK, Berkowitz K, Kjos S, Xiang A, Buchanan TA. TRIPOD (TRoglitazone In the Prevention Of Diabetes): a randomized, placebo-controlled trial of troglitazone in women with prior gestational diabetes mellitus. *Control Clin Trials* 1998; 19:217–231.
43. Xiang AH, Peters RK, Kjos SL *et al.* Effect of pioglitazone on pancreatic beta-cell function and diabetes risk in Hispanic women with prior gestational diabetes. *Diabetes* 2006; 55:517–522.
44. Gerstein HC, Yusuf S, Bosch J *et al.*; DREAM (Diabetes REduction Assessment with ramipril and rosiglitazone Medication) Trial Investigators. Effect of rosiglitazone on the frequency of diabetes in patients with impaired glucose tolerance or impaired fasting glucose: a randomised controlled trial. *Lancet* 2006; 368:1096–1105.
45. Stumvoll M, Haring HU. Glitazones: clinical effects and molecular mechanisms. *Ann Med* 2002; 34:217–224.
46. Nauck MA, Wollschlager D, Werner J *et al.* Effects of subcutaneous glucagon-like peptide 1 (GLP-1 [7-36 amide]) in patients with NIDDM. *Diabetologia* 1996; 39:1546–1553.

47. Kreymann B, Williams G, Ghatei MA, Bloom SR. Glucagon-like peptide-1 7-36: a physiological incretin in man. *Lancet* 1987; 2:1300–1304.
48. Holst JJ, Gromada J. Role of incretin hormones in the regulation of insulin secretion in diabetic and nondiabetic humans. *J Physiol Endocrinol Metab* 2004; 287:E199–E206.
49. Vilsbøll T, Holst JJ. Incretins, insulin secretion and type 2 diabetes mellitus. *Diabetologia* 2004; 47:357–366.
50. Ørskov C, Holst JJ, Knuhtsen S, Baldissera FG, Poulsen SS, Nielsen OV. Glucagon-like peptides GLP-1 and GLP-2, predicted products of the glucagon gene, are secreted separately from pig small intestine but not pancreas. *Endocrinology* 1986; 119:1467–1475.
51. Holst JJ. Glucagon-like Peptide 1 (GLP-1): an intestinal hormone, signalling nutritional abundance, with an unusual therapeutic potential. *Trends Endocrinol Metab* 1999; 10:229–235.
52. Drucker DJ. Glucagon-like peptides. *Diabetes* 1998; 47:159–169.
53. Zander M, Madsbad S, Madsen JL, Holst JJ. Effect of 6-week course of glucagon-like peptide 1 on glycaemic control, insulin sensitivity, and β-cell function in type 2 diabetes: a parallel-group study. *Lancet* 2002; 359:824–830.
54. Parkes DG, Pittner R, Jodka C, Smith P, Young AA. Insulinotropic actions of exendin-4 and glucagon-like peptide-1 in vivo and in vitro. *Metabolism* 2001; 50:583–589.
55. Rayner CK, Samsom M, Jones KL, Horowitz M. Relationships of upper gastrointestinal motor and sensory function with glycemic control. *Diabetes Care* 2001; 24:371–381.
56. Schwartz JG, Green GM, Guan D, McMahan CA, Phillips WT. Rapid gastric emptying of a solid pancake meal in type II diabetic patients. *Diabetes Care* 1996; 19:468–471.
57. Flint A, Raben A, Astrup A, Holst JJ. Glucagon-like peptide 1 promotes satiety and suppresses energy intake in humans. J *Clin Invest* 1998; 101:515–520.
58. Naslund E, Barkeling B, King N *et al.* Energy intake and appetite are suppressed by glucagon-like peptide-1 (GLP-1) in obese men. *Int J Obes Relat Metab Disord* 1999; 23:304–311.
59. Gutzwiller JP, Drewe J, Göke B *et al.* Glucagon-like peptide-1 promotes satiety and reduces food intake in patients with diabetes mellitus type 2. *Am J Physiol* 1999; 276:R1541–R1544.
60. Tourrel C, Bailbe' D, Meile M-J, Kergoat M, Portha B. Glucagon-like peptide-1 and exendin-4 stimulate β-cell neogenesis in streptozotocin-treated newborn rats resulting in persistently improved glucose homeostasis at adult age. *Diabetes* 2001; 50:1562–1570.
61. Tourrel C, Bailbe' D, Lacorne M, Meile M-J, Kergoat M, Portha B. Persistent improvement of type 2 diabetes in the Goto-Kakizaki rat model by expansion of the β-cell mass during the prediabetic period with glucagon-like peptide-1 or exendin-4. *Diabetes* 2002; 51:1443–1452.
62. Kieffer TJ, Habener JF. The glucagon-like peptides. *Endocr Rev* 1999; 20:876–913.
63. Zhou J, Wang X, Pineyro MA, Egan JM. Glucagon-like peptide 1 and exendin-4 convert pancreatic AR42J cells into glucagon- and insulin-producing cells. *Diabetes* 1999; 48:2358–2366.
64. Perfetti R, Zhou J, Doyle ME, Egan JM. Glucagon-like peptide-1 induces cell proliferation and pancreatic-duodenum homeobox-1 expression and increases endocrine cell mass in the pancreas of old, glucose-intolerant rats. *Endocrinology* 2000; 141:4600–4605.
65. Kieffer TJ, McIntosh CHS, Pederson RA. Degradation of glucose-dependent insulinotropic polypeptide and truncated glucagon-like peptide 1 in vitro and in vivo by dipeptidyl peptidase IV. *Endocrinology* 1995; 136:3585–3596.
66. Deacon CF, Nauck MA, Toft-Nielsen M, Pridal L, Willms B, Holst JJ. Both subcutaneously and intravenously administered glucagon-like peptide I are rapidly degraded from the NH2-terminus in type II diabetic patients and in healthy subjects. *Diabetes* 1995; 44:1126–1131.
67. Drucker DJ. Minireview: the glucagon-like peptides. *Endocrinology* 2001;142:521–527.
68. Keating GM. Exenatide. *Drugs* 2005; 65:1681–1692.
69. Fehse F, Trautmann M, Holst JJ *et al.* Exenatide augments first- and second-phase insulin secretion in response to intravenous glucose in subjects with type 2 diabetes. *J Clin Endocrinol Metab* 2005; 90:5991–5997.
70. Eng J, Kleinman WA, Singh L, Singh G, Raufman J-P. Isolation and characterization of exendin-4, an exendin-3 analogue, from Heloderma suspectum venom. *J Biol Chem* 1992; 267:7402–7405.
71. Kaptiza C, Heise T, Klein O *et al.* BIM51077, a novel GLP-1 analog, showed linear PK and dose-response relationship over 7 days of treatment. *Diabetes* 2006; 55(suppl 1):A119.
72. Giannoukakis N. CJC-1131. ConjuChem. *Curr Opin Investig Drugs* 2003; 4:1245–1249.

73. Agersø H, Jensen LB, Elbrønd B, Rolan P, Zdravkovic M. The pharmacokinetics, pharmacodynamics, safety and tolerability of NN2211, a new long-acting GLP-1 derivative, in healthy men. *Diabetologia* 2002; 45:195–202.
74. Degn KB, Juhl CB, Sturis J *et al.* One week's treatment with the long-acting glucagon-like peptide 1 derivative liraglutide (NN2211) markedly improves 24-h glycemia and alpha- and β-cell function and reduces endogenous glucose release in patients with type 2 diabetes. *Diabetes* 2004; 53:1187–1194.
75. Young AA. Glucagon-like peptide-1, exendin and insulin sensitivity. In: Hansen B, Shafrir E (eds). *Insulin Resistance and Insulin Resistance Syndrome*. New York: Harwood Academic Press, 2002; pp 235–262.
76. Chen YE, Drucker DJ. Tissue-specific expression of unique mRNAs that encode proglucagon-derived peptides or exendin 4 in the lizard. *J Biol Chem* 1997; 272:4108–4115.
77. Kolterman OG, Kim DD, Shen L *et al.* Pharmacokinetics, pharmacodynamics, and safety of exenatide in patients with type 2 diabetes mellitus. *J Health Syst Pharm* 2005; 62:173–181.
78. Egan JM, Clocquet AR, Elahi D. The insulinotropic effect of acute exendin 4 administered to humans: comparison of nondiabetic state to type 2 diabetes. *J Clin Endocrinol Metab* 2002; 87:1282–1290.
79. Kolterman OG, Buse JB, Fineman MS *et al.* Synthetic exendin 4 (exenatide) significantly reduces postprandial and fasting plasma glucose in subjects with type 2 diabetes. *J Clin Endocrinol Metab* 2003; 88:3082–3089.
80. Gedulin B, Jodka L, Hoyt J. Exendin-4 (AC2993) decreases glucagon secretion during hyperglycemic clamps in diabetic fatty Zucker rats. *Diabetes* 1999; 48(suppl 1):A199.
81. Nielsen LL, Young AA, Parkes DG. Pharmacology of exenatide (synthetic exendin-4): a potential therapeutic for improved glycemic control of type 2 diabetes. *Regul Pept* 2004; 117:77–88.
82. Szayna M, Doyle ME, Betkey JA *et al.* Exendin-4 decelerates food intake, weight gain, and fat deposition in Zucker rats. *Endocrinology* 2000; 141:1936–1941.
83. Young AA, Gedulin BR, Bhavsar S *et al.* Glucose-lowering and insulin-sensitizing actions of exendin-4: studies in obese diabetic (ob/ob, db/db) mice, diabetic fatty Zucker rats, and diabetic rhesus monkeys (Macaca mulatta). *Diabetes* 1999; 48:1026–1034.
84. Xu G, Stoffers DA, Habener JF, Bonner-Weir S. Exendin-4 stimulates both β-cell replication and neogenesis, resulting in increased β-cell mass and improved glucose tolerance in diabetic rats. *Diabetes* 1999; 48:2270–2276.
85. Degn KB, Brock B, Juhl CB *et al.* Effect of intravenous infusion of exenatide (synthetic exendin-4) on glucose-dependent insulin secretion and counterregulation during hypoglycemia. *Diabetes* 2004; 53:2397–2403.
86. Buse JB, Henry RR, Han J, Kim DD, Fineman MS, Baron AD. For the exenatide 113 clinical study group: Effects of exenatide (exendin-4) on glycemic control over 30 weeks in sulfonylurea-treated patients with type 2 diabetes. *Diabetes Care* 2004; 27:2628–2635.
87. DeFronzo RA, Ratner RE, Han J, Kim DD, Fineman MS, Baron AD. Effects of exenatide (exendin-4) on glycemic control and weight over 30 weeks in metformin-treated patients with type 2 diabetes. *Diabetes Care* 2005; 28:1092–1100.
88. Kendall DM, Riddle MC, Rosenstock J *et al.* Effects of exenatide (exendin-4) on glycemic control over 30 weeks in patients with type 2 diabetes treated with metformin and a sulfonylurea. *Diabetes Care* 2005; 28:1083–1091.
89. Klonoff DC, Buse JB, Nielsen LL *et al.* Exenatide effects on diabetes, obesity, cardiovascular risk factors and hepatic biomarkers in patients with type 2 diabetes treated for at least 3 years. *Curr Med Res Opin* 2008; 24:275–286.
90. Kendall D, Bhole D, Guan X *et al.* Exenatide treatment for 82 weeks reduced C-reactive protein, HbA1C, and body weight in patients with type 2 diabetes mellitus. *Diabetologia* 2006; 49(suppl 1):S475.
91. Zinman B, Hoogwerf B, Duran Garcia S *et al.* The effect of adding exenatide to a thiazolidinedione in suboptimally controlled type 2 diabetes: a randomized trial. *Ann Intern Med* 2007; 146:477–485.
92. Heine RJ, Van Gaal LF, Johns D, Mihm MJ, Widel MH, Brodows RG; GWAA study group. Exenatide versus insulin glargine in patients with suboptimally controlled type 2 diabetes: a randomized trial. *Ann Intern Med* 2005; 143:559–569.
93. Medina J, Fernandez-Salazar LI, Garcia-Buey L, Moreno-Otero R. Approach to the pathogenesis and treatment of nonalcoholic steatohepatitis. *Diabetes Care* 2004; 27:2057–2066.
94. Kim DD, MacConell L, Zhuang D *et al.* Effects of once-weekly dosing of a long-acting release formulation of exenatide on glucose control and body weight in subjects with type 2 diabetes. *Diabetes Care* 2007; 30:1487–1493.

95. Fineman MS, Shen LZ, Taylor K, Kim DD, Baron AD. Effectiveness of progressive dose-escalation of exenatide (exendin-4) in reducing dose-limiting side effects in subjects with type 2 diabetes. *Diabetes Metab Res Rev* 2004; 20:411–417.
96. Guivarc'h P-H, Castaigne J-P, Gagnon C, Peslherbe L, Dreyfus JH, Drucker DJ. CJC-1131, a long acting GLP-1 analog safely normalizes post-prandial glucose excursion and fasting glycemia in type 2 diabetes mellitus. *Diabetes* 2004a; 53(suppl 2):A127.
97. Benquet C, Le'ger R, Huang X, Thibaudeau K, Bridon D, Castaigne J-P. CJC-1131 (DAC:GLP-1) binds covalently in vivo to endogenous albumin: update on the DAC technology. *Diabetes* 2004; 53(suppl 2):A116.
98. Guivarc'h P-H, Dreyfus J-F, Mathi S, Castaigne J-P, Drucker DJ. CJC-1131, a long acting GLP-1 analog for Type 2 diabetes mellitus: clinical development update. *Diabetologia* 2004b; 47(suppl 1):A282.
99. Vilsbøll T, Zdravkovic M, Le-Thi T *et al.* Liraglutide significantly improves glycemic control, and lowers body weight without risk of either major or minor hypoglycemic episodes in subjects with type 2 diabetes. *Diabetes* 2006; 55(suppl 1):A27.
100. Chang AM, Jakobsen G, Sturis J *et al.* The GLP-1 derivative NN2211 restores β-cell sensitivity to glucose in type 2 diabetic patients after a single dose. *Diabetes* 2003; 52:1786–1791.
101. Harder H, Nielsen L, Thi TDT, Astrup A. The effect of liraglutide, a long-acting glucagon-like peptide 1 derivative, on glycemic control, body composition, and 24-h energy expenditure in patients with type 2 diabetes. *Diabetes Care* 2004; 27:1915–1921.
102. Juhl CB, Hollingdal M, Sturis J *et al.* Bedtime administration of NN2211, a long-acting GLP-1 derivative, substantially reduces fasting and postprandial glycemia in type 2 diabetes. *Diabetes* 2002; 51:424–429.
103. Madsbad S, Schmitz O, Ranstam J, Jakobsen G, Matthews DR; on behalf of the NN2211-1310 International Study Group. Improved glycemic control with no weight increase in patients with type 2 diabetes after once-daily treatment with the long-acting glucagon-like peptide 1 analog liraglutide (NN2211): a 12-week, double-blind, randomized, controlled trial. *Diabetes Care* 2004; 27:1335–1342.
104. Nauck MA, Hompesch M, Filipczak R, Le TD, Zdravkovic M, Gumprecht J; NN2211-1499 Study Group. Five weeks of treatment with the GLP-1 analogue liraglutide improves glycaemic control and lowers body weight in subjects with type 2 diabetes. *Exp Clin Endocrinol Diabetes* 2006; 114:417–423.
105. Feinglos MN, Saad MF, Pi-Sunyer FX, An B, Santiago O; on behalf of the Liraglutide Dose-Response Study Group. Effects of liraglutide (NN2211), a long-acting GLP-1 analogue, on glycaemic control and bodyweight in subjects with Type 2 diabetes. *Diabet Med* 2005; 22:1016–1023.
106. Courreges J-P, Zdravkovic M, Le-Thi T *et al.* Liraglutide treatment, blood pressure and biomarkers of cardiovascular risk in patients with type 2 diabetes: 14 weeks monotherapy study. *Diabetologia* 2006; 49(suppl 1):S4.
107. Holst JJ. Therapy of type 2 diabetes mellitus based on the actions of glucagon-like peptide-1. *Diabetes Metab Res Rev* 2002; 18:430–441.
108. Ahren B, Landin-Olsson M, Jansson P-A, Svensson M, Holmes D, Schweizer A. Inhibition of dipeptidyl peptidase-4 reduces glycemia, sustains insulin levels, and reduces glucagon levels in type 2 diabetes. *J Clin Endocrinol Metab* 2004; 89:2078–2084.
109. Herman GA, Stevens C, Van Dyck K *et al.* Pharmacokinetics and pharmacodynamics of sitagliptin, an inhibitor of dipeptidyl peptidase IV, in healthy subjects: Results from two randomized, double-blind, placebo-controlled studies with single oral doses. *Clin Pharmacol Ther* 2005; 78:675–688.
110. Herman GA, Zhao P-L, Dietrich B *et al.* The DPP-IV inhibitor MK-0431 enhances active GLP-1 and reduces glucose following an OGTT in type 2 diabetics. *Diabetes* 2004; 53(suppl 2):A82.
111. Aschner P, Kipnes MS, Lunceford JK, Sanchez M, Mickel C, Williams-Herman DE; Sitagliptin Study 021 Group. Effect of the dipeptidyl peptidase-4 inhibitor sitagliptin as monotherapy on glycemic control in patients with type 2 diabetes. *Diabetes Care* 2006; 29:2632–2637.
112. Raz I, Hanefeld M, Xu L, Caria C, Williams-Herman D, Khatami H; Sitagliptin Study 023 Group. Efficacy and safety of the dipeptidyl peptidase-4 inhibitor sitagliptin as monotherapy in patients with type 2 diabetes mellitus. *Diabetologia* 2006; 49:2564–2571.
113. Charbonnel B, Karasik A, Liu J, Wu M, Meininger G; Sitagliptin Study 020 Group. Efficacy and safety of the dipeptidyl peptidase-4 inhibitor sitagliptin added to ongoing metformin therapy in patients with type 2 diabetes inadequately controlled with metformin alone. *Diabetes Care* 2006; 29:2638–2643.
114. Rosenstock J, Brazg R, Andryuk PJ, Lu K, Stein P; Sitagliptin Study 019 Group. Efficacy and safety of the dipeptidyl peptidase-4 inhibitor sitagliptin added to ongoing pioglitazone therapy in patients with

type 2 diabetes: a 24-week, multicenter, randomized, double-blind, placebo-controlled, parallel-group study. *Clin Ther* 2006; 28:1556–1568.

115. Goldstein BJ, Feinglos MN, Lunceford JK, Johnson J, Williams-Herman DE; Sitagliptin 036 Study Group. Effect of initial combination therapy with sitagliptin, a dipeptidyl peptidase-4 inhibitor, and metformin on glycemic control in patients with type 2 diabetes. *Diabetes Care* 2007; 30:1979–1987.
116. Hermansen K, Kipnes M, Luo E, Fanurik D, Khatami H, Stein P; Sitagliptin Study 035 Group. Efficacy and safety of the dipeptidyl peptidase-4 inhibitor, sitagliptin, in patients with type 2 diabetes mellitus inadequately controlled on glimepiride alone or on glimepiride and metformin. *Diabetes Obes Metab* 2007; 9:733–745.
117. Nauck MA, Meininger G, Sheng D, Terranella L, Stein PP; Sitagliptin Study 024 Group. Efficacy and safety of the dipeptidyl peptidase-4 inhibitor, sitagliptin, compared with the sulfonylurea, glipizide, in patients with type 2 diabetes inadequately controlled on metformin alone: a randomized, double-blind, non-inferiority trial. *Diabetes Obes Metab* 2007; 9:194–205.
118. Ristic S, Byiers S, Foley J, Holmes D. Improved glycaemic control with dipeptidyl peptidase-4 inhibition in patients with type 2 diabetes: vildagliptin (LAF237) dose response. *Diabetes Obes Metab* 2005; 7:692–698.
119. Ahren B, Pacini G, Foley JE, Schweizer A. Improved meal-related β-cell function and insulin sensitivity by the dipeptidyl peptidase-IV inhibitor vildagliptin in metformin-treated patients with type 2 diabetes over 1 year. *Diabetes Care* 2005; 28:1936–1940.
120. Bosi E, Camisasca RP, Collober C, Rochotte E, Garber AJ. Effects of vildagliptin on glucose control over 24 weeks in patients with type 2 diabetes inadequately controlled with metformin. *Diabetes Care* 2007; 30:890–895.
121. Pi-Sunyer FX, Schweizer A, Mills D, Dejager S. Efficacy and tolerability of vildagliptin monotherapy in drug-naive patients with type 2 diabetes. *Diabetes Res Clin Pract* 2007; 76:132–138.

List of Abbreviations

4S	Scandinavian Simvastatin Survival Study
A to Z	Aggrastat to Zocor study
ACCORD	Action to Control Cardiovascular Risk in Diabetes (trial)
ACE	angiotensin-converting enzyme
ACSM	American College of Sports Medicine
ADA	American Diabetes Association
ADMA	asymmetric dimethylarginine
AGI	alpha glucosidase inhibitor
AHA	American Heart Association
AIM-HIGH	Atherosclerosis Intervention in Metabolic Syndrome with Low HDL/High Triglycerides and Impact on Global Health Outcomes (study)
AIRE	Acute Infarction Ramipril Efficacy (trial)
ALLHAT	Antihypertensive and Lipid Lowering treatment to prevent Heart Attack Trial
ALPINE	Antihypertensive treatment and Lipid Profile In a North of Sweden Efficacy
ALT	alanine aminotransferase
AMI	acute myocardial infarction
ANBP-2	Second Australian National Blood Pressure Study
Ang II	angiotensin II
AP-1	activator protein 1
apoB	apoliprotein B
ARB	angiotensin receptor blocker
ASA	acetylsalicylic acid
ASCOT-BPLA	Anglo Scandinavian Cardiac Outcomes Trial Blood Pressure Lowering Arm
AST	aspartate aminotransferase
AT_1	angiotensin II receptor type 1
AT_2	angiotensin II receptor type 2
ATP III	Adult Treatment Panel III (of the NCEP)
AURORA	A study to evaluate the Use of Rosuvastatin in subjects On Regular haemodialysis: an Assessment of survival and cardiovascular events
BIGPRO	Biguanides and Prevention of Risks in Obesity trial
BIP	Bezafibrate Infarction Prevention (study)
BMI	body mass index
BP	blood pressure
CABG	coronary artery bypass graft
CAD	coronary artery disease
cAMP	cyclic adenosine 3',5'-monophosphate
CAPP	Captopril Prevention Project
CARMEN	Carbohydrate Ratio Management in European National diets study

CB	cannabinoid receptor
CCA-IMT	common carotid arteries intimal-media thickness
CDP	Coronary Drug Project
CETP	cholesteryl ester transfer protein
cGMP	cyclic guanosine monophosphate
CHARM	Candesartan in Heart Failure Assessment of Reduction in Mortality and Morbidity study
CHD	coronary heart disease
CHF	congestive heart failure
CI	confidence interval
CIMT	carotid intimal-medial thickness
CK	creatine kinase
CNS	central nervous system
CONSENSUS	Cooperative New Scandinavian Enalapril Survival Study
CRP	C-reactive protein
CT	computed tomography
CV	cardiovascular
CVD	cardiovascular disease
CVE	cerebrovascular event(s)
DAIS	Diabetes Atherosclerosis Intervention Study
DASH	Dietary Approaches to Stop Hypertension
DCCT/EDIC	Diabetes Control and Complications Trial/Epidemiology of Diabetes Interventions and Complications
DEA	Drug Enforcement Administration
DHA	docasahexaenoic acid
DM	diabetes mellitus
DPP	Diabetes Prevention Program
DPP-IV	dipeptidyl peptidase-IV
DREAM	Diabetes Reduction Assessment with Ramipril and Rosiglitazone Medication trial
dsDNA	double-stranded DNA
ECM	extracellular matrix
Egr-1	early growth response factor-1
ELITE II	Evaluation of Losartan In The Elderly II study
eNOS	endothelial nitric oxide synthase
EPA	eicosapentaenoic acid
EPIC-Norfolk	European Prospective Investigation of Cancer, Norfolk study
ESRD	end-stage renal disease
FDA	Food and Drug Administration
FDPS	Finnish Diabetes Prevention Study
FFA	free fatty acids
FGF	fibroblast growth factor
FIELD	Fenofibrate Intervention and Event Lowering in Diabetes (trial)
FPG	fasting plasma glucose
GIP	glucose-dependent insulinotropic peptide
GISSI-3	Gruppo Italiano per lo Studio della Sopravivenza nell'Infarto Miocardica III
GLP-1	glucagon-like peptide-1
GLUT 4	glucose transporter 4
HATS	HDL Atherosclerosis Treatment Study
HbA1c	glycosylated hemoglobin
HDL	high-density lipoprotein
HERITAGE	Health, Risk Factors, Exercise Training, and Genetics study

HIF-1a	hypoxia-inducible factor-1a
HL	hepatic lipase
HMG-CoA	3-hydroxy-3-methylglutaryl coenzyme A
HOMA	homeostasis model assessment (index)
HOMA-B	homeostasis model assessment – pancreatic B-cell function
HOMA-IR	homeostasis model assessment – insulin resistance
HOPE	Heart Outcomes Prevention Evaluation (study)
HRmax	maximal heart rate
HR	hazard ratio
hs-CRP	highly-sensitive C-reactive protein
HTN	hypertension
ICAM-1	intracellular adhesion molecule-1
ICU	intensive care unit
IDEAL	Incremental Decrease in Endpoints through Aggressive Lipid lowering (trial)
IDF	International Diabetes Federation
IDL	intermediate-density lipoprotein
IDNT	Irebesartan in Diabetic Nephropathy trial
IFG	impaired fasting glucose
IFN	interferon
IGT	impaired glucose tolerance
IKK	I kappa B kinase
IKKβ	I kappa B kinase beta subunit
IL-6	interleukin-6
ILLUMINATE	Investigation of Lipid Level Management to Understand its Impact in Atherosclerotic Events trial
IMT	intima-media thickness
iNOS	inducible nitric oxide synthase
IRMA	Irbesartan in Patients with Type 2 Diabetes and Microalbuminuria study
IRS	insulin resistance syndrome
IRS-1	insulin receptor substrate 1
ISIS-4	International Study of Infarct Survival 4
Iκ-Ba	inhibitor kappa B a
JNK	Jun N-terminal kinase
LDL	low-density lipoprotein
LIFE	Losartan Intervention For Endpoint Reduction in Hypertension study
Look AHEAD	Action for Health in Diabetes (trial)
Lp(a)	lipoprotein (a)
LPL	lipoprotein lipase
LVD	left ventricular dysfunction
LVH	left ventricular hypertension
MAPK	mitogen activated protein kinase
MCP-1	monocyte chemoattractant/chemotactic protein-1
MI	myocardial infarction
MIF	migration inhibitory factor
MMP	matrix metalloproteinase
MRI	magnetic resonance imaging
MS	metabolic syndrome
NADPH	nicotinamide adenine dinucleotide phosphate
NAVIGATOR	Nateglinide And Valsartan in Impaired Glucose Tolerance Outcomes Research
NCEP	National Cholesterol Education Program

NF-κB	nuclear factor kappa B
NGT	normal glucose tolerance
NHANES	National Health and Nutrition Examination Survey
NIH	National Institutes of Health
NMR	nuclear magnetic resonance
NO	nitric oxide
NSAID	non-steroidal anti-inflammatory drug
NYHA	New York Heart Association
ONTARGET	Ongoing Telmisartan Alone and in Combination with Ramipril Global Endpoint Trial
OPTIMAAL	Optimal Therapy in Myocardial Infarction with the Angiotensin II Antagonist Losartan study
ORIGIN	Outcome Reduction with an Initial Glargine Intervention
OTC	over-the-counter
PAI-1	plasminogen-activator inhibitor type 1
PAR	population attributable risk
PCOS	polycystic ovary syndrome
PDGF	platelet-derived growth factor
PEACE	Prevention of Events with Angiotensin Converting Enzyme inhibition
PG	prostaglandin
PI-3K	phosphotidyl inositol 3 kinase
PIA-1	plasminogen activator inhibitor type 1
PIPOD	Pioglitazone in the Prevention of Diabetes
PKCb	protein kinase C b
PPAR-a	peroxisome proliferator-activated receptor-a
PPAR-g	peroxisome proliferator-activated receptor-g
PROVE-IT	Pravastatin or Atorvastatin Evaluation and Infection Therapy
RAAS	renin-angiotensin-aldosterone system
RENAAL	Reduction of Endpoints in NIDDM with the Angiotensin II Antagonist Losartan
RMR	resting metabolic rate
ROS	reactive oxygen species
RR	relative risk
SAA	serum amyloid A
SAFARI	San Antonio Family Assessment of Metabolic Risk Indicators in Youth study
SAVE	Survival and Ventricular Enlargement (trial)
SBP	systolic blood pressure
SCD	sudden cardiovascular death
SCOPE	Study of Cognition and Prognosis in the Elderly
SCr	serum creatinine
SENDCAP	St Mary's, Ealing, Northwick Park Diabetes Cardiovascular Disease Prevention (trial)
SLE	systemic lupus erythematosus
SMILE	Survival of Myocardial Infarction Long-Term Evaluation (trial)
SOCS-3	suppressor of cytokine signaling
SOLVD	Studies on Left Ventricular Dysfunction
SREBP-1	sterol regulatory element binding protein
STAT-3	signal transducer and activator of transcription 3
STOP-NIDDM	STOP-Non-Insulin Dependent Diabetes Mellitus trial
STORM	Sibutramine Trial of Obesity Reduction and Maintenance

STRRIDE	Studies of a Targeted Risk Reduction Intervention through Defined Exercise study
T2DM	type 2 diabetes mellitus
TCF7L2	transcription factor 7-like 2 gene
TEF	thermogenic effect of food
TF	tissue factor
TG	triglyceride
THRIVE	Treatment of HDL to Reduce the Incidence of Vascular Events trial
TLC	therapeutic lifestyle change
TLR	toll-like receptor
TNF-α	tumor necrosis factor alpha
TNT	Treat to New Target trial
tPA	tissue plasminogen activator
TRACE	Trandolapril Cardiac Evaluation (trial)
TRANSCEND	Telmisartan Randomized Assessment Study in ACE Intolerant Subjects with Cardiovascular Disease
TRB3	mammalian tribbles homolog 3
TRIPOD	Troglitazone in the Prevention of Diabetes
TZD	thiazolidinedione
UKPDS	United Kingdom Prospective Diabetes Study
VA-HIT	Veterans Affairs High-Density Lipoprotein Cholesterol Intervention Trial
VALIANT	VALsartan In Acute myocardial iNfarcTion trial
VALUE	Valsartan Antihypertensive Long-term Use Evaluation trial
VCAM	vascular cell adhesion molecule
VEGF	vascular endothelial growth factor
V-HeFTII	Vasodilator-Heart Failure Trial II
VLDL	very low-density lipoprotein
VSMC	vascular smooth muscle cell
WHO	World Health Organization
WHR	waist-to-hip ratio

Index

abdominal fat, effect of exercise 30, 32
abdominal obesity 56–7, 138
acarbose 44–5, 63
ACCORD trial 106–7, 141
acetylsalicylic acid (ASA, aspirin) 131–2, 141
activator protein-1 (AP-1) 114, 130
acute coronary syndromes 97
acute-phase response 128
adherence, exercise program 39
adipocytes 14, 47, 113–14, 138
adipokines 14, 47, 57, 138
adiponectin 47, 126
  dietary influences 14, 15
  RAAS inhibition and 83–4
  thiazolidinediones and 48
adipose tissue 57, 127, 138–9
aerobic exercise 37–8
  intensity 37
  rate of progression 38
  recommendations 31, 32
  volume 37–8
aerobic fitness 32
AIM-HIGH trial 107
AIRE study 75
ALLHAT study 79, 81
alpha glucosidase inhibitors (AGI) 44–5, 47, 63
ALPINE study 79
American College of Sports Medicine (ACSM) 31, 32, 37, 39
American Diabetes Association (ADA) 15, 104
American Heart Association (AHA) 15, 126
  exercise guidelines 31, 32, 37, 39
amlodipine 78
amphetamines 60
amylin analog 63
angiotensin II (Ang II) 71–2
  effects of inhibition 83
  insulin resistance and 73–4
angiotensin receptor blockers (ARBs) 75–81
  diabetes prevention 78–81
  mechanism of diabetes prevention 83–4
angiotensin-converting enzyme (ACE) 71, 72, 73
angiotensin-converting enzyme (ACE) inhibitors 74–5
  diabetes prevention 78–83
  mechanism of diabetes prevention 83–4
angiotensinogen 71, 128
antidiabetes (hypoglycemic) medications 43–50
  cardiometabolic risk factors 47–50
  diabetes prevention 43–5, 46, 142–3
  incretin mimetics/DPP-IV inhibitors 144–51
  inflammation and 128–32
  metabolic syndrome 43–7, 141–3
  role in obesity 62–3
anti-inflammatory agents, specific 131–2
antimalarial agents 132
apolipoprotein B (apoB) 94–5
aspirin 131–2, 141
atherosclerosis 126
atorvastatin 96–7, 98
A-to-Z study 97, 98
AURORA trial 107
autonomic neuropathy, diabetic 34

bariatric surgery 63–5
behavior modification, weight loss 58–9
β-cell function
  incretin/incretin mimetic actions 144, 145–6, 149
  interleukin-1 receptor antagonist 132
  mechanisms of loss 116–17
bezafibrate 101–2, 130
Bezafibrate Infarction Prevention (BIP) study 101
BIGPRO trial 62
BIM-51077 145, 148
body fat distribution 56–7

body mass index (BMI) 55, 56, 140
bradykinin 72, 83

calorie restriction 22–3, 25, 116
candesartan 77, 78, 79
cannabinoid-1 (CB-1) receptor antagonists 61–2, 140–1
captopril 75
carbohydrate, dietary 13, 17–23
  development of metabolic syndrome and 18–19
  glycemic index or glycemic load 21–2
  low-calorie diets 22–3
  recommended intake 19, 25
  restricted intake 19–20, 25
  simple vs complex 20–1
cardiovascular disease (CVD)
  glycemic control in diabetes and 6–7
  hypoglycemic agents and 44
  lifestyle interventions in diabetes 3–6
  lipid-lowering therapy 95–107
  pre-exercise evaluation 33, 34
  primary prevention in prediabetes 8
  RAAS blockade 75–8
  risk in diabetes 1–2
  risk in prediabetes 2–3, 93
  role of RAAS activation 71–2
  targets for risk reduction 4
CARMEN study 20–1
carotid artery intima-media thickness (IMT, CIMT)
  hypoglycemic agents 44–5, 49
  lipid-lowering therapy 98, 102, 105
CD40 ligand 114, 130
CD69 114–15
Centers for Disease Control and Prevention 126
central obesity 56–7, 138
cereal fiber 24
CHARM studies 77, 78, 79
chlorthalidone 79, 81
cholesterol
  non-HDL 95
  see also high-density lipoprotein cholesterol; low-density lipoprotein cholesterol
cholesteryl ester transfer protein (CETP) 93, 101
  inhibitors 106
CJC-1131/CJC-1134 145, 148–9
CONSENSUS study 74–5
corn-based syrups 18–19
coronary artery bypass grafting (CABG) 113
Coronary Drug Project (CDP) 105
coronary heart disease (CHD)
  hypertriglyceridemia and 99–100
  lipid-lowering trials 95–7, 101–3, 105
  pre-exercise evaluation 33
  risk factors 93, 94
C-reactive protein (CRP) 111–13, 125–7
  highly sensitive (hs-CRP) 126
  IL-6 and 128
  insulin actions 113, 114
  lifestyle interventions and 16–17
  pharmacologic modulation 45, 48, 130
cytokines, pro-inflammatory 47–8, 127–8, 138
  dietary influences 14, 15, 114
  RAAS and 72
  thiazolidinediones and 48

Da Qing study 7, 70
DAIS study 101, 102
DASH (Dietary Approaches to Stop Hypertension) diet 22–3
Diabetes Control and Complications Trial (DCCT) 6
diabetes mellitus
  chronic complications 1–2
  exercise 34
  glycemic control and CVD risk 6–7
  lifestyle interventions 3–6
  mechanisms of CVD risk 2
  medications *see* antidiabetes medications
  obesity surgery 64–5
  prevalence 69
  see also type 1 diabetes; type 2 diabetes
diabetes prevention
  barriers 70
  dietary modification 7–8, 16–17
  hypoglycemic agents 43–5, 46, 142–3
  lifestyle interventions 7–8, 70–1, 139–40
  mechanisms of RAAS inhibition 83–4
  RAAS inhibition 78–83
  thiazolidinediones 46, 81–3, 143
  vs delaying onset 84–5
Diabetes Prevention Program (DPP) 7–8, 70–1, 139
  diet modification 15–17
  exercise 31
  metformin 45, 62–3, 130, 142
  weight loss 58, 59
diabetic nephropathy, angiotensin receptor blockers 75, 76, 78
diabetic retinopathy, exercise 34
diet 13–25

pathogenic role 14–15, 18–19, 23–4
patterns 23–4, 25
pro-inflammatory effects 114–16
dietary modification 139–40
CVD prevention in diabetes 5–6
diabetes prevention 7–8, 16–17
glycemic control and 7
metabolic syndrome management 15–17, 19–23, 25
diethylpropion 60
dipeptidyl peptidase-IV (DPP-IV) 144, 145
inhibitors 47, 144, 145, 149–51
DREAM study 46, 81–3, 84, 143
dyslipidemia 93–107, 141
combination therapy 104–6
efficacy and safety of statins 97–8
exercise 30
hypoglycemic agents 45, 47, 49–50
LDL-lowering (statin) trials 95–7
major ongoing trials 106–7
novel interventions 106
pathophysiology 94, 95
pro-inflammatory cytokines and 128
thiazolidinediones and 49–50, 106
treatment recommendations 104
triglyceride- and HDL-interventions 99–103

Early growth response-1 (Egr-1) 113, 114
ELITE II study 75, 77
enalapril 74–5, 79
endothelial (dys)function
exercise effects 30
insulin actions 113
pro-inflammatory cytokines and 127–8
RAAS inhibition and 83–4
role of RAAS activation 72–4
thiazolidinediones and 48–9
endothelin 49, 72
energy balance 57–8
energy expenditure 31, 57
EPIC-Norfolk study 3, 4
epigenetic factors 8–9
E-selectin 130
exenatide 47, 63, 64, 144–8
exendin-4 145
exercise (physical activity) 29–40, 139–40
aerobic 31, 32, 37–8
benefits 30–1
CVD prevention in diabetes 5–6
energy expenditure table 31
glycemic control and 7
guidelines 32
optimal type/volume 31–2
pre-exercise evaluation 32–3, 34
prescription 33–9
adherence 39
beyond walking 36–9
initiating a walking program 34–6
monitoring progress 36, 39
primary prevention of diabetes 7–8
resistance 31, 32, 37, 39
weight loss and 30–1
ezetimibe 98, 107

fast food meals 115
fasting plasma glucose (FPG) 138
fat, dietary 13, 14–17
pathogenic role 14–15, 115
recommended intake 17, 25
restricted intake 15–17
fatty acids
dietary, types 15
free (FFA), plasma 15, 93, 115
fenofibrate
clinical trials 101, 102, 103
combination therapy 104, 107, 141
modulation of inflammation 130
fiber, dietary 24, 25
fibrates 101–3, 141
combination therapy 104–6
guidelines on use 104
ongoing trials 107
fibrinogen 127, 130
FIELD study 101, 103
Finnish Diabetes Prevention Study (FDPS) 7, 8, 15–16, 17, 70
fish oils 106
fitness, aerobic 32
Framingham Offspring Study 21, 23–4
free fatty acids (FFA), plasma 15, 93, 115
fructose 18–19

gastric bypass surgery 64–5
gastric inhibitory polypeptide (GIP) *see* glucose-dependent insulinotropic peptide
gemfibrozil 101, 102–3, 130
ghrelin 64
GLP-1 *see* glucagon-like peptide-1
glucagon 145, 146
glucagon-like peptide-1 (GLP-1) 46–7, 143–4
based therapies 47, 63, 144–9
DPP-IV inhibitors and 150
gastric bypass surgery and 64
receptor 145

Glucerna® 58
glucocorticoids 131
glucose
  fasting plasma (FPG) 138
  intolerance *see* impaired fasting glucose; impaired glucose tolerance
  pro-inflammatory effects 114–16
glucose-dependent insulinotropic peptide (GIP) 46–7, 143
glucotoxicity 116
GLUT 4 glucose transporter 83
glycemic control
  CVD risk reduction 6–7
  DPP-IV inhibitors 150
  incretin mimetics 146, 147–8, 149
  weight loss and 141
  see also antidiabetes medications
glycemic index 21–2, 24, 25
glycemic load 21–2, 25

HATS study 105
HDL *see* high-density lipoprotein
heart failure 75, 77, 79, 82
heart rate, maximum (HR_{max}) 37, 38
Helsinki Heart Study (HHS) 101
hemoglobin, glycosylated (HbA1c) 3, 4
  DPP-IV inhibitors 150
  incretin mimetics 146, 147, 148, 149
hepatic lipase (HL) 93
HERITAGE study 30
high-density lipoprotein (HDL)
  atherogenesis and 101
  particle size 94
high-density lipoprotein (HDL) cholesterol 93, 138
  benefits of raising 99–103
  effect of thiazolidinediones 49–50, 106
  therapies targeting 106
HMG-CoA reductase inhibitors *see* statins
homocysteine 103
HOPE study 75, 78–9, 81
hydroxychloroquine 132
hyperglycemia 1–2
  control *see* glycemic control
  treatment *see* antidiabetes medications
hypertension 138, 141
  exercise 30, 34
  lifestyle interventions 8
  RAAS inhibitors 75, 76, 79, 80–1
  thiazolidinediones and 49
hypertriglyceridemia 93, 99–103, 106, 138
hypoglycemic agents *see* antidiabetes medications
hypoxia-inducible factor-1α (HIF-1α) 130

IDEAL study 97, 98
IDNT study 76, 78
IKKβ 128, 131, 132
ILLUMINATE trial 106
impaired fasting glucose (IFG) 2–3
  ACE inhibitors 82
  dietary modification 16, 17
  insulin therapy 118
  thiazolidinediones 46, 82–3
impaired glucose tolerance (IGT) 2–3, 138–9
  ACE inhibitors 82
  CVD prevention 8
  dietary modification 16–17
  epigenetic factors in progression 8–9
  hypoglycemic agents 43–5, 46
  insulin therapy 118
  lifestyle interventions 7–8, 70–1
  thiazolidinediones 46, 84–5
  treatments targeting 141–51
incretin effect 143–4
incretin hormones 46–7, 143–4
incretin mimetics 47, 144–9
inflammation 111–12, 125–32
  chemical markers 125–7
  diabetes treatments and 48, 128–32
  dietary influences 14, 15, 114–16
  insulin actions 113–14
  lifestyle interventions and 128–9
  pathogenic role 116–17, 125, 126, 129
  RAAS activation and 72
  see also cytokines, pro-inflammatory
inhibitor kappa B (Iκ-B) 113, 114, 115, 128, 132
insulin 111–18
  anti-inflammatory effect 113–14
  biological effects 112
  intensive therapy, CVD risk reduction 6–7
  role in management 118
  signal transduction 116–17
  weight gain 142
insulin glargine 118, 148
insulin receptor substrate 1 (IRS-1) 116
insulin resistance 2, 112
  angiotensin II and 73–4
  dietary factors 14, 20
  dyslipidemia 93–5
  effect of exercise 30

pathogenic role of inflammation 116–17, 125, 126, 128, 129
RAAS blockade and 83–4
Insulin Resistance Atherosclerosis Study 127
insulin secretagogues 43–4, 142
intercellular adhesion molecule-1 (ICAM-1) 113, 130
Interheart study 100
interleukin-1 (IL-1) 48, 127–8
interleukin-1 (IL-1) receptor antagonist 132
interleukin-6 (IL-6) 48, 113–14, 127–8
dietary influences 14, 15, 114
pathogenic role 116
pharmacologic modulation 130
interleukin-18 (IL-18) 15
intermediate-density lipoprotein (IDL) 93
International Diabetes Federation (IDF) 138
intima-media thickness *see* carotid artery intima-media thickness
irbesartan 76, 78
IRMA study 76, 78
ISIS-4 study 75

Jenny Craig program 59

LAF237 (vildagliptin) 149–50
lap-band procedure 64
LDL *see* low-density lipoprotein
left ventricular dysfunction (LVD) 75
left ventricular hypertrophy (LVH) 75, 76, 79
leptin 47, 128, 138
LIFE study 75, 76, 78–9, 81
lifestyle interventions 1–9, 111, 139–40
CVD prevention in diabetes 3–6
CVD prevention in prediabetes 8
diabetes prevention 7–8, 70–1
modulation of inflammation 128–9
molecular mechanisms 8–9
obesity 58–9
see also dietary modification; exercise
lipid abnormalities *see* dyslipidemia
lipid-lowering therapy 95–107, 141
combination 104–6
major ongoing trials 106–7
modulation of inflammation 130
novel approaches 106
recommendations 104
lipoprotein (a) (Lp(a)) 106
lipoprotein lipase (LPL) 93
lipotoxicity 116
liraglutide 145, 148, 149
lisinopril 75, 79, 81
LOOK-Ahead project 5–6, 140
losartan 75, 76, 77, 79, 81
lovastatin 105
Lovaza 106
low-calorie diets 22–3, 25, 116
low-carbohydrate diets 19–20, 25
low-density lipoprotein (LDL)
particle size 94
small, dense particles 93, 106
low-density lipoprotein (LDL) cholesterol 15, 94
lowering trials 95–8
targets 97
thiazolidinediones and 50
low-fat diets 15–17

macronutrients, pro-inflammatory effects 114–16
macrophage migration inhibitory factor (MIF) 130
macrophages 127–8
management of metabolic syndrome 118, 139–51
anti-obesity medications 59–62, 140–1
dietary modification 15–17, 19–23, 25, 139–40
exercise 33–9
hypoglycemic agents 43–7, 62–3, 141–51
incretin-based therapies 144–51
lifestyle interventions 1–9, 58–9, 111, 139–40
lipid-lowering therapy 95–107
modulation of inflammation 128–32
obesity surgery 63–5
potential role of insulin 118
RAAS inhibitors 74 83
targeting CVD risk factors 141
matrix metalloproteinase-9 (MMP-9) 113
meal replacement diets 22, 23, 58
Mediterranean diet 5, 24
metabolic syndrome
definitions 2, 111, 137–8
prevalence 137–8
metformin 45, 47, 142
modulation of inflammation 130
obesity 62–3
vs lifestyle interventions 8, 16
metiglinides 43–4
mitogen activated protein kinase (MAPK) pathway 73–4
MK-0431 (sitagliptin) 149–50
MK-0524 106

monocyte chemoattractant protein-1 (MCP-1) 113, 128, 130
monocytes 127–8
monounsaturated fats 17
myocardial infarction (MI) 75–8
- anti-inflammatory effect of insulin 113, 114
- lipid-lowering trials 95, 102, 103, 105
- risk factors 100

myopathy, statin- and fibrate-associated 104–5
myristic acid 15

nateglinide 43–4
National Cholesterol Education Program, Adult Treatment Panel III (NCEP, ATP III) 2, 15, 69, 95, 104, 137–8
National Health and Nutrition Examination Surveys (NHANES) 55, 126, 139
National Health and Nutrition Survey (Germany) 126–7
National Strength and Conditioning Association 39
NAVIGATOR trial 43–4, 85
niacin (nicotinic acid) 104, 105–6, 107
nitric oxide (NO) 72, 73, 83
- insulin actions 113, 114

nitric oxide synthase (NOS)
- endothelial (eNOS) 113, 114
- inducible (iNOS) 113

non-steroidal anti-inflammatory drugs (NSAIDs) 131–2
nuclear factor kappa B (NF-κB) 128, 129
- insulin actions 113
- nutrients influencing 114, 115
- pharmacologic modulation 130, 131, 132

Nurse's Health Study 15, 18, 93

obesity 55–65
- behavior modification/lifestyle change 58–9
- central or abdominal 56–7, 138
- definition and concepts 56–7
- diabetes medications 62–3
- dietary factors in development 14–15, 17–18
- extreme (class III) 55, 56, 64
- food-induced inflammation 115
- high vs low glycemic index diets 22
- inflammatory markers 126
- low-carbohydrate diets 19, 20
- medical complications 56, 69
- metabolic effects 111–13
- pathogenic role 116–17, 138–9
- pharmacologic treatment 59–62, 140–1
- prevalence 43, 55
- simple vs complex carbohydrates 20–1
- surgery 63–5
- treatment options 58–65
- *see also* weight gain; weight loss

omega-3 fatty acids 15, 106
ONTARGET study 84–5
OPTIMAAL study 75, 76
ORIGIN study 118
orlistat 59, 60–1, 140
osteoporosis 34
overweight 55, 56
- inflammatory markers 126
- *see also* obesity

oxidative stress
- nutrient intake and 114, 116
- pathogenic role 116–17
- *see also* reactive oxygen species

p47^{phox} 113, 114
P70 S6 kinase 74
palmitic acid 15
pathogenesis of metabolic syndrome 117, 129
- dietary factors 14–15, 18–19, 23–4
- impaired insulin action 113–14, 115
- inflammation 114–17, 125–8
- obesity and glucose intolerance 138–9
- RAAS activation 71–4

PEACE trial 79–80
pedometer-based walking program 35, 36
peripheral neuropathy, exercise 34, 35
peroxisome proliferator activator receptor-gamma (PPAR-γ) agonists 84, 130–1
- *see also* thiazolidinediones

phentermine 60, 140
phosphatidyl inositol kinase (PI-3K) pathway 73, 74
physical activity *see* exercise
pioglitazone 48–50, 106, 142–3
PIPOD study 143
plasminogen-activator inhibitor type 1 (PAI-1) 47, 48, 111–13, 127, 128
platelets 114, 131–2
polyunsaturated fats 17
pramlintide 63
prediabetes
- cardiovascular risk 2–3, 93
- dietary modification 16–17
- epigenetic factors in progression 8–9

lifestyle interventions 7–8
primary prevention of CVD 8
role for insulin therapy 118
PROVE-IT trial 97, 98, 100
PYY-3-36 64

quinapril 83–4

RAAS *see* renin–angiotensin–aldosterone system
ramipril 75, 81–3, 84–5
reactive oxygen species (ROS) 49, 113
nutrient intake and 114, 115, 116
see also oxidative stress
remnant particles 93
RENAAL study 75, 76
renin–angiotensin–aldosterone system (RAAS) 71–85
mechanism of blockade in diabetes prevention 83–4
preventing vs delaying diabetes onset 84–5
role of activation 71–4
as therapeutic target 74–83
resistance exercise 31, 32, 37, 39
resistin 128
retinol-binding-4 128
rimonabant 61–2, 140–1
Rio-Europe trial 62
Rio-Lipids trial 62
Rio-North America trial 62
risk factors, cardiometabolic 137
cumulative effects 93, 94
exenatide actions 47, 146–7
impact of diabetes treatments 47–50
inflammatory markers and 126–7
lifestyle interventions 3–6, 7–8
management strategies 139
obesity and 55
targeted treatment 141
type 2 diabetes 2
rosiglitazone 46, 142–3
diabetes prevention 46, 81–3, 143
impact on risk factors 48–9, 142–3
lipid effects 106
rosuvastatin 107

SAFARI trial 104
salicylates 131–2
saturated fat 15, 17, 115
SAVE study 75
Scandinavian Simvastatin Survival Study (4S) 96, 99
SENDCAP study 101–2
serum amyloid A (SAA) 113, 128
sibutramine 59, 60, 61, 140, 141
simvastatin 96, 98, 99, 141
combination therapy 104, 105
ongoing trials 107
sitagliptin 149–50
SlimFast® 58
small, dense low-density lipoprotein (LDL) particles 93, 106
smoking cessation 4–5
SOLVD study 74–5, 79
STAT-3 113–14
statins 95–8, 141
cardiovascular outcomes 95–7
combination therapy 104–6
efficacy and safety 97–8
guidelines on use 104
modulation of inflammation 130
ongoing trials 107
stearic acid 15
sterol regulatory element binding protein (SREBP-1) 93
STOP-NIDDM trial 6–7, 44–5
strength and endurance training 32, 37, 39
stroke, lipid-lowering trials 95, 97, 102, 105
STORM trial 60
STRRIDE trial 31–2
sulfonylureas (SU) 43, 47, 142, 148
suppressor of cytokine signaling (SOCS-3) 116
Swedish Obesity Study 64

telmisartan 84–5
thiazolidinediones (TZDs) 142–3
anti-inflammatory effects 131
diabetes prevention 46, 81–3, 143
effect on metabolic syndrome 46, 47
impact on risk factors 48–50
lipid effects 49–50, 106
THRIVE trial 107
tissue factor (TF) 113, 114
TNT trial 96–7, 98, 99–100
torcetrapib 106
trandolapril 75, 79–80
trans fatty acids 15
TRANSCEND study 85
transcription factor 7-like 2 (*TCF7L2*) gene variants 8–9
treatment of metabolic syndrome *see* management of metabolic syndrome

triglycerides, serum 93, 138
  benefits of intervention 99–103
  thiazolidinediones and 49–50
TRIPOD study 143
troglitazone 48, 49–50, 82, 143
tumor necrosis factor-α (TNF-α) 47–8, 127–8, 138
  dietary influences 14, 15, 114
  gene polymorphisms 8
  inhibition 128
  lipid-lowering therapy and 130
  pathogenesis of insulin resistance 116
type 1 diabetes (T1DM) 1–2
type 2 diabetes (T2DM) 1, 137
  anti-inflammatory agents 131
  chronic complications 1–2
  delaying onset 84–5
  dietary factors in development 18
  dyslipidemia 93–5
  incretin-based therapies 47, 145–51
  inflammation and pathogenesis 116–17, 127, 128, 129
  mechanisms of CVD risk 2
  medical management 141–51
  medications *see* antidiabetes medications
  obesity surgery 64–5
  prevalence 69
  prevention *see* diabetes prevention
  risk factors 69

UK Prospective Diabetes Study (UKPDS) 6, 45
unsaturated fats 15, 17

VA-HIT study 101, 102–3
VALIANT study 77, 78
valsartan 43–4, 75–8, 79
VALUE study 76, 78, 79
vascular endothelial function *see* endothelial function
vascular endothelial growth factor (VEGF) 113
vascular wall abnormalities, thiazolidinediones and 48–9
very low-calorie diets 22, 23, 25
very low-density lipoprotein (VLDL) 93, 94
V-HeFT II study 75, 77
vildagliptin 149–50
visceral fat 14
  effect of exercise 30, 32
visfatin 128

walking program 34–6
  step (pedometer)-based 35, 36
  time-based 35–6
weight gain
  dietary influences 14, 18–19
  medications causing 43, 50, 142, 143
weight loss 13, 55–65, 139–40
  anti-inflammatory effects 116
  anti-obesity medications 59–62, 140–1
  calorie-controlled portions 22, 23, 58
  commercial programs 58–9
  diabetes medications 62–3
  exercise 30–1
  incretin mimetics 146–7, 148, 149
  lifestyle change 58–9
  low-calorie diets 22, 23
  low-carbohydrate diets 20
  low-fat diets 16, 17
  obesity surgery 63–5
  prediabetes 7–8
  recommended 25
  simple vs complex carbohydrates 21
  strategies 57–8
Weight Watchers 58–9
Women's Health Survey 127
World Health Organization (WHO) 137–8

zofenopril 75